A–Z Guide to Drug-Herb-Vitamin Interactions

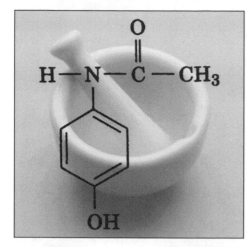

Schuyler W. Lininger, Jr. DC, Editor-in-Chief

Alan R. Gaby MD

Steve Austin ND

Forrest Batz PharmD

Eric Yarnell ND

Donald J. Brown ND

George Constantine RPh, PhD

A-Z
GUIDE TO
DRUG-HERB-VITAMIN
INTERACTIONS

How to Improve Your Health and Avoid Problems

When Using Common Medications and Natural Supplements Together

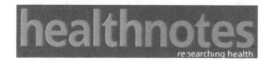

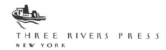

THREE RIVERS PRESS
NEW YORK

Published by Three Rivers Press, New York, New York.
Member of the Crown Publishing Group, a division of Random House, Inc.
www.randomhouse.com

THREE RIVERS PRESS and the Tugboat design are registered trademarks of Random House, Inc.

Originally published by Prima Publishing, Roseville, California, in 1999.

Disclaimer: Random House, Inc., has designed this book to provide information in regard to the subject matter covered. It is sold with the understanding that the publisher and the author are not liable for the misconception or misuse of information provided. Every effort has been made to make this book as complete and as accurate as possible. The purpose of this book is to educate. The author and Random House, Inc., shall have neither liability nor responsibility to any person or entity with respect to any loss, damage, or injury caused or alleged to be caused directly or indirectly by the information contained in this book. The information presented herein is in no way intended as a substitute for medical counseling.

All products mentioned in this book are trademarks of their respective companies.

Published in association with Healthnotes Online, Inc.

HEALTHNOTES is a registered trademark of Healthnotes, Inc.

Cover photos copyright © EyeWire

Printed in the United States of America

Library of Congress Cataloging-in-Publication Data
   A-z guide to drug-herb-vitamin interactions : how to improve your health and avoid problems
   when using common medications and natural supplements together/Schuyler W. Lininger . . . [et al.].
     p. cm.
   Includes bibliographical information and index.
   1. Drug-herb interactions. 2. Drug-nutrient interactions. I. Lininger, Schuyler W.
RM666.H33D78   1999
615'7045—dc21   99-39218
                                                                           CIP

ISBN 0-7615-1599-2

10 9 8

First Edition

For the pioneers and champions of complementary
and integrative medicine and the Healthnotes team

Contents

Contents

Foreword

In the hyper-speed of today's pressure-cooker world, people are now taking a major interest in participating in and maintaining their own health and wellness. There is a major concern in the mixing of health systems, such as alternative or natural medicine and orthodox western medicine. As this is now becoming the "norm," we must gain true knowledge of this wonderful new emerging field of integrated medicine.

Dr. Skye Lininger and the Healthnotes team, in their first book, *The Natural Pharmacy*, became pioneers by compiling one of the best, single-source reference books on "alternative medicine." Now, with this new book, the *A–Z Guide to Drug-Herb-Vitamin Interactions*, the best experts in the new field of integrated medicine have created a clear, concise, user-friendly reference book for everyday use for the new millennium.

This book lists by drug—then class and family—both over-the-counter and prescription medications. It breaks compound mixtures into component parts while making the information easily accessible by using both brand and generic names. Not only are the drug-nutrient interactions with dietary supplements addressed, but also interactions with herbs, foods, and alcohol. Interactions—both positive and negative—include nutrient depletions, side-effect risk reduction, potential adverse reactions, reduced drug absorption and bioavailability, and supportive interactions.

The *A–Z Guide to Drug-Herb-Vitamin Interactions* is the only comprehensive book to take into consideration that drug depletions can be a severe problem and that we sometimes need to replace what the medications take out of our system and put our bodies back in balance. Integrative or complementary therapies, when understood, are synergistic and offer potentially more benefits than any single system. However, if misused, they have the potential for harmful results.

The use of this excellent book can do so much to improve a person's general health and knowledge. Putting into practice the easy-to-use information in this book can help avoid many potential problems and can greatly increase good health and well-being.

—**James M. Brodsky, R.Ph.**
Instructor, University of
Southern California College of Pharmacy

Acknowledgments

No innovative book of this scope comes into existence without the inspiration and help of many people—most of whom labor behind the scenes.

For taking a conversational concept and moving it forward into its first iteration and then into its current form, appreciation and acknowledgment are due Steve Austin, N.D., the Chief Science Officer at Healthnotes, Inc. Dr. Austin is, quite simply, the best.

For his attention to detail and commitment to excellence, the fine work of Forrest Batz, Pharm.D.—this book would not have been possible without his expertise and experience. The work of George Constantine, R.Ph., Ph.D., is also appreciated.

The information on herbal interactions is one of the areas about which the least is known and for which real expertise is demanded. We are fortunate that two of the best in this field contributed to making this book the best on the subject ever created. Eric Yarnell, N.D., and Don Brown, N.D., have served variously as expert product advisers to industry and college-level instructors on evidence-based natural medicine. As you will see as you read this book, there is good reason Drs. Yarnell and Brown are held in high esteem by both their students and their colleagues.

Providing critical editorial review and additional content from his database of over 30,000 scientific and medical journal articles was our friend and mentor Alan Gaby, M.D. His revisions and comments made this book much better.

Special thanks to Victoria Dolby Toews, M.P.H., for her diligent and professional job in serving as managing editor to all editions of Healthnotes Online software and the first edition of this book.

Thanks to my family for their love and putting up with long hours, a demanding travel schedule, and an exciting yet stressful period in our lives; to all the team at Healthnotes, Inc. who are the best at what they do of any I have ever worked with; to our Chief Technical Officer Rick Wilkes (and his team); to those talented people who helped make the original Healthnotes Online software a reality from a graphics and programmatic perspective, Marcia Barrentine and Loren Jenkins; to those who were there at the beginning (and helped inspire, motivate, and create), Michael Peet and his sister, Margaret, Stan Amy, Cheryl Bottger, and Eileen Brady; to our friends from Catalyst II, Jill Higgins and David Cole, for their support, encouragement, and mentoring.

To our publishing partners at Prima; to Dr. Joe Pizzorno, the President of Bastyr University; to all the retailers in health and natural food stores, grocery stores, and pharmacies and departments who offer high-quality supplements; and to the pioneers and innovators in natural medicine who have kept as their credo the care of their patients . . . naturally.

Introduction

After the publication of our first book, *The Natural Pharmacy* (Prima, 1998), it became clear to us that the "new" users of vitamins and herbs were often taking prescription and non-prescription medicines along with their supplements. At the same time, overall usage of supplements soared and pharmacists and medical doctors began receiving questions from their patients about whether or not they could safely mix their supplements with their medications.

To our surprise, this safety information had never been compiled in one resource.

Our writing team, which is responsible for the "Healthnotes Online" electronic database (the most relied upon database in the industry) and *The Natural Pharmacy, 2nd Edition* (Prima Health and Healthnotes, Inc., 1999) was tasked with reviewing over 25,000 scientific articles from over 550 journals. Their job: To find all the safety and interaction information they could on the top 100 prescription and top 100 non-prescription drugs.

The result of that effort is in your hands.

Two decades ago, many scientific articles had been written about most of the vitamins and a few of the herbs, but getting hold of that information was challenging. It is only in recent years that medicine has become interested in the use of nutritional supplements as a complement to conventional medicine. In most cases, the subject is just now being added to the curriculum in some medical schools.

In the 1970s, books about supplements were of mixed quality. Despite being poorly referenced and filled with errors, the books provided enough information (much of which later proved true) to help millions of people with their health problems.

Beginning in the early 1980s, a steady stream of articles about antioxidants and other dietary supplements began appearing in the medical literature. By the late 1980s, the stream had become a flood and some 15,000 articles began forming a solid foundation for nutritional therapies. Books appearing in those years began to take advantage of the scientific underpinnings and gradually became more reliable and useful. However, they were still aimed squarely at those who accepted the premise that only natural was good.

Our expert scientific and evidence-based medical team consists of M.D.s (Dr. Gaby), pharmacists (Batz and Constantine), N.D.s—naturopaths—(Drs. Austin, Brown, and Yarnell), and D.C.s (myself). Our goal was to create a book that covered the essential information a person would need to determine whether he or she should take a vitamin or herb with their medicine. The answer is often surprising, and always helpful.

This book has numerous unique characteristics.

- All statements that might be controversial have been documented with a reference from the scientific literature (from some of those 25,000 articles I mentioned).

- Thousands of citations are included so the serious reader can retrieve the article and review the material we relied on.
- In addition, we have tried to use primarily human studies; although in the area of interactions, animal or test tube trials are the only resource available.
- All of our key contributors have actually been in practice with real patients. They are not biochemists or researchers writing theoretically or from an ivory tower—but from real-life experience in their clinics.

In short, we have created the most useful, authoritative, and balanced book that has ever been made available on this topic and is the only place you can currently turn to for a comprehensive look at this information.

All the authors join me in wishing you good health.

**—Schuyler W. Lininger, Jr.,
D.C., Editor-in-Chief**

How to Use This Book

The *A–Z Guide to Drug-Herb-Vitamin Interactions* reviews more than 4,500 known major interactions between pharmaceutical drugs and food, specific nutrients, and herbs—for example, inhibition of vitamin K caused by antibiotics or iron deficiency triggered by long-term use of aspirin. This handy reference book gives you information about how some herbs or nutritional supplements help drugs work better; which drugs deplete your body of crucial nutrients; which drugs and supplements should never be taken together; and which drug side effects can be reduced by taking the right nutritional supplement or herb.

IMPORTANT FEATURES

All the prescription drugs and over-the-counter medications covered in *A–Z Guide to Drug-Herb-Vitamin Interactions* are listed alphabetically in the table of contents by generic name. Near the end of *A–Z Guide to Drug-Herb-Vitamin Interactions* you will find the following useful appendices:

- **Appendix 1:** Combination Drugs, lists almost 250 vitamins, minerals, herbs, and other nutritional supplements.
- **Appendix 2:** Drug Interactions by Herb or Supplement, lists supplements and herbs that might interact (positively or negatively) with specific drugs.

- **Appendix 3:** Pharmacist Classification, lists drugs by classification, such as cardiovascular drugs or hormones and synthetic substitutes.

Each generic drug article includes a "Summary of Interactions" table, which rates each nutrient with which the drug reacts and provides a quick reference. The nutrients are divided into one or more of the following categories:

- **Depletion or Interference:** This indicates that the drug may deplete or interfere with the absorption or function of the supplement or herb.
- **Adverse Interaction:** This indicates that the supplement or herb used together with the drug may result in undesirable effects.
- **Side Effect Reduction/Prevention:** This indicates that the supplement or herb may reduce the likelihood and/or severity of a potential side effect caused by the drug.
- **Supportive Interaction:** This indicates that the supplement or herb may support or aid the function of the drug.
- **Reduced Drug Absorption/ Bioavailability:** This indicates that the supplement or herb may decrease the absorption and/or activity of the drug in the body.

WHAT IS NOT COVERED IN THIS BOOK?

The following types of interactions are not discussed in *A–Z Guide to Drug-Herb-Vitamin Interactions*:

- Side effects that may be caused by drug interactions between two or more drugs
- Interactions between alcohol and specific nutrients
- Interactions between drugs and water (for example, drugs inducing dehydration)

Although this book is extensive, it does not include every drug-nutrient or drug-herb interaction. Therefore, if a drug is not mentioned in this section, there still may be drug-food, drug-nutrient, or drug-herb interactions.

For these reasons, it is not sufficient to rely solely on the information presented here. It is always wise for people seeking information about interactions between a prescription drug and food, specific nutrients, or herbs to talk with their pharmacist, prescribing physician, or both.

In addition, the information in this book is not intended to replace information supplied by a doctor or pharmacist; neither is it intended to replace package inserts or other printed material that may be available or accompany a particular drug.

Table Key

For the convenience of the reader, the information in the summary is categorized as follows:

Depletion or interference — *indicates the drug may deplete or interfere with the absorption or function of the supplement or herb*

Adverse interaction — *indicates that the supplement or herb used together with the drug may result in undesirable effects*

Side effect reduction/ prevention — *indicates the supplement or herb may reduce the likelihood and/or severity of a potential side effect caused by the drug*

Supportive interaction — *indicates the supplement or herb may support or aid the function of the drug*

Reduced drug absorption/bioavailability — *indicates that the supplement or herb may decrease the absorption and/or activity of the drug in the body*

An asterisk (*) next to an item in the summary indicates that the interaction is supported only by weak, fragmentary, and/or contradictory scientific evidence.

A–Z Guide to Drug-Herb-Vitamin Interactions

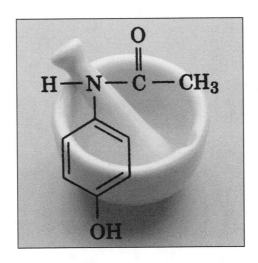

ANGIOTENSIN-CONVERTING ENZYME (ACE) INHIBITORS

Angiotensin-converting enzyme (ACE) inhibitors constitute a family of drugs used to treat high blood pressure and some types of heart failure. ACE inhibitors are also used to slow the progression of kidney disease in people with diabetes. ACE inhibitors include **captopril** (page 35) (Capoten) and **enalapril** (page 82) (Vasotec).

INTERACTIONS WITH DIETARY SUPPLEMENTS

Potassium

ACE inhibitors may increase blood potassium levels.[1] Potassium supplements, potassium-containing salt substitutes (No Salt, Morton Salt Substitute, and others), and even high-potassium foods (primarily fruit) can be problematic.

Zinc

Preliminary research has found significant loss of zinc in urine triggered by taking captopril.[2] In this trial, depletion of zinc reduced red blood cell levels of zinc—a test that can be ordered by a doctor. Although details remain unclear, it now appears that chronic use of the ACE inhibitor captopril may lead to a zinc deficiency.[3] It makes sense for people taking captopril long term to consider taking a zinc supplement or a multimineral tablet containing zinc as a precaution. (Such multiminerals usually contain no more than 99 mg of potassium, probably not enough to trigger the above-mentioned interaction.) Supplements containing zinc should also contain copper, to protect against a zinc-induced copper deficiency.

SUMMARY OF INTERACTIONS FOR ACE INHIBITORS

Depletion or interference	*Zinc*
Adverse interaction	*Potassium*
Side effect reduction/prevention	*None known*
Supportive interaction	*None known*
Reduce drug absorption/bioavailability	*None known*

ACETAMINOPHEN
(APAP, Tylenol, and Others)

Acetaminophen is used to reduce pain and fever. Unlike **NSAIDs** (page 157) (nonsteroidal anti-inflammatory drugs), it lacks anti-inflammatory activity. Acetaminophen is available by itself or in nonprescription and prescription-only combination products used to relieve pain and the symptoms associated with colds and flu.

Acetaminophen is available in prescription products used to treat moderate to severe pain. Prescription acetaminophen products include the following:

- Acetaminophen/**codeine** (page 54) (Tylenol with codeine and others)
- Acetaminophen/**hydrocodone** (page 110) (Lortab, Vicodin, and others)
- Acetaminophen/**oxycodone** (page 163) (Percocet, Roxicet, and others)
- Acetaminophen/**propoxyphene** (page 179) (Darvocet, Wygesic, and others)

Acetaminophen is also available in nonprescription products used to treat cold and flu symptoms. Nonprescription acetaminophen products include the following:

- Acetaminophen/**diphenhydramine** (page 75) (Excedrin PM, Tylenol PM, and others)
- Acetaminophen/**pseudoephedrine** (page 83) (Tylenol Sinus and others)
- Acetaminophen/**pseudoephedrine** (page 83)/**chlorpheniramine** (page 45) (Alka-Seltzer Plus, Theraflu, and others)
- Acetaminophen/**pseudoephedrine** (page 83)/**chlorpheniramine** (page 45)/**dextromethorphan** (page 70) (Tylenol Cold and others)
- Acetaminophen/**pseudoephedrine** (page 83) **diphenhydramine** (page 75) (Tylenol Allergy Sinus and others)
- Acetaminophen/**pseudoephedrine** (page 83)/**doxylamine** (page 81)/**dextromethorphan** (page 70)/alcohol (Nyquil and others)

INTERACTIONS WITH DIETARY SUPPLEMENTS

N-Acetyl Cysteine (NAC)

Hospitals use oral and intravenous N-acetyl cysteine (NAC) in treating liver damage induced by acetaminophen overdose poisoning.[1] This use of NAC is administered by emergency room medical doctors and should not be attempted without medical supervision.

Vitamin C

Taking 3 grams vitamin C with acetaminophen has been shown to prolong the amount of time acetaminophen stays in the body.[2] This theoretically might allow people to use less acetaminophen, thereby reducing the risk of side effects. Consult with a doctor of natural medicine about this potential before reducing the dose of acetaminophen.

INTERACTIONS WITH HERBS

Milk Thistle *(Silybum marianum)*

Silymarin is a collection of complex flavonoids found in milk thistle that has been shown to elevate liver glutathione levels in rats.[3] Acetaminophen can cause liver damage, which is believed to involve glutathione depletion.[4] In one study involving rats, silymarin protected against acetaminophen-induced glutathione depletion.[5] While studies to confirm this action in humans have not been conducted, some doctors of natural medicine recommend silymarin supplementation with 200 mg milk thistle extract, containing 70 to 80% silymarin, 3 times per day for people taking acetaminophen in large doses for more than 1 year and/or with other risk factors for liver problems.

Schisandra *(Schisandra chinensis)*

Gomisin A is a constituent found in the Chinese herb schisandra. In a study of rats given liver-damaging doses of acetaminophen, gomisin A appeared to protect against some liver damage but did not prevent glutathione depletion[6] (unlike milk thistle, as reported above). Studies have not yet confirmed this action in humans.

INTERACTIONS WITH FOODS AND OTHER COMPOUNDS

Food

Food, especially foods high in pectin (including jellies), carbohydrates, and large amounts of cruciferous vegetables (broccoli, Brussels sprouts, cabbage, and others) can interfere with acetaminophen absorption.[7] It is unclear how much effect this interaction has on acetaminophen activity.

Alcohol

Moderate to high doses of acetaminophen have caused liver damage in people with alcoholism.[8] To prevent problems, people taking acetaminophen should avoid alcohol.

SUMMARY OF INTERACTIONS FOR ACETAMINOPHEN

Depletion or interference	*None known*
Adverse interaction	*None known*
Side effect reduction/prevention	*N-acetyl cysteine, Milk thistle**
Supportive interaction	*Vitamin C**
Reduced drug absorption/bioavailability	*None known*
Other (see text)	*Schisandra*

ALBUTEROL
(Proventil, Ventolin)

Albuterol is a short-acting, beta-adrenergic bronchodilator drug used for relief and prevention of bronchospasm. It is also used to prevent exercise-induced bronchospasm. While albuterol is available in tablet form, it is most commonly used by oral inhalation into the lungs.

INTERACTIONS WITH DIETARY SUPPLEMENTS

Minerals

Therapeutic doses of intravenous (IV) salbutamol (albuterol) in four healthy people were associated with decreased plasma levels of calcium, magnesium, phosphate, and potassium.[1] Decreased potassium levels have been reported with oral,[2] intramuscular (IM), and subcutaneous (SQ) albuterol administration.[3] How frequently this effect occurs is not known, nor is the relationship between these changes in laboratory findings and dietary or supplemental mineral levels.

INTERACTIONS WITH HERBS

Digitalis (Digitalis lanata, Digitalis purpurea)

Digitalis refers to a family of plants commonly called foxglove that contain digitalis glycosides, chemicals with actions and toxicities similar to the prescription drug **digoxin** (page 71).

In a small study of salbutamol (albuterol) in people receiving digoxin, albuterol was associated with decreased serum digoxin levels.[4] No interactions between albuterol and digitalis have been reported. Until more is known, albuterol and digitalis-containing products should be used only under the direct supervision of a doctor trained in their use.

INTERACTIONS WITH FOODS AND OTHER COMPOUNDS

Food

Albuterol may be taken with food to prevent stomach upset.[5]

SUMMARY OF INTERACTIONS FOR ALBUTEROL

Depletion or interference	*Calcium,*[*] *Magnesium,*[*] *Phosphate,*[*] *Potassium*[*]
Adverse interaction	*None known*
Side effect reduction/prevention	*None known*
Supportive interaction	*None known*
Reduced drug absorption/bioavailability	*None known*
Other (see text)	*Digitalis*

ALENDRONATE
(Fosamax)

Alendronate is a member of the bisphosphonate family of drugs used to treat/ prevent osteoporosis. It is also used to treat some bone diseases and some cases of cancer that have spread to bones.

INTERACTIONS WITH DIETARY SUPPLEMENTS

Calcium

Calcium supplements may interfere with alendronate absorption.[1] However, one researcher suggested that addition of large doses of supplemental calcium to alendronate therapy in people with bone metastases (with evidence of osteomalacia) related to prostate cancer might improve the clinical outcome.[2] Moreover, both calcium and alendronate are commonly used in the treatment of osteoporosis in the same people. To prevent potential interactions, alendronate should be taken 2 hours before or after calcium supplements.

Magnesium

Absorption of tiludronate, a drug related to alendronate, is reduced when taken with magnesium and/or aluminum-containing antacids.[3] This interaction has not yet been reported with alendronate. Until more is known, alendronate should be taken 2 hours before or after magnesium and/or aluminum-containing **antacids** (page 13).

INTERACTIONS WITH FOODS AND OTHER COMPOUNDS

Food

Food, coffee, and orange juice significantly reduce absorption of alendronate.[4]

Alendronate should be taken with a large glass of plain water, upon arising in the morning, and 30 minutes or more before any food, beverages, supplements, or other medications.[5] People taking alendronate should remain upright (do not lie down) for 30 minutes after taking each dose.[6]

SUMMARY OF INTERACTIONS FOR ALENDRONATE

Depletion or interference	*None known*
Adverse interaction	*None known*
Side effect reduction/prevention	*None known*
Supportive interaction	*None known*
Reduced drug absorption/bioavailability	*None known*
Other (see text)	*Calcium, Magnesium*

ALUMINUM HYDROXIDE

Aluminum hydroxide acts as an **antacid** (page 13) and is most commonly used in the treatment of heartburn, gastritis, and peptic ulcer. This drug is also sometimes used to reduce absorption of phosphorus for people with kidney failure.

Aluminum hydroxide is found in a variety of **antacids** (page 13), such as Di-Gel, Maalox, Mylanta, Riopan, and others. People should read the ingredient label for over-the-counter (OTC) drugs carefully before purchase to know exactly what they contain.

INTERACTIONS WITH DIETARY SUPPLEMENTS

Alginates

A thick gel derived from algae has been used together with aluminum antacids to treat heartburn. Together, alginate gel and antacid were more effective at relieving symptoms[1] and improving healing.[2] Alginate is believed to work by physically blocking stomach acid from touching the esophagus. According to these studies, two tablets containing 200 mg alginic acid should be chewed before each meal and at bedtime.

Calcium

Aluminum hydroxide may increase urinary and stool loss of calcium.[3] Also, aluminum is a toxic mineral, and a limited amount of aluminum absorption from aluminum-containing antacids does occur.[4] As a result, most nutritionally oriented doctors do not recommend routine use of aluminum-containing **antacids** (page 13).[5] Other types of antacids containing calcium or **magnesium** (page 135) instead of aluminum are available.

Citrate

Several studies have shown that combination of citrate, either as calcium citrate supplements or from orange and lemon juice, with aluminum-containing antacids increases aluminum levels in the body.[6] [7] [8] Calcium in forms other than calcium citrate has been shown to not increase aluminum absorption.[9] Drinking 7 to 10 ounces of orange juice provides sufficient citrate to be problematic.[10] [11] Intake of 950 mg calcium citrate greatly elevates aluminum absorption.[12] People with renal failure may be at particular risk of kidney damage due to elevated aluminum levels if they combine aluminum hydroxide with citrate.[13]

Phosphorus

Depletion of phosphorus may occur as a result of taking aluminum hydroxide. For those with kidney failure, reducing phosphorus absorption is the purpose of taking the drug, as excessive phosphorus levels can result from kidney failure. However, when people with normal kidney function take aluminum hydroxide for extended periods of time, it is possible to deplete phosphorus to unnaturally low levels.

SUMMARY OF INTERACTIONS FOR ALUMINUM HYDROXIDE

Depletion or interference	*Calcium, Phosphorus*
Adverse interaction	*Citrate*
Side effect reduction/prevention	*None known*
Supportive interaction	*Alginates*
Reduced drug absorption/bioavailability	*None known*

AMILORIDE
(Midamor)

AMILORIDE/HYDROCHLOROTHIAZIDE
(Moduretic)

Amiloride is a potassium-sparing (prevents excess loss of potassium) **diuretic** (page 76) drug. Diuretics increase urinary water loss from the body and are used to treat high blood pressure, congestive heart failure, and some kidney or liver conditions. Amiloride is available as a single agent and in the combination of amiloride/hydrochlorothiazide (Moduretic).

INTERACTIONS WITH DIETARY SUPPLEMENTS

Magnesium

Preliminary research in animals suggests that amiloride, besides preventing excess potassium loss, may also prevent excess magnesium loss.[1] It is unknown if this same effect would occur in humans. Nevertheless, persons taking more than 300 mg of magnesium per day and amiloride should consult with a nutritionally oriented doctor, as this may lead to potentially dangerous levels of magnesium in the body. The combination of amiloride and hydrochlorothiazide would likely eliminate this problem, as **hydrochlorothiazide** (page 202) may deplete magnesium.

Potassium

As a potassium-sparing drug, amiloride reduces urinary loss of potassium. This can cause potassium levels to build up in the body. People taking this drug should avoid use of potassium chloride–containing products, such as Morton Salt Substitute, No Salt, Lite Salt, and others. Even eating several pieces of fruit per day can sometimes cause problems for people taking potassium-sparing diuretics, due to the high potassium content of fruit.

Sodium

Diuretics, including amiloride, cause increased loss of sodium in urine. By removing sodium from the body, diuretics cause water to leave the body as well. This reduction of water in the body is the purpose of taking amiloride. Therefore, there is usually no reason to replace lost sodium, although strict limitation of salt intake in combination with the action of diuretics can sometimes cause excessive sodium depletion. On the other hand, people who restrict sodium intake and in the process reduce blood pressure may need to have their dose of diuretics lowered.

SUMMARY OF INTERACTIONS FOR AMILORIDE

Depletion or interference	*None known*
Adverse interaction	*Magnesium,* * *Potassium*
Side effect reduction/prevention	*None known*
Supportive interaction	*None known*
Reduced drug absorption/bioavailability	*None known*
Other (see text)	*Sodium*

AMIODARONE
(Cordarone)

Amiodarone is a drug occasionally used to treat life-threatening arrhythmias of the heart.

INTERACTIONS WITH DIETARY SUPPLEMENTS

Vitamin E

Limited research in human lung tissue suggests that vitamin E might reduce lung toxicity caused by amiodarone.[1] When vitamin E is given to people with heart disease, many nutritionally oriented doctors recommend 400 to 800 IU per day.

SUMMARY OF INTERACTIONS FOR AMIODARONE

Depletion or interference	*None known*
Adverse interaction	*None known*
Side effect reduction/prevention	*Vitamin E*
Supportive interaction	*None known*
Reduced drug absorption/bioavailability	*None known*

AMLODIPINE
(Norvasc)

Amlodipine is a calcium channel blocker used to treat angina pectoris and high blood pressure.

INTERACTIONS WITH FOODS AND OTHER COMPOUNDS

Grapefruit Juice

Ingestion of grapefruit juice has been shown to increase the absorption of felodipine (a drug similar in structure and action to that of amlodipine) and to increase the adverse effects of the medication in people with hypertension. Until more is known, it seems that grapefruit juice should not be ingested at the same time as amlodipine or similar drugs.[1] The same effects might be seen from eating grapefruit as from drinking its juice.

Food

Amlodipine may be taken with or without food.[2]

SUMMARY OF INTERACTIONS FOR AMLODIPINE

Depletion or interference	*None known*
Adverse interaction	*None known*
Side effect reduction/prevention	*None known*
Supportive interaction	*None known*
Reduced drug absorption/bioavailability	*None known*
Other (see text)	*Grapefruit juice*

AMOXICILLIN
(Amoxil, Polymox, and Others)

Amoxicillin is a member of the penicillin family of **antibiotics** (page 14). Amoxicillin is used to treat bacterial infections, including infections of the middle ear. The combination of amoxicillin/clavulanate (Augmentin) is an extended-spectrum antibiotic used to treat bacterial infections resistant to amoxicillin alone.

INTERACTIONS WITH DIETARY SUPPLEMENTS

Bromelain

When taken with amoxicillin, bromelain was shown to increase absorption of amoxicillin in humans.[1] When 80 mg of bromelain was taken together with amoxicillin and **tetracycline** (page 199), blood levels of both drugs increased, though how bromelain acts on drug metabolism remains unknown.[2] An older report found bromelain also increased the actions of other antibiotics, including penicillin, chloramphenicol, and **erythromycin** (page 86), in treating a variety of infections. In that trial, twenty-two out of twenty-three people who had previously not responded to these antibiotics did so after adding bromelain taken 4 times per day.[3] Doctors of natural medicine will sometimes prescribe enough bromelain to equal 2,400 gelatin dissolving units (listed as GDU on labels) per day. This amount would equal approximately 3,600 MCU (milk clotting units), another common measure of bromelain activity.

Probiotics

A nonpathogenic yeast known as *Saccharomyces boulardii* has been shown in two double-blind studies to decrease frequency of diarrhea in people taking amoxicillin as well as other penicillin-type drugs compared to placebo.[4] [5] There were overall few people in these studies using amoxicillin specifically, so there is no definitive proof that *Saccharomyces boulardii* will be beneficial for everyone when it is combined with amoxicillin. The studies used 1 gram of *Saccharmoyces boulardii* per day.

A separate double-blind study found that taking a combination of *Lactobacillus acidophilus* and *Lactobacillus bulgaricus,* two normal gut bacteria, with amoxicillin did not protect children from developing diarrhea.[6] The authors of the study point out some problems such as the parents' inability to consistently define diarrhea. However, at this time, it is unknown if lactobacillus products will reduce diarrhea due to amoxicillin.

SUMMARY OF INTERACTIONS FOR AMOXICILLIN

Depletion or interference	*None known*
Adverse interaction	*None known*
Side effect reduction/prevention	*Probiotics*
Supportive interaction	*Bromelain*
Reduced drug absorption/bioavailability	*None known*

AMPHOTERICIN B
(Fungizone)

Amphotericin B is an antifungal drug. Topically, it is used to treat skin yeast infections. Intravenously, it is used to treat a variety of life-threatening fungal infections.

INTERACTIONS WITH DIETARY SUPPLEMENTS

Magnesium

Amphotericin B has been reported to increase urinary excretion of magnesium.[1] It remains unclear whether it is important for people taking this drug to supplement magnesium.

SUMMARY OF INTERACTIONS FOR AMPHOTERICIN B

Depletion or interference	*Magnesium**
Adverse interaction	*None known*
Side effect reduction/prevention	*None known*
Supportive interaction	*None known*
Reduced drug absorption/bioavailability	*None known*

ANESTHETICS, MAJOR

Major general anesthetics are used to make people unconscious during surgery. They are very different from minor (local) anesthetics (such as lidocaine) used in dentistry. Major anesthetics circulate through the entire body and have stronger actions on the nervous system.

INTERACTIONS WITH HERBS

Ginger (Zingiber officinale)

Major anesthetics commonly cause nausea upon waking. Administration of 1 gram of powdered ginger root in capsules 1 hour before surgery has led to reduction in nausea and vomiting as effectively as the antinausea drug metoclopramide in a double-blind study.[1] These results have been independently confirmed.[2] Due to ginger's potential effect on blood clotting, a surgeon should be informed about ginger use prior to surgery.

Milk Thistle (Silybum marianum)

Major anesthetics infrequently cause liver damage. Some herbally oriented doctors suggest taking milk thistle extract containing 70 to 80% silymarin to protect against such problems. The suggested dose is 140 mg of silymarin 3 times per day beginning a week before the surgery and continuing for at least 2 weeks after surgery.

SUMMARY OF INTERACTIONS FOR MAJOR ANESTHETICS

Depletion or interference	*None known*
Adverse interaction	*None known*
Side effect reduction/prevention	*Ginger*
Supportive interaction	*None known*
Reduced drug absorption/bioavailability	*None known*
Other (see text)	*Milk thistle*

ANTACIDS

See also: **aluminum hydroxide** (page 6) and **magnesium hydroxide** (page 135)

Antacids neutralize stomach acid and are recommended by medical doctors to relieve symptoms of heartburn (gastroesophageal reflux), ulcers, and stomach irritation. Calcium-containing antacids are sometimes recommended by medical doctors as a source of supplemental calcium to treat and prevent osteoporosis. Antacid products contain **aluminum hydroxide** (page 6), **magnesium hydroxide** (page 135), calcium carbonate, or other ingredients individually or in various combinations. People should read antacid labels carefully before purchasing to know exactly what they contain.

INTERACTIONS WITH DIETARY SUPPLEMENTS

Vitamins and Minerals

Antacids may interfere with the absorption of other drugs and nutrients, including folic acid and possibly copper and phosphate.[1] [2] [3] It makes sense for people who take antacids long term to supplement with a multivitamin/mineral. People can reduce/prevent nutrient malabsorption problems associated with antacids by talking with their prescribing doctor or pharmacist before using antacids.

SUMMARY OF INTERACTIONS FOR ANTACIDS

Depletion or interference	*Folic acid*
Adverse interaction	*None known*
Side effect reduction/prevention	*None known*
Supportive interaction	*None known*
Reduced drug absorption/bioavailability	*None known*
Other (see text)	*Copper, Phosphate*

ANTHRALIN
(Dithranol, Drithocreme, Micanol Cream)

Anthralin is a drug applied only to affected skin areas to treat psoriasis.

INTERACTIONS WITH DIETARY SUPPLEMENTS

Vitamin E

Anthralin can cause inflammation of the skin. A preliminary study found that topical use of vitamin E was able to protect against this side effect.[1] This report used a tocopherol form of the vitamin rather than tocopheryl. This makes sense, as there is no conclusive proof that the tocopheryl forms (which require an enzyme to split vitamin E from the fatty acid to which it is attached) have any activity on the skin.

SUMMARY OF INTERACTIONS FOR ANTHRALIN

Depletion or interference	*None known*
Adverse interaction	*None known*
Side effect reduction/prevention	*Vitamin E (topical)*
Supportive interaction	*None known*
Reduced drug absorption/bioavailability	*None known*

ANTIBIOTICS

(See also specific listings by drug name.)

Antibiotics constitute a broad range of drugs that are used to treat infections caused by bacteria (antibacterials), viruses (antivirals), fungi (antifungals), and protozoa (antiprotozoals).

INTERACTIONS WITH DIETARY SUPPLEMENTS

Lactobacillus

When antibiotics disturb bacteria in the colon, diarrhea can result. Diarrhea reduces the absorption of all nutrients. Many doctors of natural medicine recommend that people taking antibiotics supplement *Lactobacillus acidophilus,* a "friendly" bacteria that helps reestablish normal conditions in the colon and has been shown to protect against antibiotic-induced diarrhea.[1] Placebo controlled studies have shown clinically and statistically significant results using *Lactobacillus casei* and *Lactobacillus acidophilus* as well as other probiotic microorganisms.[2] Bifidobacteria are sometimes used similarly. A reasonable supplemental amount of friendly (also called probiotic) bacteria is believed to be at least one billion colony forming units (CFU) per day.

Saccharomyces

Saccharomyces boulardii, a harmless yeast, has been shown to prevent diarrhea due to a variety of antibiotics in a double-blind study.[3] A total of 500 mg twice per day of the yeast was used in this study.

One study found that a combination of the antibiotic vancomycin and *Saccharomyces boulardii* (500 mg twice per day) was effective at preventing recurrence of a severe form of diarrhea due to antibiotics known as pseudomembranous colitis.[4] Another study used a related yeast known as brewer's yeast *(Sacchardomyces cerevisiae)* alone to effectively treat this form of antibiotic-induced diarrhea.[5] The amount used was specified only as 3 tablets 3 times per day. People with severe immune compromise (advanced cancer, AIDS, etc.) should use yeast products only under careful supervision, as they may develop infections due to the yeast itself.

Vitamin C

One study has shown that 500 mg of vitamin C could increase the absorption of **tetracycline** (page 199).[6] Another study found that 2,000 mg vitamin C in combination with the antibiotics **trimethoprim-sulfamethoxazole** (page 218) improved the efficacy of the antibiotics in people with cystic fibrosis.[7] Given the preliminary nature of these studies and the differences in how different antibiotics may act when administered with vitamin C, people should consult with a doctor of natural medicine before combining them.

Vitamin K

Vitamin K is important for healthy blood clotting. Antibiotics may interfere with the action of vitamin K in the body or, especially when taken by mouth, may kill friendly bacteria in the large intestine that produce vitamin K. With short-term (a few weeks or less) antibiotic use, the antibiotic actions on vitamin K are usually mild and cause no problems. Vitamin K_1 (phylloquinone) is now found in some multivitamins.

SUMMARY OF INTERACTIONS FOR ANTIBIOTICS

Depletion or interference	*Lactobacillus, Vitamin K*
Adverse interaction	*None known*
Side effect reduction/prevention	*Lactobacillus, Saccharomyces boulardii, Sacchardomyces cerevisiae*
Supportive interaction	*Saccharomyces boulardii, Vitamin C**

Reduced drug absorption/bioavailability   *None known*

ANTICONVULSANTS

Anticonvulsants are a class of drugs used primarily to control (prevent) seizures in people with epilepsy. They are also used to treat seizures in some people with brain cancer, head injury, stroke, and other conditions.

Anticonvulsants include carbamazepine (Tegretol), phenytoin (Dilantin), phenobarbital, primidone (Mysoline), and others. Note: Primidone is an inactive drug that requires conversion by the body to phenobarbital, which has antiseizure activity. See also: **Valproic acid** (page 220) (Depakene) and **divalproex** (page 220) (valproic acid/valproate, Depakote).

INTERACTIONS WITH DIETARY SUPPLEMENTS

Biotin

One study has shown that long-term anticonvulsant treatment may decrease biotin levels in the body.[1] A later study in children found some evidence that anticonvulsant drugs depleted biotin as well.[2] Though the evidence was somewhat mixed in this study, it suggested that anticonvulsants excessively increased the body's breakdown of biotin.

Carnitine

Administration of **valproic acid** (page 220), alone or in combination with other anticonvulsants, lowers carnitine levels.[3] [4] One double-blind study found that when children taking valproic acid or carbamazepine were given 100 mg/kg body weight of carnitine, they did not have significantly better quality of life than when given placebo.[5] Another small study suggested that 15 mg/kg body weight of carnitine could help children on valproic acid who specifically have problems with fatigue and excessive sleepiness.[6] It also appears that rarely children taking valproic acid will develop a condition similar to Reye's syndrome or liver damage due to low carnitine levels.[7] It is unknown if giving carnitine would decrease these problems. At the present time it appears only children with fatigue, symptoms of Reye's syndrome, or liver damage due to valproic acid are likely to benefit from carnitine supplementation. Consult with a doctor immediately if anyone taking valproic acid develops new symptoms of fatigue, yellowing of the skin (jaundice), severe nausea and vomiting, confusion, or forgetfulness.

Folic Acid

Carbamazepine (Tegretol), **valproic acid** (page 220) (Depakene), and phenytoin (Dilantin) have been reported to reduce folic acid absorption in humans.[8][9][10] Homocysteine, a potential marker for folic acid deficiency and for increased risk of heart disease, has been reported to increase in people taking anticonvulsant medications.[11] Drug-induced depletion of folic acid could explain this finding. Anticonvulsant drug therapy in pregnant women has been associated with increased risk of birth defects in their babies. Folic acid supplementation in pregnant women greatly reduces the risk of neural tube defects (a serious, preventable form of birth defects) in their children. Preliminary research, in pregnant women taking anticonvulsant drugs with or without folic acid, found a lower likelihood of birth defects in babies whose mothers took folic acid.[12] Another study involving six fertile women reported that Dilantin taken alone caused a drop in blood folic acid levels while Dilantin plus folic acid resulted in increased blood folic acid levels.[13] While supplementing 1 mg per day of folic acid with anticonvulsant drugs appears to protect against folic acid deficiency, taking higher doses may decrease the efficacy of these drugs, leading to more seizures.[14]

Dilantin therapy causes gum disease (gingival hyperplasia) in some people. A regular program of dental care has been reported to limit or prevent gum disease in people taking Dilantin.[15][16][17] Additional human research suggests that daily mouth rinses with a liquid folic acid preparation may also inhibit Dilantin-induced gum disease.[18]

Melatonin

Evening administration of **valproic acid** (page 220) has been shown to decrease blood levels of melatonin, unlike placebo.[19] Whether valproic acid may cause problems due to melatonin suppression when used as an anticonvulsant drug is presently unknown.

Vitamin D

Anticonvulsant drug therapy can interfere with vitamin D activity, leading to bone loss (osteomalacia).[20] One study of 450 people living in Florida, who took anticonvulsants, found minimal evidence of anticonvulsant-induced bone disease, suggesting that regular exposure to sunlight may be protective.[21]

Vitamin K

Anticonvulsant drug therapy in pregnant women has been associated with vitamin K deficiency in the babies at birth.[22] Research suggests that high-dose (10 mg per day) vitamin K_1 supplementation in pregnant women taking anticonvulsant drugs can prevent vitamin K deficiency in their babies.[23]

SUMMARY OF INTERACTIONS FOR ANTICONVULSANTS

Depletion or interference	*Biotin, Carnitine, Folic Acid, Melatonin, Vitamin D, Vitamin K*
Adverse interaction	*Folic acid (high dose)*
Side effect reduction/prevention	*Folic acid*
Supportive interaction	*None known*
Reduced drug absorption/bioavailability	*None known*

ASPIRIN
(Acetylsalicylic Acid, ASA)

Aspirin is a drug that reduces swelling, pain, and fever. In recent years, long-term low-dose aspirin has been recommended to reduce the risk of heart attacks and strokes. In the future aspirin may be recommended to reduce the risk of some cancers. Reye's syndrome, a rare but serious illness affecting children and teenagers, has been associated with aspirin use. To prevent Reye's syndrome, people should consult their doctor and/or pharmacist before giving aspirin, aspirin-containing products, or herbs containing salicylates to children and teenagers.

INTERACTIONS WITH DIETARY SUPPLEMENTS

Folic Acid

Increased loss of folic acid in urine has been reported in people with rheumatoid arthritis.[1] Reduced blood levels of the vitamin have also been reported in people with arthritis who take aspirin.[2] Some doctors of natural medicine recommend for people with arthritis who regularly take aspirin to supplement 400 mcg of folic acid per day—an amount frequently found in multivitamins.

Iron

Gastrointestinal (GI) bleeding is a common side effect of taking aspirin. A person with aspirin-induced GI bleeding may not always have symptoms (like stomach pain) or obvious signs of blood in their stool. Such bleeding causes loss of iron from the body. Long-term blood loss due to regular use of aspirin can lead to iron deficiency anemia. Lost iron can be replaced with iron supplements. Iron supplementation should be used only in cases of iron deficiency verified with laboratory tests.

Vitamin C

Taking aspirin has been associated with increased loss of vitamin C in urine and has been linked to depletion of vitamin C.[3] People who take aspirin regularly should consider supplementing at least a few hundred milligrams of vitamin C per day. Such an amount is often found in a multivitamin.

Vitamin E

Although vitamin E is thought to act like a blood thinner, very little research has supported this idea. In fact, a double-blind study found that very high amounts of vitamin E do not increase the effects of the powerful blood-thinning drug **warfarin** (page 224).[4] Nonetheless, a double-blind trial found that the combination of aspirin plus 50 IU vitamin E led to a statistically significant increase in bleeding gums compared with taking aspirin alone (affecting one person in three versus one in four with just aspirin).[5] The authors concluded that vitamin E might, especially if combined with aspirin, increase the risk of bleedings.

Zinc

Intake of 3 grams of aspirin per day has been shown to decrease blood levels of zinc.[6] Aspirin appeared to increase loss of zinc in the urine in this study, and the effect was noted beginning 3 days after starting aspirin.

INTERACTIONS WITH HERBS

Cayenne (*Capsicum annuum, Capsicum frutescens*)

Cayenne contains the potent chemical capsaicin, which acts on special nerves found in the stomach lining. In two rat studies, researchers reported that stimulation of these nerves by capsaicin might protect against the damage aspirin can cause to the stomach.[7] [8] In a study of eighteen healthy human volunteers, a single dose of 600 mg aspirin taken after ingestion of 20 grams of chili pepper was found to cause less damage to the lining of the stomach and duodenum (part of the small intestine) than aspirin without chili pepper.[9] However, cayenne may cause stomach irritation in some individuals with stomach inflammation (gastritis) or ulcers and should be used with caution.

Licorice (*Glycyrrhiza glabra*)

The flavonoids found in the extract of licorice known as DGL (deglycyrrhizinated licorice) are helpful for avoiding the irritating actions aspirin has on the stomach and intestines. One study found that 350 mg of chewable DGL taken together with each dose of aspirin reduced gastrointestinal bleeding caused by the aspirin.[10] DGL has been shown in controlled human research to be as effective as drug therapy (**cimetidine** [page 46]) in healing stomach ulcers.[11] One animal study also showed that DGL and the acid-blocking drug **Tagamet** (page 46) (cimetidine) work together more effectively than either alone for preventing negative actions of aspirin.[12]

SUMMARY OF INTERACTIONS FOR ASPIRIN

Depletion or interference	*Folic acid,* * Iron, Vitamin C, Zinc*
Adverse interaction	*Vitamin E*
Side effect reduction/prevention	*None known*
Supportive interaction	*Cayenne, Licorice*
Reduced drug absorption/bioavailability	*None known*

ATENOLOL
(Tenormin and Others)

ATENOLOL/CHLORTHALIDONE
(Tenoretic and Others)

Atenolol is a beta-blocker drug used to treat some heart conditions, reduce the symptoms of angina pectoris (chest pain), lower blood pressure in people with hypertension, and treat people after heart attacks. Atenolol is available alone (Tenormin and others) and in the combination atenolol/chlorthalidone (Tenoretic and others) used to lower blood pressure.

INTERACTIONS WITH FOODS AND OTHER COMPOUNDS

Food

Atenolol may be taken with or without food.[1]

Alcohol

Atenolol may cause drowsiness, dizziness, lightheadedness, or blurred vision.[2] Alcohol may intensify these effects and increase the risk of accidental injury. To prevent problems, people taking atenolol should avoid alcohol.

Tobacco

In a double-blind study of ten cigarette smokers with angina treated with atenolol for 1 week, angina episodes were significantly reduced during the nonsmoking phase compared to the smoking phase.[3] People with angina taking atenolol who do not smoke should avoid starting. Those who smoke should consult with their prescribing doctor about quitting.

SUMMARY OF INTERACTIONS FOR ATENOLOL

Depletion or interference	*None known*
Adverse interaction	*Tobacco*
Side effect reduction/prevention	*None known*
Supportive interaction	*None known*
Reduced drug absorption/bioavailability	*None known*

ATORVASTATIN
(Lipitor)

Atorvastatin is a member of the HMG-CoA reductase inhibitor family of drugs that blocks the body's production of cholesterol. Atorvastatin is used to lower elevated cholesterol.

INTERACTIONS WITH DIETARY SUPPLEMENTS

Coenzyme Q₁₀

In a randomized, double-blind trial, blood levels of coenzyme Q_{10} (CoQ_{10}) were found in forty-five people with high cholesterol treated with **lovastatin** (page 133) or **pravastatin** (page 175) (drugs related to atorvastatin) for 18 weeks.[1] A significant decline in blood levels of CoQ_{10} occurred with either drug. One study found that supplementation with 100 mg of CoQ_{10} prevented declines in CoQ_{10} when taken with **simvastatin** (page 189) (another HMG-CoA reductase inhibitor drug).[2] Many nutritionally oriented doctors recommend that people taking HMG-CoA reductase inhibitor drugs such as atorvastatin also supplement with approximately 100 mg CoQ_{10} per day, although lower doses, such as 10 to 30 mg per day, might conceivably be effective in preventing the decline in CoQ_{10} levels.

Magnesium-Containing Antacids

A magnesium- and aluminum-containing **antacid** (page 13) was reported to interfere with atorvastatin absorption.[3] People can avoid this interaction by taking atorvastatin 2 hours before or after any aluminum/ magnesium-containing antacids. Some magnesium supplements such as **magnesium hydroxide** (page 135) are also antacids.

Niacin

Niacin is the form of vitamin B_3 used to lower cholesterol. High-dose niacin taken with **lovastatin** (page 133) (a drug closely related to atorvastatin) or with atorvastatin itself may cause muscle disorders (myopathy) that can become serious (rhabdomyolysis).[4] [5] Such problems appear to be uncommon.[6] [7] Moreover, niacin has been successfully combined with statin drugs to reduce cholesterol more effectively than using these drugs without niacin.[8] [9] People taking both atorvastatin and niacin should be monitored for muscle disorders by the prescribing physician.

Vitamin A

A study of thirty-seven people with high cholesterol treated with diet and HMG-CoA reductase inhibitors found blood vitamin A levels increased over 2 years of therapy.[10] Until more is known, people taking HMG-CoA reductase inhibitors, including atorvastatin, should have blood levels of vitamin A monitored if they intend to supplement vitamin A.

INTERACTIONS WITH FOODS AND OTHER COMPOUNDS

Food

Atorvastatin is best absorbed when taken without food[11] in the morning.[12] However, it has been reported to be equally well absorbed when taken with or without food.[13]

SUMMARY OF INTERACTIONS FOR ATORVASTATIN

Depletion or interference	*Coenzyme Q$_{10}$*
Adverse interaction	*Vitamin A**
Side effect reduction/prevention	*None known*
Supportive interaction	*None known*
Reduced drug absorption/bioavailability	*None known*
Other (see text)	*Magnesium-containing antacids, Niacin*

ATROPINE

Atropine is an alkaloid (a family of chemicals with pharmocologic activity and a common structure) that affects the nervous system. It is found in deadly nightshade (*Atropa belladona*) and other plants. Some effects of atropine include blurred vision, dilated pupils, constipation, dry mouth, and dry eyes.

Atropine is available as a prescription drug, synthesized in the laboratory. It is used to help restore or control heart function. It is used in combination with other drugs to treat other health problems including diarrhea and excessive salivation (saliva production). Atropine drops (Isopto Atropine and others) are used to dilate pupils for eye exams.

INTERACTIONS WITH HERBS

Tannin-Containing Herbs

Tannins are a group of unrelated chemicals that give plants an astringent taste. Herbs containing high amounts of tannins, such as green tea *(Camellia sinensis)*, black tea, uva ursi *(Arctostaphylos uva-ursi)*, black walnut *(Juglans nigra)*, red raspberry *(Rubus idaeus)*, oak *(Quercus* spp.), and witch hazel *(Hamamelis virginiana)*, may interfere with the absorption of atropine taken by mouth.[1]

SUMMARY OF INTERACTIONS FOR ATROPINE

Depletion or interference	*None known*
Adverse interaction	*None known*
Side effect reduction/prevention	*None known*
Supportive interaction	*None known*
Reduced drug absorption/bioavailability	*Tannin-containing herbs* * such as green tea, black tea, uva ursi, black walnut, red raspberry, oak, and witch hazel*

AZITHROMYCIN
(Zithromax)

Azithromycin is a macrolide **antibiotic** (page 13) used to treat a variety of bacterial infections.

INTERACTIONS WITH DIETARY SUPPLEMENTS

Magnesium

A magnesium- and aluminum-containing **antacid** (page 13) was reported to interfere with azithromycin absorption in a study of ten healthy people.[1] People can avoid this interaction by taking azithromycin 2 hours before or after any aluminum/magnesium-containing products. It has not yet been shown that magnesium compounds typically found in supplements affect absorption of this drug.

INTERACTIONS WITH HERBS

Digitalis (*Digitalis lanata, Digitalis purpurea*)

Digitalis refers to a family of plants commonly called foxglove that contain digitalis glycosides, chemicals with actions and toxicities similar to the prescription drug **digoxin** (page 71).

Erythromycin (page 86) and **clarithromycin** (page 51) (drugs closely related to azithromycin) can increase the serum level of digitalis glycosides, increasing the therapeutic effects as well as the risk of side effects.[2] While this interaction has not been reported with azithromycin, until more is known, azithromycin and digitalis-containing products should be used only under the direct supervision of a doctor trained in their use.

INTERACTIONS WITH FOODS AND OTHER COMPOUNDS

Food

Azithromycin suspension should be taken on an empty stomach, 1 hour before or 2 hours after food.[3] Azithromycin tablets may be taken with or without food and should be swallowed whole, without cutting, chewing, or crushing.[4]

SUMMARY OF INTERACTIONS FOR AZITHROMYCIN

Depletion or interference	*None known*
Adverse interaction	*None known*
Side effect reduction/prevention	*None known*
Supportive interaction	*None known*
Reduced drug absorption/bioavailability	*None known*
Other (see text)	*Magnesium, Digitalis*

AZT
(*Azidothymidine, Zidovudine, Retrovir*)

AZT inhibits reproduction of retroviruses, including the human immunodeficiency virus (HIV). HIV is the virus that infects people, causing acquired immunodeficiency syndrome (AIDS), also called HIV disease. AZT is one of a number of drugs used to treat HIV infection and HIV disease.

INTERACTIONS WITH DIETARY SUPPLEMENTS

General Nutrition

Preliminary human research suggests AZT therapy may cause a reduction in copper and zinc blood levels. Animal studies suggest that vitamin E may improve the efficacy of AZT.[1] The practical importance of these findings remains unclear.

Carnitine

There is some preliminary information suggesting that muscle damage sometimes caused by AZT is at least partially due to depletion of carnitine in the muscles by the drug.[2]

Vitamin B_{12}

Vitamin B_{12} deficiency in HIV-infected persons may be more common in those taking AZT.[3] HIV-infected people with low vitamin B_{12} levels were shown in one study to be more likely to develop blood-related side effects (particularly anemia) from taking AZT.[4]

Thymopentin

Thymopentin is a small protein that comes from a natural hormone in the body known as thymopoietin. This hormone stimulates production of the white blood cells known as T lymphocytes. Combination of thymopentin with AZT tended to decrease the rate at which HIV-infected persons progressed to AIDS.[5] Thymopentin alone did not seem to have a benefit in this study. Since thymopentin is administered by injections into the skin, people should consult with a doctor of medicine as to the availability of this substance.

Zinc

A study found that adding 200 mg zinc per day to AZT treatment decreased the number of *Pneumocystis carinii* pneumonia and *Candida* infections in people with AIDS compared with people treated with AZT alone.[6] The zinc also improved weight and CD4 cell levels. The amount of zinc used in this study was very high and should be combined with 1 to 2 mg of copper to reduce the risk of immune problems from the zinc long term.

SUMMARY OF INTERACTIONS FOR AZT

Depletion or interference	*Carnitine,* Copper, Vitamin B_{12}*
Adverse interaction	*None known*
Side effect reduction/prevention	*None known*
Supportive interaction	*Thymopentin, Zinc*
Reduced drug absorption/bioavailability	*None known*
Other (see text)	*Vitamin E*

BENAZEPRIL
(Lotensin)

Benazepril is an **angiotensin-converting enzyme (ACE) inhibitor** (page 1) drug used to treat high blood pressure.

INTERACTIONS WITH DIETARY SUPPLEMENTS

Potassium

ACE inhibitors may increase blood potassium levels.[1] This problem is more likely to occur with advanced kidney disease. Potassium supplements, potassium-containing salt substitutes (No Salt, Morton Salt Substitute, and others), and even foods that are uncommonly high in potassium (primarily fruit) will increase the chances of potentially dangerous elevations in blood potassium. People taking ACE inhibitors should avoid unnecessary potassium supplementation.

Zinc

In a study of thirty-four people with hypertension, 6 months of **captopril** (page 35) or **enalapril** (page 82) (ACE inhibitors related to benazepril) treatment led to decreased zinc levels in certain white blood cells,[2] raising concerns about possible ACE inhibitor–induced zinc depletion. While zinc depletion has not been reported with benazepril, until more is known, it makes sense for people taking benazepril long term to consider, as a precaution, taking a zinc supplement or a multimineral tablet containing zinc. (Such multiminerals usually contain no more than 99 mg of potassium, probably not enough to trigger the above-mentioned interaction.) Supplements containing zinc should also contain copper, to protect against a zinc-induced copper deficiency.

INTERACTIONS WITH FOODS AND OTHER COMPOUNDS

Food

Benazepril may be taken with or without food.[3]

SUMMARY OF INTERACTIONS FOR BENAZEPRIL

Depletion or interference	Zinc[*]
Adverse interaction	Potassium[*]
Side effect reduction/prevention	None known
Supportive interaction	None known
Reduced drug absorption/bioavailability	None known

BENZODIAZEPINES

Benzodiazepines are used to treat insomnia, anxiety, panic attacks, seizures, and other conditions.

Benzodiazepines are a family of drugs that include alprazolam (Xanax), chlordiazepoxide (Librium), clonazepam (Klonopin), diazepam (Valium), flurazepam (Dalmane), lorazapam (Ativan), temazepam (Restoril), triazolam (Halcion), and others.

INTERACTIONS WITH DIETARY SUPPLEMENTS

Melatonin

Combination of melatonin and the benzodiazepine triazolam in healthy people has been shown to have some beneficial effects on sleep in a small study.[1] A very high dose of melatonin (100 mg) was used in this study and is generally unnecessary.

INTERACTIONS WITH HERBS

Kava *(Piper methysticum)*

Kava was once thought to act in a related way to benzodiazepines, but this has not been borne out by science.[2] Instead, kava appears to work in the limbic system, a part of the brain involved in regulating mood and wakefulness.[3] Kava has been used by some doctors of natural medicine as an alternative to benzodiazepines.

In one report, a man taking the benzodiazepine alprazolam (Xanax) plus other prescription drugs and kava was hospitalized in a lethargic and disoriented state; however, kava was not proven to be the cause of this reaction.[4] One of the drugs he was taking was **cimetidine** (page 46) (Tagamet), which can alter the metabolism of other drugs and possibly herbs.

SUMMARY OF INTERACTIONS FOR BENZODIAZEPINES

Depletion or interference	*None known*
Adverse interaction	*Kava**
Side effect reduction/prevention	*None known*
Supportive interaction	*Melatonin**
Reduced drug absorption/bioavailability	*None known*

BILE ACID SEQUESTRANTS
(Cholestyramine, Questran; Colestipol, Colestid)

Cholestyramine (Questran) and **colestipol** (page 56) (Colestid) are bile acid sequestrants—a class of drugs that binds bile acids, prevents their reabsorption from the digestive system, and reduces cholesterol levels. Cholestyramine and colestipol are two of many drugs used to lower cholesterol levels in people with high cholesterol.

Bile acids are produced in the liver from cholesterol and secreted into the small intestine to help with the absorption of dietary fat and cholesterol. Bile acid sequestrants bind bile acids in the small intestine and carry them out of the body. This causes the body to use more cholesterol to make more bile acids, which are secreted into the small intestine, bound to bile acid sequestrants, and carried out of the body. The end result is lower cholesterol levels. Bile acid sequestrants also prevent absorption of some dietary cholesterol.

INTERACTIONS WITH DIETARY SUPPLEMENTS

Vitamins

Bile acid sequestrants may prevent absorption of folic acid and the fat-soluble vitamins A, D, E, and K.[1] [2] Other medications and vitamin supplements should be taken 1 hour before or 4 to 6 hours after bile acid sequestrants for optimal absorption.[3] Animal studies suggest calcium and zinc may also be depleted by taking cholestyramine.[4]

Carotenoids

Use of colestipol for 6 months has been shown to significantly lower blood levels of carotenoids including beta-carotene.[5]

INTERACTIONS WITH FOODS AND OTHER COMPOUNDS

Food

Bile acid sequestrants should be taken with plenty of water before meals.[6]

SUMMARY OF INTERACTIONS FOR BILE ACID SEQUESTRANTS

Depletion or interference	Calcium,* Carotenoids, Folic acid, Vitamin A, Vitamin D, Vitamin E, Vitamin K, Zinc*
Adverse interaction	None known

Side effect reduction/prevention	*None known*
Supportive interaction	*None known*
Reduced drug absorption/bioavailability	*None known*

BISACODYL
(Dulcolax)

Bisacodyl, a stimulant-type laxative used to treat constipation, is available as a nonprescription product. All laxatives, including bisacodyl, should be used for a maximum of 1 week to prevent laxative dependence and loss of normal bowel function.

INTERACTIONS WITH DIETARY SUPPLEMENTS

Potassium and Other Nutrients

Prolonged and frequent use of stimulant laxatives, including bisacodyl, may cause excessive and unwanted loss of water, potassium, and other nutrients from the body.[1] [2] Bisacodyl should be used for a maximum of 1 week, or as directed on the package label. Excessive use of any laxative can cause depletion of many nutrients. In order to protect against multiple nutrient deficiencies, it is important to not overuse laxatives.[3] People with constipation should consult with their doctor or pharmacist before using bisacodyl.

INTERACTIONS WITH FOODS AND OTHER COMPOUNDS

Food

Bisacodyl tablets are enteric coated to pass through the stomach and dissolve in the small intestine. Milk, dairy products, vegetables, almonds, chestnuts, and other foods can cause the enteric coating to dissolve in the stomach, leading to irritation and cramping.[4] People should take bisacodyl 1 hour before or 2 hours after meals to avoid this problem.

SUMMARY OF INTERACTIONS FOR BISACODYL

Depletion or interference	*Potassium*
Adverse interaction	*None known*
Side effect reduction/prevention	*None known*
Supportive interaction	*None known*
Reduced drug absorption/bioavailability	*None known*

BISMUTH SUBSALICYLATE
(BSS, Pepto-Bismol, Bismatrol, and Others)

Bismuth subsalicylate is a nonprescription drug used to relieve indigestion without constipation, nausea, and abdominal cramps. It is also used to control diarrhea and traveler's diarrhea. Bismuth subsalicylate is used together with prescription **antibiotics** (page 14) and stomach acid-blocking drugs to treat gastric and duodenal ulcers associated with *Helicobacter pylori* infection.

INTERACTIONS WITH HERBS

Salicylate-Containing Herbs

Bismuth subsalicylate contains salicylates. Various herbs including meadowsweet *(Filipendula ulmaria)*, poplar *(Populus tremuloides)*, willow *(Salix* spp.), and wintergreen *(Gaultheria procumbens)* contain salicylates as well. Though similar to **aspirin** (page 18), plant salicylates have been shown to have different actions in test tube studies.[1] Furthermore, salicylates are poorly absorbed and likely do not build up to levels sufficient to cause negative interactions that aspirin might.[2] No reports have been published of negative interactions between salicylate-containing plants and aspirin or aspirin-containing drugs.[3] Therefore concerns about combining salicylate-containing herbs remain theoretical, and the risk of causing problems appears to be low.

SUMMARY OF INTERACTIONS FOR BISMUTH SUBSALICYLATE

Depletion or interference	*None known*
Adverse interaction	*Salicylate-containing herbs* * *such as meadowsweet, poplar, willow, and wintergreen*
Side effect reduction/prevention	*None known*
Supportive interaction	*None known*
Reduced drug absorption/bioavailability	*None known*

BISOPROLOL
(Zebeta)

BISOPROLOL/HYDROCHLOROTHIAZIDE
(Ziac)

Bisoprolol is a beta-blocker drug used to lower blood pressure in people with hypertension. Bisoprolol is available alone (Zebeta) and in the combination bisoprolol/**hydrochlorothiazide** (page 202) (Ziac).

INTERACTIONS WITH FOODS AND OTHER COMPOUNDS

Food

Bisoprolol may be taken with or without food.[1]

Alcohol

Bisoprolol may cause drowsiness, dizziness, lightheadedness, or blurred vision.[2] Alcohol may intensify these effects and increase the risk of accidental injury. To prevent problems, people taking bisoprolol should avoid alcohol.

SUMMARY OF INTERACTIONS FOR BISOPROLOL

Depletion or interference	*None known*
Adverse interaction	*None known*
Side effect reduction/prevention	*None known*
Supportive interaction	*None known*
Reduced drug absorption/bioavailability	*None known*

BROMPHENIRAMINE
(Dimetapp Allergy and Others)

BROMPHENIRAMINE/PHENYLPROPANOLAMINE
(Dimetapp, DayQuil Allergy Relief, and Others)

Brompheniramine is an antihistamine used to relieve allergic rhinitis (seasonal allergy) symptoms including sneezing, runny nose, itching, and watery eyes. It is also used to treat immediate allergic reactions. Brompheniramine is available in nonprescription products alone (Dimetapp Allergy and others), in the combination brompheniramine/**phenylpropanolamine** (page 172) (Dimetapp, DayQuil Allergy Relief, and others), and in combination with other nonprescription drugs to treat symptoms of allergy, colds, and upper respiratory infections.

INTERACTIONS WITH HERBS

Henbane *(Hyoscyamus niger)*

Antihistamines, including brompheniramine, can cause "anticholinergic" side effects such as dryness of mouth and heart palpitations. Henbane also has anticholinergic activity and side effects. Therefore, use with brompheniramine could increase the risk of anticholinergic side effects,[1] though apparently no interactions have yet been reported with brompheniramine and henbane. Henbane should not be taken except by prescription from a physician trained in herbal medicine, as it is extremely toxic.

INTERACTIONS WITH FOODS AND OTHER COMPOUNDS

Alcohol

Brompheniramine causes drowsiness.[2] Alcohol may intensify this effect and increase the risk of accidental injury.[3] To prevent problems, people taking brompheniramine or brompheniramine-containing products should avoid alcohol.

SUMMARY OF INTERACTIONS FOR BROMPHENIRAMINE

Depletion or interference	*None known*
Adverse interaction	*Henbane*[*]
Side effect reduction/prevention	*None known*
Supportive interaction	*None known*
Reduced drug absorption/bioavailability	*None known*

BUSPIRONE

(Buspar)

Buspirone is used to treat anxiety disorders and less commonly to treat symptoms of premenstrual syndrome.

INTERACTIONS WITH HERBS

Kava *(Piper methysticum)*

Although no direct interactions have been reported, busiprone should not be used together with kava.

INTERACTIONS WITH FOODS AND OTHER COMPOUNDS

Food

Food reduces metabolism of buspirone, increasing serum buspirone levels.[1] Buspirone should be taken at the same time each day, always with food or always without food.

Alcohol

Buspirone may cause drowsiness and dizziness.[2] Alcohol may compound these effects and increase the risk of accidental injury. To prevent problems, people taking buspirone should avoid alcohol.

SUMMARY OF INTERACTIONS FOR BUSPIRONE

Depletion or interference	*None known*
Adverse interaction	*Kava*
Side effect reduction/prevention	*None known*
Supportive interaction	*None known*
Reduced drug absorption/bioavailability	*None known*

CAFFEINE
(Caffedrine, NoDoz, Quick Pep, Vivarin)

CAFFEINE/ASPIRIN
(Anacin and Others)

Caffeine is a central nervous system stimulant drug used as an aid to stay awake, for mental alertness due to fatigue, and as an adjunct with other drugs for pain relief. Caffeine is available alone as a nonprescription drug (Caffedrine, NoDoz, Quick Pep, Vivarin). It is also available in combination with other nonprescription drugs (caffeine/aspirin, Anacin and others) and in prescription drug combinations for relief of pain and headache.

INTERACTIONS WITH DIETARY SUPPLEMENTS

Calcium

In 205 healthy postmenopausal women, caffeine consumption (3 cups of coffee per day) was associated with bone loss in women with calcium intake of less than 800 mg per day.[1] In a group of 980 postmenopausal women, lifetime caffeine intake equal to 2 cups of coffee per day was associated with decreased bone density in those who did not drink at least 1 glass of milk daily during most of their life.[2] However, in 138 healthy postmenopausal women, long-term dietary caffeine (coffee) intake was not associated with bone density.[3] Until more is known, postmenopausal women should limit caffeine consumption and consume a total of approximately 1,500 mg of calcium per day (from diet and supplements).

INTERACTIONS WITH HERBS

Guaraná (Paullinia cupana)

Guaraná is a plant with a high caffeine content. Combining caffeine drug products and guaraná increases caffeine-induced side effects.

Ephedra sinica (Ma huang)

Many herbal weight loss and quick energy products combine caffeine or caffeine-containing herbs with ma huang (Ephedra sinica). This combination may lead to dangerously increased heart rate and blood pressure and should be avoided by people with heart conditions, hypertension, diabetes, or thyroid disease.[4]

INTERACTIONS WITH FOODS AND OTHER COMPOUNDS

Food

Caffeine is found in coffee, tea, soft drinks, and chocolate. To reduce side effects, people taking caffeine-containing drug products should limit their intake of caffeine-containing foods/beverages.

Tobacco

Smoking can increase caffeine metabolism,[5] decreasing effectiveness. Smokers who use caffeine-containing drug products may require higher doses of caffeine to achieve effectiveness.

SUMMARY OF INTERACTIONS FOR CAFFEINE

Depletion or interference	*Calcium*
Adverse interaction	*Ephedra, Tobacco*

Side effect reduction/prevention	*None known*
Supportive interaction	*None known*
Reduced drug absorption/bioavailability	*None known*
Other (see text)	*Guaraná*

CAPTOPRIL
(Capoten)

Captopril is an **angiotensin-converting enzyme (ACE) inhibitor** (page 1)—a family of drugs used to treat high blood pressure and some types of heart failure. Captopril is also used to slow the progression of kidney disease in people with diabetes.

INTERACTIONS WITH DIETARY SUPPLEMENTS

Potassium

ACE inhibitors may increase blood potassium levels.[1] Potassium supplements, potassium-containing salt substitutes (No Salt, Morton Salt Substitute, and others), and even high-potassium foods (primarily fruit) can be problematic.

Zinc

Preliminary research has found significant loss of zinc in urine triggered by taking captopril.[2] In this trial, depletion of zinc reduced red blood cell levels of zinc—a test that can be ordered by a doctor. Although details remain unclear, it now appears that chronic use of captopril may lead to a zinc deficiency.[3] It makes sense for people taking captopril long term to consider taking a zinc supplement or a multimineral tablet containing zinc as a precaution. (Such multiminerals usually contain no more than 99 mg of potassium, probably not enough to trigger the above-mentioned interaction.) Supplements containing zinc should also contain copper, to protect against a zinc-induced copper deficiency.

SUMMARY OF INTERACTIONS FOR CAPTOPRIL

Depletion or interference	*Zinc*
Adverse interaction	*Potassium*
Side effect reduction/prevention	*None known*
Supportive interaction	*None known*
Reduced drug absorption/bioavailability	*None known*

CARBIDOPA
(Lodosyn)

CARBIDOPA/LEVODOPA
(Sinemet)

Carbidopa is used together with the drug **levodopa** (page 124) to reduce symptoms of Parkinson's disease.

INTERACTIONS WITH DIETARY SUPPLEMENTS

Iron

Iron supplements taken with carbidopa may interfere with the action of the drug.[1]

5-Hydroxytryptophan (5-HTP)

5-HTP and carbidopa have been reported to improve intention myoclonus (a neuromuscular disorder) in some human cases but not others.[2][3][4] Several cases of scleroderma-like illness have been reported in people using carbidopa and 5-HTP for intention myoclonus.[5][6][7]

SUMMARY OF INTERACTIONS FOR CARBIDOPA

Depletion or interference	*None known*
Adverse interaction	*None known*
Side effect reduction/prevention	*None known*
Supportive interaction	*None known*
Reduced drug absorption/bioavailability	*Iron*
Other (see text)	*5-HTP*

CARBIDOPA/LEVODOPA
(Sinemet)

Levodopa (page 124) is required by the brain to produce dopamine, an important neurotransmitter (chemical messenger). People with Parkinson's disease have depleted levels of dopamine, leading to debilitating symptoms. Levodopa is given to increase production of dopamine and reduce the symptoms of Parkinson's disease. When taken by mouth, levodopa is broken down by the body before it reaches the brain. Sinemet combines levodopa with **carbidop**a (page 36), a drug that prevents the breakdown, allowing levodopa to reach the brain to increase dopamine levels.

INTERACTIONS WITH DIETARY SUPPLEMENTS

Vitamin B$_6$

Levodopa is broken down in the body by a process requiring vitamin B$_6$. Breakdown of the large doses of levodopa used to treat Parkinson's disease may use up available vitamin B$_6$, possibly leading to vitamin B$_6$ deficiency. Carbidopa blocks levodopa breakdown and prevents vitamin B$_6$ depletion. People taking Sinemet (carbidopa/levodopa) have no risk for levodopa-induced vitamin B$_6$ deficiency.[1]

Iron

Iron supplements taken with carbidopa interfere with the action of the drug.[2] People taking carbidopa should not supplement iron without consulting with the prescribing physician.

5-Hydroxytryptophan (5-HTP)

5-HTP and carbidopa have been reported to improve intention myoclonus (a neuromuscular disorder) in some human cases but not others.[3][4][5] Several cases of scleroderma-like illness have been reported in people using carbidopa and 5-HTP for intention myoclonus.[6][7][8]

INTERACTIONS WITH FOODS AND OTHER COMPOUNDS

Food

Food, especially foods high in protein, can alter levodopa absorption.[9][10] However, Sinemet is often taken with food to avoid stomach upset. Sinemet and Sinemet CR should be taken at the same time, always with or always without food, every day.

SUMMARY OF INTERACTIONS FOR CARBIDOPA/LEVODOPA

Depletion or interference	*None known*
Adverse interaction	*None known*
Side effect reduction/prevention	*None known*
Supportive interaction	*None known*
Reduced drug absorption/bioavailability	*Iron*
Other (see text)	*5-HTP, Vitamin B$_6$*

CARISOPRODOL
(Soma and Others)

CARISOPRODOL/ASPIRIN
(Soma Compound and Others)

CARISOPRODOL/ASPIRIN/CODEINE
(Soma Compound with Codeine)

Carisoprodol is a drug used as an adjunct to rest and physical therapy for relief of muscle pain. Carisoprodol is available alone by prescription (Soma and others). It is also available in the combinations carisoprodol/**aspirin** (page 18) (Soma Compound and others) and carisoprodol/**aspirin** (page 18)/**codeine** (page 54) (Soma Compound with Codeine).

INTERACTIONS WITH FOODS AND OTHER COMPOUNDS

Food

Carisoprodol may be taken with food to prevent stomach upset.[1]

Alcohol

Carisoprodol may cause dizziness or drowsiness.[2] Alcohol may intensify these effects and increase the risk of accidental injury. To prevent problems, people taking carisoprodol or carisoprodol-containing products should avoid alcohol.

SUMMARY OF INTERACTIONS FOR CARISOPRODOL

Depletion or interference	*None known*
Adverse interaction	*None known*
Side effect reduction/prevention	*None known*
Supportive interaction	*None known*
Reduced drug absorption/bioavailability	*None known*

CEPHALOSPORINS

Cephalosporins are a family of **antibiotics** (page 14), related to penicillins, that are used to treat a wide variety of bacterial infections. Cephalosporins include cefixime (Suprax), cefpodoxime (Vantin), cefprozil (Cefzil), ceftriaxone

(Rocephin), cefuroxime (Ceftin), cephaclor (Ceclor), cephadroxil (Duricef), cephalexin (Keflex, Keftab), loracarbef (Lorabid), and many others.

INTERACTIONS WITH DIETARY SUPPLEMENTS

Vitamin K

Cephalosporins and other antibiotics may interfere with the action of vitamin K in the body, or especially when taken by mouth may kill friendly bacteria in the large intestine, which produces vitamin K.[1] With short-term (a few weeks or less) cephalosporin use, the actions on vitamin K are usually mild and typically cause no problems. After finishing cephalosporin therapy, vitamin K activity returns to normal. Vitamin K_1 (phylloquinon) is now found in some multivitamins.

SUMMARY OF INTERACTIONS FOR CEPHALOSPORINS

Depletion or interference	*Vitamin K*
Adverse interaction	*None known*
Side effect reduction/prevention	*None known*
Supportive interaction	*None known*
Reduced drug absorption/bioavailability	*None known*

CETIRIZINE
(Zyrtec)

Cetirizine is a selective antihistamine used to relieve allergic rhinitis (seasonal allergy) symptoms including sneezing, runny nose, itching, and watery eyes. It is also used to treat people with idiopathic urticaria.

INTERACTIONS WITH FOODS AND OTHER COMPOUNDS

Food

Cetirizine may be taken with or without food.[1]

Alcohol

Selective antihistamines, including cetirizine, may cause drowsiness or dizziness, although it is less likely than with nonselective antihistamines.[2] Alcohol can intensify drowsiness and dizziness, increasing the risk of accidental injury. People taking cetirizine should use alcohol only with caution.

SUMMARY OF INTERACTIONS FOR CETIRIZINE

Depletion or interference	*None known*
Adverse interaction	*None known*
Side effect reduction/prevention	*None known*
Supportive interaction	*None known*
Reduced drug absorption/bioavailability	*None known*

CHEMOTHERAPY

Chemotherapy is used primarily to treat people with cancer, although certain chemotherapy drugs have other functions. For example, **methotrexate** (page 140) is also used with some people with rheumatoid arthritis. Certain chemotherapy drugs have interactions with specific nutrients. For drug-specific information, see the sections on **doxorubicin** (page 78) (Adriamycin), **cisplatin** (page 50), **cyclophosphamide** (page 64), **methotrexate** (page 140), and **paclitaxel** (page 164). What follows is general information about chemotherapy and nutrition.

Nausea

The newer antinausea drugs prescribed for people taking chemotherapy lead to greatly reduced nausea and vomiting for most people. Nonetheless, these drugs often do not totally eliminate all nausea. Natural substances used to reduce nausea should not be used instead of prescription antinausea drugs. Rather, under the guidance of a nutritionally oriented doctor, they should be added to those drugs if needed. At least one trial suggests that N-acetyl cysteine (NAC), at 1,800 mg per day may reduce nausea and vomiting caused by chemotherapy.[1] NAC is an amino acid–like supplement that produces antioxidant activity. Ginger can also be helpful in alleviating nausea and vomiting caused by chemotherapy.[2] [3] Ginger, as tablets, capsules, or liquid herbal extracts, can be taken in 500 mg amounts every 2 or 3 hours, for a total of 1 gram per day.

Mouth Sores

Chemotherapy frequently causes mouth sores. In one trial, people were given approximately 400,000 IU of beta-carotene per day for 3 weeks and then 125,000 IU per day for an additional 4 weeks.[4] Those taking beta-carotene still suffered mouth sores, but the mouth sores developed later and tended to be less severe than mouth sores that formed in people receiving the same chemotherapy without beta-carotene.

In a study of chemotherapy-induced mouth sores, six of nine people who applied vitamin E directly to their mouth sores had complete resolution of the sores compared with one of nine people who applied placebo.[5] Others have confirmed the potential for vitamin E to help people with chemotherapy-induced mouth sores.[6] Applying vitamin E only once per day was helpful to only some groups of people in another trial,[7] and not all studies have found vitamin E to be effective.[8] Until more is known, if vitamin E is used in an attempt to reduce chemotherapy-induced mouth sores, it should be applied topically twice per day and should probably be in the tocopherol (versus tocopheryl) form.

The role of glutamine for mouth sores is explained in more detail in a subsequent section.

Food Aversions

Often, people who undergo chemotherapy develop aversions to certain foods, sometimes making it permanently difficult to eat those foods. Exposing people to what researchers have called a "scapegoat stimulus" just before the administration of chemotherapy can direct the food aversion to the "scapegoat" food instead of more important parts of the diet. In one trial, fruit drinks administered just before chemotherapy were most effective in protecting against aversions to other foods.[9]

INTERACTIONS WITH DIETARY SUPPLEMENTS

Vitamin A and Late-Stage Disease

A controlled French trial reported that when women with post-menopausal late-stage breast cancer were given very large amounts of vitamin A (350,000 to 500,000 IU per day) along with chemotherapy, remission rates were significantly better than when the chemotherapy was not accompanied by vitamin A.[10] Similar results were not found in premenopausal women. The large doses of vitamin A used in the study are toxic and require clinical supervision.

Antioxidants

Chemotherapy can injure cancer cells by creating oxidative damage. As a result, some oncologists (cancer specialists) recommend that people avoid supplementing antioxidants if they are undergoing chemotherapy. Limited test tube research occasionally does support the idea that an antioxidant can interfere with oxidative damage to cancer cells.[11] However, most scientific research does not support this supposition.

A modified form of vitamin A has been reported to work synergistically with chemotherapy in test tube research.[12] Vitamin C appears to increase the effectiveness of chemotherapy in animals[13] and with human breast cancer cells in test tube research.[14] In a double-blind study, Japanese researchers found that the combination of vitamin E, vitamin C, and N-acetyl cysteine (NAC)—all antioxidants—protected against chemotherapy-induced heart damage without interfering with the action of the chemotherapy.[15] A comprehensive review of antioxidants and chemotherapy leaves open the question of whether supplemental antioxidants definitely help people with chemotherapy side effects, but it clearly shows that antioxidants need not be avoided for fear that the actions of chemotherapy are interfered with.[16] Although research remains incomplete, the idea that people taking chemotherapy should avoid antioxidants is not supported by scientific research.

Glutamine

Though cancer cells use glutamine as a fuel source, studies in humans have not found that glutamine stimulates growth of cancers in people taking chemotherapy.[17] [18] In fact, animal studies show that glutamine may actually decrease tumor growth while increasing susceptibility of cancer cells to radiation and chemotherapy,[19] [20] though such effects have not yet been studied in humans.

Glutamine has successfully reduced chemotherapy-induced mouth sores.[21] In this trial, people were given 4 grams of glutamine in an oral rinse, which was swished around the mouth and then swallowed twice per day. Thirteen of fourteen people in the study had fewer days with mouth sores as a result. These excellent results have been duplicated in randomized double-blind research.[22]

It has been suggested by one double-blind study that 6 grams of glutamine taken 3 times per day can decrease diarrhea caused by chemotherapy.[23] However, other studies using higher amounts or intravenous glutamine have not reported this effect.[24] [25]

Intravenous use of glutamine in people undergoing bone marrow transplants, a procedure sometimes used to allow very high doses of chemotherapy to be used, has led to reduced hospital stays, leading to a savings of over $21,000 for each person given glutamine instead of placebo.[26]

N-Acetyl Cysteine (NAC)

NAC has been used in four human studies to decrease the kidney and bladder toxicity of the chemotherapy drug ifosfamide.[27] [28] [29] [30] These studies used 1 to 2 grams NAC 4 times per day. There was no sign that NAC interfered with the efficacy of ifosfamide in any of these studies. Intakes of NAC over 4 grams per day may cause nausea and vomiting.

Melatonin

High doses of melatonin have been combined with a variety of chemotherapy drugs to reduce their side effects or improve drug efficacy. One study gave melatonin at night in combination with the drug triptorelin to men with metastatic prostate.[31] All of these men had previously become unresponsive to triptorelin. The combination decreased PSA levels—a marker of prostate cancer progression—in eight of fourteen people, decreased some side effects of triptorelin, and helped nine of fourteen to live longer than 1 year. The outcome of this preliminary study suggests that melatonin may improve the efficacy of triptorelin even after the drug has apparently lost effectiveness.

Nutrient Malabsorption

Many chemotherapy drugs can cause diarrhea, lack of appetite, vomiting, and damage to the gastrointestinal tract. Recent antinausea prescription medications are often effective. Nonetheless, nutritional deficiencies still occur.[32] It makes sense for people undergoing chemotherapy to take a high-potency multivitamin/mineral to protect against deficiencies.

Apparently unrelated to vomiting, taurine has been shown to be depleted in people taking chemotherapy.[33] It remains unclear how important this effect is or if people taking chemotherapy should take taurine supplements.

INTERACTIONS WITH HERBS

PSK (Coriolus versicolor)

The mushroom *Coriolus versicolor* contains an immune-stimulating substance called polysaccharide krestin, or PSK. PSK has been shown in several studies to help people with cancer undergoing chemotherapy. One study involved women with estrogen receptor-negative breast cancer. PSK combined with chemotherapy significantly prolonged survival time compared with chemotherapy alone.[34] Another study followed women with breast cancer who were given chemotherapy with or without PSK. The PSK-plus-chemotherapy group had a 25% better chance of survival after 10 years compared with those taking chemotherapy without PSK.[35] Another study looked at people who had surgically removed colon cancer. They were given chemotherapy with or without PSK. Those given PSK had a longer disease-free period and longer survival time.[36] Three grams of PSK were taken orally each day in these studies.

Although PSK is rarely available in the United States, hot-water extract products made from *Coriolus versicolor* mushrooms are available. These products may have activity related to that of PSK, but their use with chemotherapy has not been studied.

Echinacea (Echinacea purpurea, Echinacea angustifolia)

Echinacea is a popular immune-boosting herb that has been investigated for use with chemotherapy. One study looked at the actions of **cyclophosphamide** (page 64), echinacea, and thymus gland extracts to treat people with advanced cancer. Although small and uncontrolled, this trial suggested that the combination modestly extended the life span of some people with inoperable cancers.[37] Signs of restoration of immune function were seen in these people.

Milk Thistle (Silybum marianum)

Milk thistle's major bioflavonoids, known collectively as silymarin, have shown synergistic actions with the chemotherapy drugs **cisplatin** (page 50) and **doxorubicin** (page 78) (Adriamycin) in test tubes.[38] Silymarin also offsets the kidney toxicity of cisplatin in animals.[39] Silymarin has not yet been studied in humans treated with cisplatin. There is some evidence that silymarin may not interfere with some chemotherapy in humans with cancer.[40]

Eleuthero (Eleutherococcus senticosus)

Russian research has looked at using eleuthero with chemotherapy. One study of people with melanoma found that chemotherapy was less toxic when eleuthero was given simultaneously. Similarly, women with inoperable breast cancer given eleuthero were reported to tolerate more chemotherapy.[41] Eleuthero treatment was also associated with improved immune function in women with breast cancer treated with chemotherapy and radiation.[42]

Thymus Peptides

Peptides or short proteins derived from the thymus gland, an important immune organ, have been used in conjunction with chemotherapy drugs for people with cancer. One study using thymosin fraction V in combination with chemotherapy, compared with chemotherapy alone, found significantly longer survival times in the thymosin fraction V group.[43] A related substance, thymostimulin, decreased some side effects of chemotherapy and increased survival time compared with chemotherapy alone.[44] A third product, thymic extract TP1, was shown to improve immune function in people treated with chemotherapy compared with effects of chemotherapy alone.[45] Thymic peptides need to be administered by injection. People interested in their combined use with chemotherapy should consult a doctor of natural medicine.

SUMMARY OF INTERACTIONS FOR CHEMOTHERAPY

Depletion or interference	*Multiple nutrients (malabsorption), Taurine*
Adverse interaction	*See **methotrexate** (page 140) (folic acid)*
Side effect reduction/prevention	*Beta-carotene* (mouth sores), Eleuthero, Ginger, Glutamine* (mouth sores), Glutamine (diarrhea), Melatonin, N-acetyl*

cysteine (NAC), Thymus peptides, Vitamin E, topical (mouth sores)

Supportive interaction — Antioxidants,* Melatonin, Milk thistle, PSK

Reduced drug absorption/bioavailability — None known

Other (see text) — Echinacea, Multivitamin/mineral, Vitamin A, Vitamin C

CHLORPHENIRAMINE
(Chlor-Trimeton Allergy and Others)

Chlorpheniramine is an antihistamine used to relieve allergic rhinitis (seasonal allergy) symptoms including sneezing, runny nose, itching, and watery eyes. It is also used to treat immediate allergic reactions. Chlorpheniramine is available in nonprescription products alone (Chlor-Trimeton Allergy and others) and in combination with other nonprescription drugs, to treat symptoms of allergy, colds, and upper respiratory infections, including:

- Chlorpheniramine/**phenylpropanolamine** (page 172) (Contac 12 Hour, Triaminic-12, and others)
- Chlorpheniramine/**pseudoephedrine** (page 83) (Chlor-Trimeton 12 Hour and others)
- Chlorpheniramine/**pseudoephedrine** (page 83)/**acetaminophen** (page 2) (Alka-Seltzer Plus Cold Liqui-Gels, Theraflu Flu and Cold, and others)
- Chlorpheniramine/**pseudoephedrine** (page 83)/**acetaminophen** (page 2)/**dextromethorphan** (page 70) (Tylenol Multi-Symptom Hot Medication and others)

INTERACTIONS WITH HERBS

Henbane (Hyoscyamus niger)

Antihistamines, including chlorpheniramine, can cause "anticholinergic" side effects such as dryness of mouth and heart palpitations. Henbane also has anticholinergic activity and side effects. Therefore, use with chlorpheniramine could increase the risk of anticholinergic side effects,[1] though apparently no interactions have yet been reported with chlorpheniramine and henbane. Henbane should not be taken except by prescription from a physician trained in herbal medicine, as it is extremely toxic.

INTERACTIONS WITH FOODS AND OTHER COMPOUNDS

Alcohol

Chlorpheniramine causes drowsiness.[2] Alcohol may intensify this effect and increase the risk of accidental injury.[3] To prevent problems, people taking chlorpheniramine or chlorpheniramine-containing products should avoid alcohol.

SUMMARY OF INTERACTIONS FOR CHLORPHENIRAMINE

Depletion or interference	*None known*
Adverse interaction	*Henbane**
Side effect reduction/prevention	*None known*
Supportive interaction	*None known*
Reduced drug absorption/bioavailability	*None known*

CIMETIDINE
(Tagamet, Tagamet HB)

Cimetidine is a member of the H-2 blocker (histamine blocker) family of drugs that prevents the release of acid into the stomach. Cimetidine is used to treat stomach and duodenal ulcers, reflux of stomach acid into the esophagus, and Zollinger-Ellison syndrome. Cimetidine is available as the prescription drug Tagamet. It is also available as a nonprescription over-the-counter product, Tagamet HB, for relief of heartburn.

INTERACTIONS WITH DIETARY SUPPLEMENTS

Iron

Stomach acid may facilitate iron absorption. H-2 blocker drugs reduce stomach acid and are associated with decreased dietary iron absorption.[1] People with ulcers may also be iron deficient due to blood loss and benefit from iron supplementation. Iron levels in the blood can be checked with lab tests.

Magnesium

In healthy volunteers, a **magnesium hydroxide** (page 135)/**aluminum hydroxide** (page 6) **antacid** (page 13), taken with cimetidine, decreased cimetidine absorption by 20 to 25%.[2] People can avoid this interaction by taking cimetidine 2 hours before or after any aluminum/magnesium-containing antacids, including magnesium hydroxide found in some vitamin/mineral supplements. However, the available studies do not clearly indicate if magnesium hydroxide was the problem and may not need to be avoided.

Vitamin B$_{12}$

Hydrochloric acid is needed to release vitamin B$_{12}$ from food so it can be absorbed by the body. Cimetidine, which reduces stomach acid, may decrease the amount of vitamin B$_{12}$ available for the body to absorb.[3] The vitamin B$_{12}$ found in supplements is available to the body without the need for stomach acid. Lab tests can determine vitamin B$_{12}$ levels in people.

Vitamin D

Cimetidine may reduce vitamin D activation by the liver.[4] Lab tests can measure activated vitamin D levels in the blood. Forms of vitamin D that do not require liver activation are available, but only by prescription.

INTERACTIONS WITH FOODS AND OTHER COMPOUNDS

Food

Cimetidine may be taken with or without food.

Caffeine

Caffeine (page 33) is found in coffee, tea, soft drinks, chocolate, guaraná *(Paullinia cupana)*, nonprescription over-the-counter drug products, and supplement products containing caffeine or guaraná. Cimetidine may decrease the clearance of caffeine from the body, causing increased caffeine blood levels and unwanted actions.[5] People taking cimetidine may choose to limit their caffeine intake to avoid problems. They should read food, beverage, drug, and supplement labels carefully for caffeine content.

SUMMARY OF INTERACTIONS FOR CIMETIDINE

Depletion or interference	*Iron, Vitamin B$_{12}$, Vitamin D*
Adverse interaction	***Caffeine** (page 33)** *
Side effect reduction/prevention	*None known*
Supportive interaction	*None known*
Reduced drug absorption/bioavailability	*Magnesium*

CIPROFLOXACIN
(Cipro)

Ciprofloxacin is member of the fluoroquinolone family of **antibiotics** (page 14). It is used to treat bacterial infections. Ciprofloxacin penetrates many hard-to-reach tissues in the body and kills a wide variety of bacteria.

INTERACTIONS WITH DIETARY SUPPLEMENTS

Minerals

Minerals such as aluminum, calcium, copper, iron, magnesium, manganese, and zinc can bind to ciprofloxacin, greatly reducing the absorption of the drug.[1] [2] [3] [4] Because of the mineral content, people are advised to take ciprofloxacin 2 hours after consuming dairy products (milk, cheese, yogurt, ice cream, and others), antacids (Maalox, Mylanta, Tums, Rolaids, and others), and mineral-containing supplements.[5]

INTERACTIONS WITH FOODS AND OTHER COMPOUNDS

Food

Food in general[6] and yogurt in particular have been found to reduce absorption of ciprofloxacin. Ciprofloxacin should be taken 2 hours before eating.[7]

Caffeine

Caffeine (page 33) is found in coffee, tea, soft drinks, chocolate, guaraná *(Paullinia cupana)*, nonprescription drug products, and supplement products containing caffeine. Ciprofloxacin may decrease the elimination of caffeine from the body, causing increased caffeine blood levels and unwanted actions.[8] People taking ciprofloxacin may choose to limit their caffeine intake to avoid problems. They should read food, beverage, drug, and supplement labels carefully for caffeine content.

SUMMARY OF INTERACTIONS FOR CIPROFLOXACIN

Depletion or interference	*None known*
Adverse interaction	*Caffeine* (page 33)
Side effect reduction/prevention	*None known*
Supportive interaction	*None known*

Reduced drug absorption/bioavailability	Calcium, Copper, Iron, Magnesium, Manganese, Zinc (if taken at the same time)

CISAPRIDE
(Propulsid)

Cisapride is a gastrointestinal stimulant drug used to treat people with night-time heartburn due to reflux of stomach acid into the esophagus. It is also used to increase movement of gastrointestinal contents in conditions of lack of spontaneous gastrointestinal movement.

INTERACTIONS WITH HERBS

Menthol-Containing Herbs

People with esophageal reflux should avoid use of menthol-containing herbs, such as peppermint; the volatile oils in these plants may decrease the pressure in the lower esophageal sphincter and make the reflux worse.[1]

INTERACTIONS WITH FOODS AND OTHER COMPOUNDS

Alcohol

Alcohol consumption is associated with nighttime heartburn and may interfere with cisapride therapy.[2] Alcohol causes sleepiness, and cisapride may intensify this effect,[3] increasing the risk of accidental injury. People taking cisapride should avoid alcohol.

Tobacco

Smoking is associated with nighttime heartburn and may interfere with cisapride therapy.[4] Smokers taking cisapride may benefit from reducing or quitting smoking.

SUMMARY OF INTERACTIONS FOR CISAPRIDE

Depletion or interference	Menthol-containing herbs such as peppermint
Adverse interaction	None known
Side effect reduction/prevention	None known
Supportive interaction	None known
Reduced drug absorption/bioavailability	Tobacco

CISPLATIN
(Platinol)

Cisplatin is a **chemotherapy** (page 40) drug used to treat some forms of cancer.

INTERACTIONS WITH DIETARY SUPPLEMENTS

Calcium and Phosphate

Cisplatin may cause depletion of calcium and phosphate due to kidney damage.[1]

Glutathione

Preliminary human research suggests that intravenous (injected into a vein) glutathione may reduce neuropathies (disorders of the nervous system) caused by cisplatin and improve quality of life.[2][3] There is no evidence that glutathione taken by mouth has the same benefits.

Magnesium and Potassium

Cisplatin may cause excessive loss of magnesium and potassium in the urine.[4][5] Two case reports and one review article suggest that both potassium and magnesium supplementation may be necessary to increase low potassium levels.[6][7] People receiving cisplatin chemotherapy should ask their prescribing doctor to closely monitor magnesium and potassium status. Some doctors of natural medicine suggest monitoring the level of magnesium in red blood cells rather than in serum. They believe the red blood cell test may be more sensitive in diagnosing magnesium deficiency.

Selenium

In one human study, administration of 4,000 mcg per day of a new selenium product, Seleno-Kappacarrageenan, reduced the kidney damage and white blood cell–lowering effects of cisplatin.[8] The level of selenium used in this study is potentially toxic and should only be used under the supervision of a doctor of natural medicine.

Sodium

Cisplatin may cause depletion of sodium due to kidney damage.[9]

SUMMARY OF INTERACTIONS FOR CISPLATIN

Depletion or interference   *Calcium,* * *Magnesium,*
                                                   Phosphate, * *Potassium, Sodium* *

Adverse interaction	*None known*
Side effect reduction/prevention	*Selenium*
Supportive interaction	*None known*
Reduced drug absorption/bioavailability	*None known*
Other (see text)	*Glutathione*

CLARITHROMYCIN
(Biaxin)

Clarithromycin is a macrolide **antibiotic** (page 14) used to treat a variety of bacterial infections.

INTERACTIONS WITH HERBS

Digitalis (Digitalis lanata, Digitalis purpurea)

Digitalis refers to a family of plants commonly called foxglove that contain digitalis glycosides, chemicals with actions and toxicities similar to the prescription drug **digoxin** (page 71).

Clarithromycin can increase the serum level of digitalis glycosides, increasing the therapeutic effects as well as the risk of side effects.[1] Clarithromycin and digitalis-containing products should be used only under the direct supervision of a doctor trained in their use.

INTERACTIONS WITH FOODS AND OTHER COMPOUNDS

Food

Clarithromycin may be taken with or without food and may be taken with milk.[2] Clarithromycin tablets should be swallowed whole, without cutting, chewing, or crushing.[3]

SUMMARY OF INTERACTIONS FOR CLARITHROMYCIN

Depletion or interference	*None known*
Adverse interaction	*None known*
Side effect reduction/prevention	*None known*
Supportive interaction	*None known*
Reduced drug absorption/bioavailability	*None known*
Other (see text)	*Digitalis*

CLEMASTINE
(Antihist-1, Tavist)

CLEMASTINE/PHENYLPROPANOLAMINE
(Tavist-D)

Clemastine is an antihistamine used to relieve allergic rhinitis (seasonal allergy) symptoms including sneezing, runny nose, itching, and watery eyes. It is also used to treat itching and swelling associated with uncomplicated allergic skin reactions. Clemastine is available in nonprescription products alone (Antihist-1, Tavist, and others) and in the combination clemastine/**phenylpropanolamine** (page 172) (Tavist-D) to treat symptoms of allergy, colds, and upper respiratory infections.

INTERACTIONS WITH HERBS

Henbane (*Hyoscyamus niger*)

Antihistamines, including clemastine, can cause "anticholinergic" side effects such as dryness of mouth and heart palpitations. Henbane also has anticholinergic activity and side effects. Therefore, use with clemastine could increase the risk of anticholinergic side effects,[1] though apparently no interactions have yet been reported with clemastine and henbane. Henbane should not be taken except by prescription from a physician trained in herbal medicine, as it is extremely toxic.

INTERACTIONS WITH FOODS AND OTHER COMPOUNDS

Alcohol

Clemastine causes drowsiness.[2] Alcohol may intensify this effect and increase the risk of accidental injury.[3] To prevent problems, people taking clemastine or clemastine-containing products should avoid alcohol.

SUMMARY OF INTERACTIONS FOR CLEMASTINE

Depletion or interference	*None known*
Adverse interaction	*Henbane**
Side effect reduction/prevention	*None known*
Supportive interaction	*None known*
Reduced drug absorption/bioavailability	*None known*

CLOFIBRATE
(Atromid-S)

Clofibrate is a drug used to lower cholesterol in people with high blood cholesterol. It is rarely used, due to the possibility of liver damage and the availability of safer, more effective drugs.

INTERACTIONS WITH DIETARY SUPPLEMENTS

Vitamin B$_{12}$

Clofibrate has been reported to reduce absorption of vitamin B$_{12}$.[1]

INTERACTIONS WITH HERBS

Milk Thistle

Although there have been no clinical studies, use of milk thistle with clofibrate may theoretically lower the risk of liver side effects associated with the drug. People may take a standardized milk thistle extract supplying 70 to 80% silymarin at a dose of 200 mg 3 times per day.

SUMMARY OF INTERACTIONS FOR CLOFIBRATE

Depletion or interference	*Vitamin B$_{12}$*[*]
Adverse interaction	*None known*
Side effect reduction/prevention	*Milk thistle*[*]
Supportive interaction	*None known*
Reduced drug absorption/bioavailability	*None known*

CLONIDINE
(Catapres, Duraclon)

CLONIDINE/CHLORTHALIDONE
(Combipres)

Clonidine is a drug that blocks signals in the brain controlling heart rate and blood pressure. It is used to lower blood pressure in people with hypertension. It is available alone in oral tablets (Catapres and others), skin patches (Catapres-TTS), in a form for intravenous (IV) injection (Duraclon), and in the oral combination clonidine/**chlorthalidone** (page 202) (Combipres). Clonidine is used with narcotics to treat severe pain and as an adjunct to alcohol with-drawal, narcotic detoxification, and quitting smoking.

INTERACTIONS WITH FOODS AND OTHER COMPOUNDS

Alcohol

Alcohol is a central nervous system depressant and can cause drowsi-ness and dizziness. Clonidine may intensify these effects, increasing the risk of accidental injury.[1] To avoid problems, people taking cloni-dine should avoid alcohol.

SUMMARY OF INTERACTIONS FOR CLONIDINE

Depletion or interference	*None known*
Adverse interaction	*None known*
Side effect reduction/prevention	*None known*
Supportive interaction	*None known*
Reduced drug absorption/bioavailability	*None known*

CODEINE

Codeine is a narcotic analgesic (pain reliever) derived from opium. It is used to treat mild to moderate pain and as a cough suppressant.

For pain relief, codeine is used by itself or in combination products such as Empirin with codeine (**aspirin** [page 18]/codeine), Tylenol with codeine (**acetaminophen** [page 2]/codeine), and others. For cough suppression, codeine is used by itself or in combination products such as Phenergan with codeine (**promethazine** [page 178]/codeine), Robi-tussin AC (codeine/**guaifenesin** [page 105]), and others.

INTERACTIONS WITH HERBS

Tannin-Containing Herbs

Tannins are a group of unrelated chemicals that give plants an astrin-gent taste. Herbs with large amounts of tannins may interfere with the absorption of codeine and should not be taken together with codeine or codeine-containing products.[1] Herbs containing high levels of tan-nins include green tea (*Camellia sinensis*), black tea, uva ursi (*Arc-tostaphylos uva-ursi*), black walnut (*Juglans nigra*), red raspberry (*Rubus idaeus*), oak (*Quercus* spp.), and witch hazel (*Hamamelis virginiana*).

INTERACTIONS WITH FOODS AND OTHER COMPOUNDS

Food

Codeine commonly causes gastrointestinal (GI) upset. Codeine and codeine-containing products may be taken with food to reduce or prevent GI upset.[2] A common side effect of narcotic analgesics, including codeine, is constipation. Increasing dietary fiber (fruits, vegetables, beans, whole-grain foods, and others) and water intake can ease constipation.

Alcohol

Alcohol causes a loss of coordination, impaired judgment, decreased alertness, drowsiness, and other actions. Narcotic analgesics, including codeine, cause similar loss of control. Combining codeine and alcohol increases the risk of accidental injury. People taking codeine-containing products should avoid alcohol.

SUMMARY OF INTERACTIONS FOR CODEINE

Depletion or interference	*None known*
Adverse interaction	*None known*
Side effect reduction/prevention	*None known*
Supportive interaction	*None known*
Reduced drug absorption/bioavailability	*Tannin-containing herbs[*] such as green tea, black tea, uva ursi, black walnut, red raspberry, oak, and witch hazel*

COLCHICINE

Colchicine reduces the inflammatory (swelling) response and pain in people with gout (high uric acid blood levels leading to painful accumulation of uric acid crystals in and around joints).

INTERACTIONS WITH DIETARY SUPPLEMENTS

Vitamin B$_{12}$

Colchicine may interfere with vitamin B$_{12}$ in the body. Research is inconsistent. Both colchicine and vitamin B$_{12}$ deficiency are reported to cause neuropathies (disorders of the nervous system), but it remains unclear whether neuropathies caused by colchicine could be due to vitamin B$_{12}$ depletion.[1] [2]

Nutrient Malabsorption

Colchicine has been associated with impaired absorption of beta-carotene, fat, lactose (milk sugar), potassium, and sodium.[3]

SUMMARY OF INTERACTIONS FOR COLCHICINE

Depletion or interference	*Beta-carotene,*[*] *Potassium,*[*] *Vitamin B$_{12}$*[*]
Adverse interaction	*None known*
Side effect reduction/prevention	*None known*
Supportive interaction	*None known*
Reduced drug absorption/bioavailability	*None known*
Other (see text)	*Sodium*

COLESTIPOL
(Colestid)

Colestipol is a **bile acid sequestrant** (page 28) (prevents absorption of bile acids in the digestive system). Bile acids may facilitate the absorption of cholesterol. Colestipol is one of many drugs used to lower cholesterol levels in people with high blood cholesterol.

INTERACTIONS WITH DIETARY SUPPLEMENTS

Vitamins

Bile acid sequestrants, including colestipol, may prevent absorption of folic acid and the fat-soluble vitamins A, D, E, K.[1] [2] People taking colestipol should consult with their prescribing doctor and/or a nutritionally oriented doctor about vitamin malabsorption and supplementation. People should take other drugs and vitamin supplements 1 hour before or 4 to 6 hours after colestipol to improve absorption.[3]

SUMMARY OF INTERACTIONS FOR COLESTIPOL

Depletion or interference	*Folic acid, Vitamin A, Vitamin D, Vitamin E, Vitamin K*
Adverse interaction	*None known*
Side effect reduction/prevention	*None known*
Supportive interaction	*None known*
Reduced drug absorption/bioavailability	*None known*

CONJUGATED ESTROGENS
(Premarin)

CONJUGATED ESTROGENS/ MEDROXYPROGESTERONE
(Prempro)

Conjugated estrogens are a combination of several natural estrogenic hormones used to treat menopausal symptoms, to prevent osteoporosis in postmenopausal women, and as replacement therapy in other conditions of inadequate estrogen production. They are also used to treat some people with advanced breast and prostate cancers. Conjugated estrogens are extracted and purified from the urine of pregnant horses. They are available alone (Premarin) and in the combination conjugated estrogens/**medroxyprogesterone** (page 137) (Prempro).

INTERACTIONS WITH DIETARY SUPPLEMENTS

Calcium

Two months of conjugated estrogen therapy in women with surgically induced menopause decreased urinary calcium loss and increased serum vitamin D levels.[1] In a 6-month placebo-controlled study of twenty-one women with postmenopausal osteoporosis, conjugated estrogens increased calcium absorption and vitamin D blood levels.[2] While estrogen may improve calcium absorption, it remains important for women taking estrogen to maintain adequate calcium intake through diet and supplementation. Many doctors of natural medicine recommend 800 to 1,200 mg of supplemental calcium in addition to the several hundred milligrams found in a typical daily diet.

Ipriflavone

Ipriflavone is a synthetic variation on isoflavones found in soybeans. It is now available as a supplement. In a group of postmenopausal women, ipriflavone (400 mg per day) plus conjugated estrogens increased vertebral bone density while calcium (500 mg per day) plus conjugated estrogens led to a decrease in bone density.[3] In a study of 133 postmenopausal women, ipriflavone (600 mg per day) plus conjugated estrogens and calcium (1 gram per day) increased bone density while conjugated estrogens plus calcium or placebo plus calcium resulted in bone loss.[4] Interpreting these results is difficult in part because other trials show that conjugated estrogens, ipriflavone, and calcium each improve bone density compared with placebo. It remains unclear whether there is a true interaction between ipriflavone and conjugated estrogens or whether each has its own unrelated effects in improving bone density.

Minerals

In a group of thirty-seven postmenopausal women treated with conjugated estrogens and **medroxyprogesterone** (page 137) for 1 year, urinary zinc and magnesium loss was reduced in those women who began the study with signs of osteoporosis and elevated zinc and magnesium excretion.[5] The clinical significance of this interaction remains unknown.

Vitamin B₆

A group of twelve women were all found to have a relative deficiency or be deficient in vitamin B_6 after 1 year of conjugated estrogens therapy without a progestin.[6] Three women who used conjugated estrogens with a progestin showed no sign of deficiency. Numerous studies have looked at the negative effects of **oral contraceptives** (page 160) (OCs) on vitamin B_6 status.[7][8] Though OCs contain different forms of estrogen than conjugated estrogens, there is possibility of a similar problem when any form of estrogen is supplemented. Some studies suggest that vitamin B_6 deficiency does not occur when low-dose OCs are used.[9] Vitamin B_6 supplements can be used in the amount of 100 mg per day.

Vitamin D

Two months of conjugated estrogens therapy in women with surgically induced menopause increased blood levels of vitamin D and decreased urinary calcium loss.[10] In a 6-month placebo-controlled study of twenty-one women with postmenopausal osteoporosis, conjugated estrogens therapy was associated with increased blood levels of vitamin D and increased calcium absorption.[11] While conjugated estrogens appear to improve vitamin D metabolism, it probably remains important for women taking such hormones to consume adequate levels of vitamin D through diet and supplements. Many nutritionally oriented doctors recommend supplementing 400 IU vitamin D per day beyond the level typically found in the diet.

Combination of 300 IU of vitamin D per day with **estradiol** (page 88) plus a progestin led to greater improvement in bone density than estradiol/progestin alone.[12] A study on the same group of women using the same combinations found that adding vitamin D to estradiol/progestin tended to reduce beneficial HDL cholesterol levels, unlike estradiol/progestin alone. The differences between estradiol and conjugated estrogens are notable and so it is unclear if the findings of these studies are applicable for conjugated estrogens. All persons taking hormone replacement therapy are advised to talk with a nutritionally oriented physician before combining vitamin D with estrogen.

INTERACTIONS WITH HERBS

Isoflavones

Herbal sources of isoflavones such as red clover may interfere with or even have an additive effect with conjugated estrogens.[13] Further studies are needed to establish the potential interaction of isoflavone supplements from red clover and soy with conjugated estrogens. Consult with your health-care professional if you are currently taking estrogen replacement therapy and wish to take a supplement high in isoflavones.

INTERACTIONS WITH FOODS AND OTHER COMPOUNDS

Tobacco

Conjugated estrogens therapy in postmenopausal women has been reported to decrease low-density lipoprotein (LDL) cholesterol levels and to increase high-density lipoprotein (HDL) cholesterol levels. However, despite the positive changes in blood levels of LDL and HDL cholesterol, there is evidence that conjugated estrogen does not reduce the risk of heart disease.[14] Nonetheless, smoking offsets the cholesterol changes induced by taking conjugated estrogens,[15] and this interference is likely to be detrimental. Women who do not smoke should avoid starting. Those who do smoke should talk with their doctor about quitting.

SUMMARY OF INTERACTIONS FOR CONJUGATED ESTROGENS

Depletion or interference	*Vitamin B₆**
Adverse interaction	*Tobacco*
Side effect reduction/prevention	*None known*
Supportive interaction	*Calcium, Ipriflavone, Vitamin D*
Reduced drug absorption/bioavailability	*Herbal sources of isoflavone supplements (red clover,* soy*)*
Other (see text)	*Magnesium, Zinc*

CORTICOSTEROIDS

Corticosteroids are a family of compounds that include the adrenal steroid hormone cortisol (hydrocortisone) and synthetic drugs, such as prednisone, that are related to cortisol. Both the natural and synthetic compounds have powerful anti-inflammatory effects. Corticosteroids are used by mouth to treat autoimmune and inflammatory diseases including asthma, bursitis, Crohn's disease, skin disorders, tendinitis, ulcerative colitis, and others. They are also used to treat severe allergic reactions and prevent organ rejection after organ transplant. Corticosteroids are inhaled by mouth to treat asthma and other conditions of restricted breathing. They are inhaled by nose to treat symptoms of seasonal allergies. Corticosteroids are combined with **antibiotics** (page 14) to treat ear infections, eye infections, and skin infections.

Corticosteroids include:

Beclomethasone (Beconase, Beclovent, Vancenase, Vanceril), Budesonide (Pulmicort, Rhinocort), Dexamethasone (Decadron, Decadron Phosphate Turbinaire, and others), Dexamethasone/Tobramycin (Tobradex), Flunisolide (AeroBid, Nasalide), Fluticasone (Cutivate, Flonase), Hydrocortisone (Cortef, Hytone, and others), Methylprednisolone (Medrol and others), Mometasone (Elocon), Prednisone (Deltasone, Orasone, and others), Prednisolone (Delta-Cortef, Pediapred, and others), and Triamcinolone (Aristocort, Azmacort, Nasacort, and others).

INTERACTIONS WITH DIETARY SUPPLEMENTS

Magnesium

Corticosteroids may increase the loss of magnesium.[1] Some nutritionally oriented doctors recommend that people taking corticosteroids for more than 2 weeks supplement with 300 to 400 mg of magnesium per day.

N-Acetyl Cysteine (NAC)

One preliminary study found that adding 600 mg N-acetyl cysteine, or NAC, 3 times per day to treatment with prednisone led to further improvement than with prednisone alone in people with fibrosing alveolitis, a rare lung disease.[2]

Potassium

Steroidal anti-inflammatory drugs increase the loss of potassium in urine.[3] For most people, this may not cause a significant problem. When potassium is to be increased, it is often best achieved by eating more fruit rather than taking potassium supplements. (Fruit contains higher levels of potassium than that found in the legally mandated supplemental level of a maximum 99 mg per pill.)

Vitamin A

In some individuals, treatment with corticosteroids can result in impaired wound healing. In one study, topical or internal administration of vitamin A improved wound healing in eight of ten people on corticosteroid therapy.[4] In theory, vitamin A might also reverse some of the beneficial effects of corticosteroids. Consult with a doctor of natural medicine to determine in which situations improved wound healing might outweigh the theoretical risk associated with concomitant vitamin A use.

Vitamin B$_6$

Corticosteroids may increase the loss of vitamin B$_6$.[5] One double-blind study failed to show any added benefit when 300 mg of pyridoxine (vitamin B$_6$) was taken along with inhaled steroids for asthma compared with placebo.[6] Therefore, while replacement of vitamin B$_6$ may be needed to prevent deficiency, additional vitamin B$_6$ may not have any added benefit. Some nutritionally oriented doctors recommend that people taking corticosteroids for longer than 2 weeks supplement with 25 to 50 mg of vitamin B$_6$ per day.

Calcium and Vitamin D

Steroidal anti-inflammatory drugs reduce the body's ability to activate vitamin D,[7] [8] increasing the risk of bone loss. Doctors can measure levels of activated vitamin D (called 1,25 dihydroxycholecalciferol) to determine whether a deficiency exists. If so, activated vitamin D is available by prescription. A study of people with rheumatoid arthritis treated with low doses of prednisone found that those who received 1,000 mg (1 gram) of calcium per day plus 500 IU of vitamin D per day maintained bone density.[9] It makes sense for people taking corticosteroids for longer than 2 weeks to ask their prescribing doctor or a nutritionally oriented doctor about calcium and vitamin D supplementation.

Dehydroepiandrosterone (DHEA)

A group of women with asthma who had been taking inhaled beclomethasone were shown to have low levels of DHEA compared with women with asthma not taking beclomethasone.[10] The authors express concern that this may be partially how corticosteroids can cause osteoporosis, but more research is needed to know for certain.

Melatonin

A single dose of the synthetic corticosteroid dexamethasone, when given to healthy volunteers, suppressed production of melatonin in nine of eleven subjects.[11] Placebo did not have a melatonin-suppressive effect. Further research is needed to determine if long-term use of corticosteroids interferes in a meaningful way with melatonin production.

Sodium

Steroidal anti-inflammatory drugs cause sodium retention. People taking corticosteroids should talk with their doctor to see if they need to restrict salt intake.

Other Nutrients

Steroidal anti-inflammatory drugs have been found to increase urinary loss of vitamin K, vitamin C, and zinc, although the clinical importance of these losses remains unclear.[12]

INTERACTIONS WITH HERBS

Aloe (Aloe vera)

Applying aloe gel topically along with a form of cortisone has enhanced the hormone's anti-inflammatory activity in the skin, according to animal research.[13]

Digitalis (Digitalis purpurea)

Digitalis refers to a family of plants commonly called foxglove that contain digitalis glycosides, chemicals with actions and toxicities similar to the prescription drug **digoxin** (page 71). Digitalis glycosides may increase the risk of side effects during corticosteroid therapy.[14]

Ephedra sinica (Ma huang)

Ephedrine (page 83) is a chemical that occurs naturally in the herb ephedra and is also available as a drug product. Ephedrine increases the clearance of dexamethasone from the body, thereby decreasing the drug's activity.[15] It is not known, however, if the herb ephedra also has this effect on dexamethasone. Until more is known, people taking dexamethasone should avoid both ephedra and ephedrine-containing products.

Licorice (Glycyrrhiza glabra)

Licorice extract was shown to decrease the clearance of prednisone in isolated rat livers.[16] If this action happens in people, it could prolong prednisone activity and possibly increase prednisone-related side effects. A single-dose study of six healthy men found that intravenous (IV) glycyrrhizin (an active constituent in licorice) given with IV prednisolone prolonged prednisolone action compared with the same dose of prednisolone given without licorice extract.[17] The authors cautioned that this effect could increase the activity and side effects of prednisolone. Intravenous glycyrrhizin is available only from some nutritionally oriented physicians in the United States and can only be legally administered by them.

An animal study has shown that glycyrrhizin prevents the immunosuppressive actions of cortisone—the natural hormone most like prednisone.[18] Further human research will be necessary to see if this action is significant in humans.

Glycyrrhetinic acid, a component related to glycyrrhizin that is also in licorice, was shown to increase the activity of hydrocortisone when applied to the skin of healthy human volunteers.[19] The authors speculate that this might allow for less hydrocortisone to be used when combined with glycyrrhetinic acid, but further study is needed before this can be confirmed.[20] People should not take licorice with corticosteroids without first consulting a nutritionally oriented doctor.

INTERACTIONS WITH FOODS AND OTHER COMPOUNDS

Food

Corticosteroids can cause stomach upset and should be taken after eating a meal, before 9:00 A.M. for best results.[21]

Protein

Steroidal anti-inflammatory drugs cause protein wasting. For this reason, medical doctors sometimes recommend a high-protein diet for people taking these drugs.[22] Considering the kidney damage associated with systemic lupus erythematosus—one of the conditions steroids are used to treat—and the link between kidney damage and high-protein diets, it remains unclear if such advice is appropriate for all people.

Alcohol

Corticosteriods can irritate the stomach, and alcohol can compound this action.[23]

SUMMARY OF INTERACTIONS FOR CORTICOSTEROIDS

Depletion or interference	*Calcium, Dehydroepiandrosterone (DHEA),* Magnesium,* Melatonin,* Potassium, Vitamin B_6,* Vitamin C,* Vitamin D, Vitamin K,* Zinc*
Adverse interaction	*Digitalis,* Sodium*
Side effect reduction/prevention	*Vitamin A*
Supportive interaction	*N-acetyl cysteine (NAC)**
Reduced drug absorption/bioavailability	*Ephedra**
Other (see text)	*Aloe, Licorice, Protein*

CYCLOBENZAPRINE
(Flexeril and Others)

Cyclobenzaprine is a drug used as an adjunct to rest and physical therapy for relief of spasm.

INTERACTIONS WITH FOODS AND OTHER COMPOUNDS

Alcohol

Cyclobenzaprine may cause dizziness, drowsiness, or blurred vision.[1] Alcohol may intensify these effects and increase the risk of accidental injury. To prevent problems, people taking cyclobenzaprine should avoid alcohol.

SUMMARY OF INTERACTIONS FOR CYCLOBENZAPRINE

Depletion or interference	*None known*
Adverse interaction	*None known*
Side effect reduction/prevention	*None known*
Supportive interaction	*None known*
Reduced drug absorption/bioavailability	*None known*

CYCLOPHOSPHAMIDE
(Cytoxan, Neosar)

Cyclophosphamide is a **chemotherapy** (page 40) drug used primarily to treat various forms of cancer. It is also used less commonly to treat some non-cancer diseases.

INTERACTIONS WITH DIETARY SUPPLEMENTS

Antioxidants

Cyclophosphamide requires activation by the liver through a process called oxidation. In theory, antioxidant nutrients (vitamin A, vitamin E, beta-carotene and others) might interfere with the activation of cyclophosphamide. There is no published research linking antioxidant vitamins to reduced cyclophosphamide effectiveness in cancer treatment. In a study of mice with vitamin A deficiency, vitamin A supplementation enhanced the anticancer action of cyclophosphamide.[1] Another animal research report indicated that vitamin C may increase the effectiveness of cyclophosphamide without producing new side effects.[2] Preliminary human research found that adding antioxidants (beta-carotene, vitamin A, and vitamin E) to cyclophosphamide therapy increased the survival of people with small-cell lung cancer treated with cyclophosphamide.[3] It is too early to know if adding antioxidants to cyclophosphamide for cancer treatment is better than cyclophosphamide alone. Vitamin A can be toxic in high doses.

INTERACTIONS WITH FOODS AND OTHER COMPOUNDS

Food

It is recommended to take cyclophosphamide on an empty stomach. If this causes severe gastrointestinal (GI) upset, cyclophosphamide may be taken with food.[4] People with questions should ask their prescribing doctor or pharmacist.

SUMMARY OF INTERACTIONS FOR CYCLOPHOSPHAMIDE

Depletion or interference	*None known*
Adverse interaction	*None known*
Side effect reduction/prevention	*Antioxidants (Vitamin C, Vitamin E, and Beta-carotene)*[*]
Supportive interaction	*None known*
Reduced drug absorption/bioavailability	*None known*

CYCLOSERINE
(Seromycin)

Cycloserine is a broad-spectrum **antibiotic** (page 14) used to treat tuberculosis. It is used rarely for treating noninfectious diseases.

INTERACTIONS WITH DIETARY SUPPLEMENTS

Calcium and Magnesium

Cycloserine may interfere with calcium and magnesium absorption.[1] The clinical significance of these interactions is unclear.

Folic Acid, Vitamin B$_6$, Vitamin B$_{12}$

Cycloserine may interfere with the absorption and/or activity of folic acid, vitamin B$_6$, and vitamin B$_{12}$.[2] [3] The clinical importance of this interaction is unclear.

Vitamin K

Many antibiotics taken by mouth, including cycloserine, may kill friendly bacteria in the large intestine that produce vitamin K.[4] With short-term (a few weeks or less) antibiotic use, the actions on vitamin K are usually mild and cause no problems. After antibiotic therapy is completed, vitamin K activity returns to normal.

INTERACTIONS WITH FOODS AND OTHER COMPOUNDS

Alcohol

Cycloserine may cause drowsiness.[5] Alcohol may intensify this drowsiness and increase the risk of accidents during activities requiring alertness. Seizures are a possible side effect of cycloserine therapy. Alcohol consumed during cycloserine therapy may increase the risk of seizures.[6] People should avoid alcohol-containing products during cycloserine therapy.

SUMMARY OF INTERACTIONS FOR CYCLOSERINE

Depletion or interference	*Calcium,* * *Folic acid,* * *Magnesium,* * *Vitamin B$_6$,* * *Vitamin B$_{12}$,* * *Vitamin K*
Adverse interaction	*None known*
Side effect reduction/prevention	*None known*
Supportive interaction	*None known*
Reduced drug absorption/bioavailability	*None known*

CYCLOSPORINE
(Sandimmune, Neoral)

Cyclosporine is a drug that suppresses the immune system. It is used in combination with other immune suppressive drugs to prevent rejection of transplanted organs by the immune system. There are two different forms of cyclosporine, Sandimmune and Neoral. These products differ in important ways and each is used in combination with different additional immunosupressant drugs. Inadequate immune suppression may result in organ rejection and serious complications. People taking cyclosporine should follow their prescribing doctor's directions exactly and discuss any changes in drug therapy, vitamins, supplements, herbal products, or any other substances with their prescribing doctor before making any changes.

INTERACTIONS WITH DIETARY SUPPLEMENTS

Magnesium

Cyclosporine has been associated with low blood magnesium levels and undesirable side effects.[1] [2] [3] Some doctors of natural medicine suggest monitoring the level of magnesium in red blood cells, rather than in serum, as the red blood cell test may be more sensitive for evaluating magnesium status.

Omega-3 Fish Oil

Several studies have shown that in people with organ transplant treated with cyclosporine, the addition of 4 to 6 grams of omega-3 fatty acids from fish oil helped reduce high blood pressure,[4][5][6] though not every study has found fish oil helpful.[7] It remains unclear to what extent fish oil supplementation will help people with high blood pressure taking cyclosporine following organ transplant.

Vitamin E

Twenty-six people with liver transplant (both adults and children) unable to achieve or maintain therapeutic cyclosporine blood levels during the early post-transplant period were given water-soluble vitamin E in the amount of 6.25 IU/2.2 pounds of body weight 2 times per day.[8] Addition of vitamin E in the early post-transplant period reduced the required dose of cyclosporine and the cost of cyclosporine therapy by 26%. These results imply that the addition of vitamin E to established cyclosporine therapy allows for a decrease in cyclosporine dosing. Combining vitamin E and cyclosporin requires medical supervision to avoid cyclosporin toxicity.

INTERACTIONS WITH HERBS

Ginkgo (*Ginkgo biloba*)

Ginkgo was reported to protect liver cells from damage caused by cyclosporine in a test tube experiment.[9] A *Ginkgo biloba* extract partially reversed cyclosporine-induced reduced kidney function in a study of isolated rat kidneys.[10] Human trials have not studied the actions of ginkgo to prevent or reduce the side effects of cyclosporine.

INTERACTIONS WITH FOODS AND OTHER COMPOUNDS

Food

Food increases the absorption of cyclosporine.[11] A change in the timing of food and cyclosporine dosing may alter cyclosporine blood levels, requiring dose adjustment.

Grapefruit Juice

In a randomized study of nine adults with cyclosporine-treated autoimmune diseases, grapefruit juice (5 ounces 2 times per day with cyclosporine, for 10 days) caused a significant increase in cyclosporine blood levels compared with cyclosporine with water.[12] The rise in cyclosporine blood levels was associated with abdominal pain, lightheadedness, nausea, and tremor in one person. Using grapefruit juice to reduce the dose of cyclosporine has not been sufficiently studied and cannot therefore be counted on to produce a predictable change in cyclosporin dose requirements. The same effects might be seen from eating grapefruit as from drinking its juice.

Milk, Apple Juice, and Orange Juice

Mixing Sandimmune solution with room-temperature milk, chocolate milk, orange juice, or apple juice may improve its flavor.[13]

Mixing Neoral solution with room temperature orange or apple juice may improve its flavor, but combining it with milk makes an unpalatable mix.[14]

SUMMARY OF INTERACTIONS FOR CYCLOSPORINE

Depletion or interference	*Magnesium*
Adverse interaction	*None known*
Side effect reduction/prevention	*Omega-3 fish oil,* Ginkgo**
Supportive interaction	*Vitamin E**
Reduced drug absorption/bioavailability	*None known*
Other (see text)	*Apple juice, Milk, Grapefruit juice, Orange juice*

DAPSONE

Dapsone is an **antibiotic** (page 14) effective against the bacteria that causes leprosy. It is an effective treatment for dermatitis herpetiformis, although it is unknown how dapsone helps with this disease. Dapsone is also used to prevent *Pneumocystis carinii* pneumonia in people infected with the human immunodeficiency virus (HIV).

INTERACTIONS WITH DIETARY SUPPLEMENTS

PABA (Para-Aminobenzoic Acid)

PABA is a compound found in foods that is considered by some to be a member of the B-vitamin family. PABA may interfere with the activity of dapsone.[1] Read supplement product labels for PABA content.

Vitamin E

In large doses, dapsone causes oxidative damage to red blood cells that may be prevented with lower doses of dapsone. Fifteen people who took dapsone for dermatitis herpetiformis were given 800 IU of vitamin

E per day for 4 weeks, followed by 4 weeks with 1,000 mg of vitamin C per day, followed by 4 weeks of vitamin E and vitamin C together.[2] The authors reported only vitamin E therapy offered some protection against dapsone-induced hemolysis.

SUMMARY OF INTERACTIONS FOR DAPSONE

Depletion or interference	*PABA**
Adverse interaction	*None known*
Side effect reduction/prevention	*Vitamin E**
Supportive interaction	*None known*
Reduced drug absorption/bioavailability	*None known*

DEFEROXAMINE
(Desferal)

Deferoxamine is a drug that binds to some metals and carries them out of the body. It is used to treat acute iron intoxication, chronic iron overload, and aluminum accumulation in people with kidney failure.

INTERACTIONS WITH DIETARY SUPPLEMENTS

Iron

People treated with deferoxamine for dangerously high levels of iron should not take iron supplements, because iron exacerbates their condition, further increasing the need for the deferoxamine. They should read all labels carefully for iron content. All people treated with deferoxamine should consult their prescribing doctor before using any iron-containing products.

SUMMARY OF INTERACTIONS FOR DEFEROXAMINE

Depletion or interference	*None known*
Adverse interaction	*Iron*
Side effect reduction/prevention	*None known*
Supportive interaction	*None known*
Reduced drug absorption/bioavailability	*None known*

DEXTROMETHORPHAN
(Benylin DM, Vicks Formula 44, and Others)

Dextromethorphan is a cough suppressant used for short-term treatment of nonproductive coughs. It is available in nonprescription products alone (Benylin DM, Vicks Formula 44, and others) and in combination with other nonprescription drugs, to treat symptoms of allergy, colds, and upper respiratory infections, including:

- Dextromethorphan/**guaifenesin** (page 105) (Robitussin DM and others)
- Dextromethorphan/**guaifenesin** (page 105)/**phenyl-propanolamine** (page 172) (Robitussin CF and others)
- Dextromethorphan/**acetaminophen** (page 2)/**doxylamine** (page 81)/**pseudoephedrine** (page 83) (Nyquil Hot Therapy Powder and others)
- Dextromethorphan/**acetaminophen** (page 2)/**chlorpheniramine** (page 45)/**pseudoephedrine** (page 83) (Tylenol Multi-Symptom Hot Medication and others)

There are currently no reported nutrient or herb interactions involving dextromethorphan.

DICYCLOMINE
(Bemote, Bentyl, Bicyclomine, Di-Spaz, and Others)

Dicyclomine is an antispasmotic drug used to treat irritable bowel syndrome.

There are currently no reported nutrient or herb interactions involving dicyclomine.

DIDANOSINE
(dideoxyinosine, ddl, Videx)

Didanosine is a drug that blocks reproduction of the human immunodeficiency virus (HIV). HIV is the virus that infects people causing acquired immunodeficiency syndrome (AIDS). Didanosine is used in combination with other drugs to treat HIV infection.

INTERACTIONS WITH HERBS

Shiitake (*Lentinas edodes*)

Lentinan is a complex sugar found in shiitake mushrooms and is recognized as an immune modulator. In an early human trial, eighty-eight HIV-positive people received didanosine (400 mg per day) plus a 2 mg lentinan injection per week.[1] Didanosine-lentinan combination therapy improved CD4 immune cell counts for a significantly longer period than didanosine alone. Lentinan is under investigation as an adjunct therapy to be used with didanosine for HIV infection.[2] Oral preparations of shiitake are available, but it is not known if they would be an effective treatment with didanosine for HIV infection.

INTERACTIONS WITH FOODS AND OTHER COMPOUNDS

Food

Didanosine should be taken on an empty stomach, 1 hour before or 2 hours after eating food.[3]

SUMMARY OF INTERACTIONS FOR DIDANOSINE

Depletion or interference	*None known*
Adverse interaction	*None known*
Side effect reduction/prevention	*None known*
Supportive interaction	*Shiitake**
Reduced drug absorption/bioavailability	*None known*

DIGOXIN

(Lanoxin)

Digoxin is a drug originally derived from the foxglove plant, *Digitalis lanata*. Digoxin is used primarily to improve the pumping ability of the heart in congestive heart failure (CHF). It is also used to help normalize some dysrhythmias (abnormal types of heartbeat).

INTERACTIONS WITH DIETARY SUPPLEMENTS

Magnesium and Potassium

People needing digoxin may have low levels of potassium or magnesium,[1] increasing the risk for digoxin toxicity. Digoxin therapy may increase magnesium elimination from the body.[2] People taking digoxin may benefit from magnesium supplementation.[3] It is less common for medical doctors to check magnesium status, and when they do, they typically use an insensitive indicator of magnesium status (serum or plasma levels). The red blood cell magnesium level may be a more sensitive indicator of magnesium status. It has been suggested that 300 to 500 mg of magnesium per day is a reasonable amount to supplement.[4] Medical doctors prescribing digoxin check for potassium depletion and prescribe potassium supplements if needed.

INTERACTIONS WITH HERBS

Digitalis (Digitalis purpurea)

Digitalis refers to a group of plants commonly called foxglove that contain chemicals with actions and toxicities similar to digoxin. Digitalis was used as an herbal medicine to treat some heart conditions before the drug digoxin was available. Some doctors of natural medicine continue to use digitalis in the United States, and it is used as an herbal medicine in other countries as well. Due to the additive risk of toxicity, digitalis and digoxin should never be used together.

Hawthorn (Crataegus oxyacantha, Crataegus monogyna)

Hawthorn (leaf with flower) extract is approved in Germany to treat mild congestive heart failure.[5] Congestive heart failure is a serious medical condition that requires expert medical management rather than self-treatment. Due to the narrow safety index of digoxin, it makes sense for people taking digoxin for congestive heart failure to consult with their prescribing doctor or an herbally oriented doctor before using hawthorn-containing products. Reports of hawthorn interacting with digitalis to potentiate its effects have not been confirmed.

Licorice (Glycyrrhiza glabra)

Low levels of potassium increase the risk of digoxin toxicity. Excessive use of licorice plant or licorice plant products may cause the body to lose potassium.[6] Artificial licorice flavoring does not cause potassium loss. People taking digoxin should read product labels carefully for licorice plant ingredients.

Senna (Cassia senna, Cassia angustifolia)

Bisacodyl (page 29), a laxative similar in action to senna, given with digoxin decreased serum digoxin levels in healthy volunteers compared with digoxin alone.[7] In people taking digoxin, laxative use was also associated with decreased digoxin levels.[8] In addition, concern has been expressed that overuse or misuse of senna may deplete potassium levels and increase both digoxin activity and risk of toxicity.[9] However, overuse of senna could also decrease digoxin activity because, as noted, laxatives can decrease the levels of the drug.

Eleuthero (*Eleutherococcus senticosus*)

People taking digoxin require regular monitoring of serum digoxin levels. In one report, addition of a product identified as Siberian ginseng to stable, therapeutic digoxin treatment was associated with dangerously high serum digoxin levels.[10] The person never experienced symptoms of digoxin toxicity. Laboratory analysis found the product was free of digoxin-like compounds but the contents were not further identified. This report may reflect an interaction of eleuthero with the laboratory test to cause a falsely elevated reading, rather than actually increasing digoxin levels.

INTERACTIONS WITH FOODS AND OTHER COMPOUNDS

Food

Many foods may interfere with the absorption of digoxin. To avoid this problem, people should take digoxin 1 hour before or 2 hours after eating food.[11] People taking digoxin should consult their prescribing doctor or pharmacist if they have questions regarding this interaction.

SUMMARY OF INTERACTIONS FOR DIGOXIN

Depletion or interference	*Magnesium, Potassium (if levels are low)*
Adverse interaction	*Digitalis, Licorice,* Senna,* Eleuthero**
Side effect reduction/prevention	*Magnesium, Potassium (if levels are low)*
Supportive interaction	*None known*
Reduced drug absorption/bioavailability	*Senna**
Other (see text)	*Hawthorn*

DILTIAZEM
(Cardizem, Dilacor XR, and Others)

Diltiazem is a calcium channel blocker used to treat angina pectoris, heart arrhythmias, and high blood pressure.

INTERACTIONS WITH FOODS AND OTHER COMPOUNDS

Food

Diltiazem may be taken with or without food.[1] Sustained-release diltiazem products should be swallowed whole, without opening, crushing, or chewing.[2]

SUMMARY OF INTERACTIONS FOR DILTIAZEM

Depletion or interference	*None known*
Adverse interaction	*None known*
Side effect reduction/prevention	*None known*
Supportive interaction	*None known*
Reduced drug absorption/bioavailability	*None known*

DIMENHYDRINATE
(Dramamine, Marmine, Nico-Vert, Triptone, and Others)

Dimenhydrinate is a combination of two drugs, diphenhydramine and chlorotheophylline. Dimenhydrinate is used to prevent and treat nausea, vomiting, dizziness, and motion sickness.

INTERACTIONS WITH HERBS

Henbane *(Hyoscyamus niger)*

Antihistamines, including dimenhydrinate, can cause "anticholinergic" side effects such as dryness of mouth and heart palpitations. Henbane also has anticholinergic activity and side effects. Therefore, use with dimenhydrinate could increase the risk of anticholinergic side effects,[1] though apparently no interactions have yet been reported with dimenhydrinate and henbane. Henbane should not be taken except by prescription from a physician trained in herbal medicine, as it is extremely toxic.

INTERACTIONS WITH FOODS AND OTHER COMPOUNDS

Alcohol

Dimenhydrinate causes drowsiness.[2] Alcohol may intensify this effect and increase the risk of accidental injury.[3] To prevent problems, people taking dimenhydrinate or dimenhydrinate-containing products should avoid alcohol.

SUMMARY OF INTERACTIONS FOR DIMENHYDRINATE

Depletion or interference	*None known*
Adverse interaction	*Henbane**
Side effect reduction/prevention	*None known*
Supportive interaction	*None known*
Reduced drug absorption/bioavailability	*None known*

DIPHENHYDRAMINE

(Benadryl, Benylin, and Others)

Diphenhydramine is an antihistamine used to relieve allergic rhinitis (seasonal allergy) symptoms including sneezing, runny nose, itching, and watery eyes and to relieve itching and swelling associated with uncomplicated allergic skin reactions. It is also used as a short-term sleep aid, to control coughs due to colds or allergy, and to prevent/treat motion sickness. Diphenhydramine is available in nonprescription products alone (Benadryl, Benylin, and others) and in combination with other nonprescription drugs, to treat symptoms of allergy, colds, and upper respiratory infections, including:

- Diphenhydramine/**acetaminophen** (page 2) (Excedrin PM, Tylenol PM Extra Strength, and others)
- Diphenhydramine/**pseudoephedrine** (page 83)/**acetaminophen** (page 2) (Tylenol Flu NightTime Maximum Strength Powder and others)

INTERACTIONS WITH HERBS

Henbane (*Hyoscyamus niger*)

Antihistamines, including diphenhydramine, can cause "anticholinergic" side effects such as dryness of mouth and heart palpitations. Henbane also has anticholinergic activity and side effects. Therefore, use with diphenhydramine could increase the risk of anticholinergic side effects,[1] though apparently no interactions have yet been reported with diphenhydramine and henbane. Henbane should not be taken except by prescription from a physician trained in herbal medicine, as it is extremely toxic.

INTERACTIONS WITH FOODS AND OTHER COMPOUNDS

Alcohol

Diphenhydramine causes drowsiness.[2] Alcohol may intensify this effect and increase the risk of accidental injury.[3] To prevent problems, people taking diphenhydramine or diphenhydramine-containing products should avoid alcohol.

SUMMARY OF INTERACTIONS FOR DIPHENHYDRAMINE

Depletion or interference	*None known*
Adverse interaction	*Henbane**
Side effect reduction/prevention	*None known*
Supportive interaction	*None known*
Reduced drug absorption/bioavailability	*None known*

DIURETICS

Diuretics constitute a class of many different drug families that all have the same action—they remove water from the body. Diuretics are used to lower blood pressure in people with hypertension and to assist the heart to pump better in people with congestive heart failure. Diuretics are also used to reduce water accumulation caused by other diseases.

Diuretics are divided into two general groups: potassium-sparing diuretics and potassium-depleting diuretics. Please refer to the following drugs for specific information.

Potassium-sparing diuretics include: **amiloride** (Midamor) (page 8), **spironolactone** (Aldactone) (page 191), and **triamterene** (Dyrenium) (page 214).

Potassium-depleting diuretics are further divided into **thiazide diuretics** (page 202), which include chlorthalidone (Hygroton and others), cholorothiazide (Diuril), hydrochlorothiazide (Esidrix, HydroDIURIL, and others), and metolazone (Zaroxolyn), and **loop diuretics** (page 129), which include bumetanide (Bumex), ethacrynic acid (Edecrin), furosemide (Lasix), and toresmide (Demadex).

DOCETAXEL

(Taxotere)

Docetaxel is a semisynthetic **chemotherapy** (page 40) drug made from an extract of needles of the yew plant. It is used to treat people with some types of late-stage cancer.

INTERACTIONS WITH DIETARY SUPPLEMENTS

Vitamin B$_6$

Docetaxel may cause a reddening, swelling, and pain in hands and feet. Two cases have been reported of people suffering these drug-induced symptoms and responding to 50 mg of vitamin B$_6$ given 3 times per day.[1] Symptoms began to resolve in 12 to 24 hours and continued to improve for several weeks.

SUMMARY OF INTERACTIONS FOR DOCETAXEL

Depletion or interference	*None known*
Adverse interaction	*None known*
Side effect reduction/prevention	*Vitamin B$_6$**
Supportive interaction	*None known*
Reduced drug absorption/bioavailability	*None known*

DORZOLAMIDE
(Trusopt)

DORZOLAMIDE/TIMOLOL
(Cosopt)

Dorzolamide is a member of the carbonic anhydrase inhibitor family of drugs used to reduce pressure in the eyes of people with ocular hypertension or open-angle glaucoma. It is available in prescription eye drops alone (Trusopt) and in the combination dorzolamide/**timolol** (page 209) (Cospot).

There are currently no reported nutrient or herb interactions involving dorzolamide or dorzolamide/timolol eye drops.

DOXAZOSIN
(Cardura)

Doxazosin is a member of the alpha blocker family of drugs used to lower blood pressure in people with hypertension. Doxazosin is also used to treat symptoms of benign prostatic hyperplasia (BPH).

There are currently no reported nutrient or herb interactions involving doxazosin.

DOXORUBICIN
(Adriamycin)

Doxorubicin is a **chemotherapy** (page 40) drug used primarily to treat people with cancer.

INTERACTIONS WITH DIETARY SUPPLEMENTS

Carnitine

Animal research suggests carnitine may prevent doxorubicin's toxicity.[1]

Coenzyme Q₁₀

Pretreating people with the antioxidant coenzyme Q_{10} before administration of doxorubicin has reduced cardiac toxicity[2]—an action also reported in animals.[3] Some doctors of natural medicine recommend 100 mg per day.

N-Acetyl Cysteine (NAC)

The antioxidant supplement N-acetyl cysteine (NAC) has protected animals from the cardiotoxicity of doxorubicin,[4] although human research has not been able to confirm these results.[5] Most doctors of natural medicine do not yet prescribe NAC for people taking doxorubicin.

Riboflavin

Animal research suggests doxorubicin may deplete riboflavin and that riboflavin deficiency promotes doxorubicin toxicity.[6]

Vitamin C

The antioxidant vitamin C has protected against cardiotoxicity (damage to the heart) of doxorubicin in an animal study.[7] In this trial, vitamin C significantly increased the life expectancy of mice and guinea pigs without interfering with anticancer action of the drug. Despite the lack of human data, some doctors of natural medicine recommend that people taking doxorubicin supplement at least 1 gram of vitamin C per day.

Vitamin E

A serious side effect sometimes caused by doxorubicin is heart failure. Animal studies show that the antioxidant activity of vitamin E protects against doxorubicin-induced cardiotoxicity.[8] [9] Test tube evidence suggests that vitamin E might also enhance the anticancer action of the drug.[10] Human trials exploring the cardioprotective action of vitamin E in people taking doxorubicin remain inconclusive, although some evidence suggests that vitamin E may allow for higher drug doses without increasing toxicity.[11]

It has been reported anecdotally that very high (1,600 IU) amounts of vitamin E may reduce the amount of hair loss accompanying use of doxorubicin.[12] However, while protection against hair loss was confirmed in a rabbit study, human research has not found this to be true.[13]

SUMMARY OF INTERACTIONS FOR DOXORUBICIN

Depletion or interference	*Riboflavin*[*]
Adverse interaction	*None known*
Side effect reduction/prevention	*Carnitine,*[*] *Coenzyme Q₁₀, Vitamin C,*[*] *Vitamin E*[*]

Supportive interaction	None known
Reduced drug absorption/bioavailability	None known
Other (see text)	N-acetyl cysteine (NAC)

DOXYCYCLINE
(Vibramycin and Others)

Doxycycline is a **tetracycline** (page 199) -like antibiotic. Doxycycline is used to treat a wide variety of infections and to prevent traveler's diarrhea.

INTERACTIONS WITH DIETARY SUPPLEMENTS

Minerals

Many minerals can decrease the absorption and reduce effectiveness of doxycycline, including calcium, magnesium, iron, zinc, and others.[1] To avoid these interactions, doxycycline should be taken 2 hours before or 2 hours after dairy products (high in calcium) and mineral-containing antacids or supplements.

Vitamin K

As with many antibiotics, doxycycline can kill friendly bacteria in the colon, potentially leading to reduced levels of vitamin K.[2] Some doctors of natural medicine believe that if doxycycline causes diarrhea for more than a few days, it makes sense to supplement vitamin K (now found in some multivitamins).

Berberine-Containing Herbs

Berberine is a chemical extracted from goldenseal (*Hydrastis canadensis*), barberry (*Berberis vulgaris*), and Oregon grape (*Berberis aquifolium*), which has antibacterial activity. However, one double-blind study found that 100 mg berberine given with tetracycline (a drug closely related to doxycycline) reduced the efficacy of tetracycline in people with cholera.[3] In that trial, berberine may have decreased tetracycline absorption. Another double-blind trial found that berberine neither improved nor interfered with tetracycline effectiveness in people with cholera.[4] Therefore, it remains unclear whether a significant interaction between berberine-containing herbs and doxycycline and related drugs exists.

INTERACTIONS WITH FOODS AND OTHER COMPOUNDS

Food

Doxycycline may be taken with or without food and should be taken with a full glass of water.[5] However, doxycycline should not be taken with milk[6] or other dairy products.

SUMMARY OF INTERACTIONS FOR DOXYCYCLINE

Depletion or interference	*Vitamin K**
Adverse interaction	*None known*
Side effect reduction/prevention	*None known*
Supportive interaction	*None known*
Reduced drug absorption/bioavailability	*Minerals**
Other (see text)	*Berberine-containing herbs such as goldenseal, barberry, and Oregon grape*

DOXYLAMINE
(Unisom)

Doxylamine is an antihistamine used for short-term treatment of insomnia. Doxylamine is available alone in the nonprescription product Unisom for sleep. It is also available in the combination doxylamine/**acetaminophen** (page 2)/**dextromethorphan** (page 70)/**pseudoephedrine** (page 83) (Nyquil Hot Therapy Powder and others) and in other combinations with nonprescription drugs to treat symptoms of allergy, colds, and upper respiratory infections.

INTERACTIONS WITH HERBS

Henbane (Hyoscyamus niger)

Antihistamines, including doxylamine, can cause "anticholinergic" side effects such as dryness of mouth and heart palpitations. Henbane also has anticholinergic activity and side effects. Therefore, use with doxylamine could increase the risk of anticholinergic side effects,[1] though apparently no interactions have yet been reported with doxylamine and henbane. Henbane should not be taken except by prescription from a physician trained in herbal medicine, as it is extremely toxic.

INTERACTIONS WITH FOODS AND OTHER COMPOUNDS

Alcohol

Doxylamine causes drowsiness.[2] Alcohol may intensify this effect and increase the risk of accidental injury.[3] To prevent problems, people taking doxylamine or doxylamine-containing products should avoid alcohol.

SUMMARY OF INTERACTIONS FOR DOXYLAMINE

Depletion or interference	*None known*
Adverse interaction	*Henbane**
Side effect reduction/prevention	*None known*
Supportive interaction	*None known*
Reduced drug absorption/bioavailability	*None known*

ECONAZOLE
(Spectazole)

Econazole is an antifungal cream used for topical (direct application to the skin) treatment of fungal skin infections. It is used most commonly to treat athlete's foot (fungal infection of the skin between the toes), jock itch (fungal infection of the skin in the groin region), and ringworm (fungal infection of nonhairy skin), and for external *Candida* infections. Econazole is for external use only.

INTERACTIONS WITH HERBS

Echinacea *(Echinacea purpurea, Echinacea angustifolia)*

The combination of oral echinacea with a topical econazole nitrate cream reduced the recurrence of vaginal yeast infections in women compared to those using the cream alone.[1]

SUMMARY OF INTERACTIONS FOR ECONAZOLE

Depletion or interference	*None known*
Adverse interaction	*None known*
Side effect reduction/prevention	*None known*
Supportive interaction	*Echinacea**
Reduced drug absorption/bioavailability	*None known*

ENALAPRIL
(Vasotec)

Enalapril is a type of **angiotensin-converting enzyme (ACE) inhibitor** (page 1), a family of drugs used to treat high blood pressure and some types of heart failure. Enalapril is also used to slow the progression of kidney disease in people with diabetes.

INTERACTIONS WITH DIETARY SUPPLEMENTS

Potassium

ACE inhibitors, including enalapril, may increase blood levels of potassium above normal[1] or reduce potassium excretion in urine.[2]

Sodium

In a short-term study of nine overweight men, enalapril plus a low-salt diet reduced blood pressure more than a low-salt diet alone.[3] Additionally, enalapril plus a low-salt diet resulted in better **insulin** (page 115) response than the low-salt diet alone. The importance of this preliminary information for overweight people with high blood pressure is unclear.

INTERACTIONS WITH FOODS AND OTHER COMPOUNDS

Food

Enalapril may be taken with or without food.[4]

SUMMARY OF INTERACTIONS FOR ENALAPRIL

Depletion or interference	*None known*
Adverse interaction	*Potassium*[*]
Side effect reduction/prevention	*None known*
Supportive interaction	*None known*
Reduced drug absorption/bioavailability	*None known*
Other (see text)	*Sodium*

EPHEDRINE AND PSEUDOEPHEDRINE

Ephedrine and pseudoephedrine are closely related drugs with actions and side effects similar to the hormone **epinephrine** (page 85) (adrenaline). Ephedrine, available in prescription and nonprescription strengths, is sometimes used to dilate bronchi (breathing tubes), making it easier for people with asthma to breathe. Drugs with better activity and fewer side effects are more commonly used. Nonprescription ephedrine nose drops (Vick Vatronol) or spray (Pretz-D) are used to relieve nasal congestion due to the flu or hay fever. Pseudoephedrine (Afrin tablets, Sudafed, and others) is a nonprescription drug taken by mouth to relieve nasal congestion due to the flu or hay fever.

INTERACTIONS WITH HERBS

Ephedra sinica (Ma huang)

Ephedra is the plant from which ephedrine was originally isolated. Ephedra, also called ma huang, is used in many herbal products including supplements promoted for weight loss. To prevent potentially serious interactions, people taking ephedrine or pseudoephedrine should avoid using ephedra-containing drug products and should read product labels carefully for ma huang or ephedra content. Native North American ephedra, sometimes called Mormon tea, contains no ephedrine.

Tannin-Containing Herbs

Tannins are a group of unrelated chemicals that give plants an astringent taste. Herbs containing high amounts of tannins may interfere with the absorption of ephedrine or pseudoephedrine taken by mouth.[1] Herbs containing high levels of tannins include green tea, black tea, uva ursi *(Arctostaphylos uva-ursi)*, black walnut *(Juglans nigra)*, red raspberry *(Rubus idaeus)*, oak *(Quercus* spp.), and witch hazel *(Hamamelis virginiana)*.

INTERACTIONS WITH FOODS AND OTHER COMPOUNDS

Food

Foods that acidify the urine may increase the elimination of ephedrine from the body, potentially reducing the action of the drug.[2] Urine-acidifying foods include eggs, peanuts, meat, chicken, vitamin C (greater than 5 grams per day), wheat-containing foods, and others.

Foods that alkalinize the urine may slow the elimination of ephedrine from the body, potentially increasing the actions and side effects of the drug.[3] Urine-alkalinizing foods include dairy products, nuts, vegetables (except corn and lentils), most fruits, and others.

Caffeine (page 33)

Caffeine, which is found in coffee, tea, chocolate, guaraná *(Paullinia cupana)*, and some nonprescription and supplement products, can amplify the side effects of ephedrine and pseudoephedrine. People should avoid combination products containing ephedrine/pseudoephedrine/ephedra and caffeine.

SUMMARY OF INTERACTIONS FOR EPHEDRINE AND PSEUDOEPHEDRINE

Depletion or interference	*None known*
Adverse interaction	***Caffeine*** *(page 33), Ephedra*
Side effect reduction/prevention	*None known*
Supportive interactionddd	*None known*
Reduced drug absorption/bioavailability	*Tannin-containing herbs* * such as green tea, black tea, uva ursi, black walnut, red raspberry, oak, and witch hazel*
Other (see text)	*Vitamin C*

EPINEPHRINE
(Brontin Mist, Primatene Mist, Bronkaid Mist, and Others)

Epinephrine, also called adrenaline, is a synthetic human hormone available as an orally inhaled, nonprescription drug to relieve temporary shortness of breath, chest tightness, and wheezing due to bronchial asthma. Epinephrine is also available as a prescription drug for injection used in emergencies, including acute asthma attacks and severe allergic reactions.

INTERACTIONS WITH DIETARY SUPPLEMENTS

Vitamins and Minerals

Intravenous administration of epinephrine to human volunteers reduced plasma concentrations of vitamin C.[1] Epinephrine and other "stress hormones" may reduce intracellular concentrations of potassium and magnesium.[2] Although there are no clinical studies in humans, it seems reasonable that individuals using epinephrine should consume a diet high in vitamin C, potassium, and magnesium or consider supplementing with these nutrients.

INTERACTIONS WITH HERBS

Ephedra sinica (Ma huang)

Ephedra is the plant from which the drug ephedrine was originally isolated. Epinephrine and ephedrine have similar effects and side effects.[3] Ephedra, also called ma huang, is used in many herbal products including supplements promoted for weight loss. While interactions between epinephrine and ephedra have not been reported, it seems likely that such interactions could occur. To prevent potential problems, people should not be taking both epinephrine and ephedra/ephedrine-containing products.

INTERACTIONS WITH FOODS AND OTHER COMPOUNDS

Caffeine (page 33)

Epinephrine can increase blood pressure and heart rate.[4] Caffeine, especially in large doses, can also increase heart rate[5] and when given with **phenylpropanolamine** (page 172), a drug with effects similar to epinephrine, produced an additive increase in blood pressure.[6] Caffeine is found in coffee, tea, soft drinks, chocolate, guaraná *(Paullinia cupana)*, nonprescription drugs, and supplements containing caffeine or guaraná. While no interactions have been reported between epinephrine and caffeine, people using epinephrine can minimize the potential for interactions by limiting or avoiding caffeine.

SUMMARY OF INTERACTIONS FOR EPINEPHRINE

Depletion or interference	*None known*
Adverse interaction	***Caffeine*** *(page 33), Ephedra*
Side effect reduction/prevention	*None known*
Supportive interaction	*None known*
Reduced drug absorption/bioavailability	*None known*
Other (see text)	*Magnesium, Potassium, Vitamin C*

ERYTHROMYCIN
(E-Mycin, Ery-Tab, Eryc, EES, Ilosone, and Others)

Erythromycin is a macrolide antibiotic used to treat a wide variety of bacterial infections. Several chemical forms of erythromycin are available for oral use to treat infections in the body. Erythromycin-containing products are also available to treat eye infections and skin infections.

INTERACTIONS WITH DIETARY SUPPLEMENTS

Bifidobacterium

Yogurt containing *Bifidobacterium longum* culture has decreased erythromycin-induced diarrhea in a single-blind study of ten healthy people.[1] Yogurt containing live cultures has also protected against other antibiotic-induced diarrhea.

Erythromycin

Bromelain

One report found bromelain improved the action of antibiotic drugs, including **penicillin** (page 168) and erythromycin, in treating a variety of infections. In that trial, twenty-two out of twenty-three people who had previously not responded to the antibiotics did so after adding bromelain 4 times per day.[2] Doctors of natural medicine will sometimes prescribe enough bromelain to equal 2,400 gelatin dissolving units (listed as GDU on labels) per day. This amount would equal approximately 3,600 MCU (milk clotting units), another common measure of bromelain activity.

Vitamins and Minerals

Erythromycin may interfere with the absorption and/or activity of calcium, folic acid, magnesium, and vitamins B_6 and B_{12},[3] which may cause problems, especially with long-term erythromycin treatment. Until more is known, it makes sense for people taking erythromycin for longer than 2 weeks to supplement with a daily multivitamin/multimineral.

INTERACTIONS WITH HERBS

Digitalis (Digitalis lanata, Digitalis purpurea)

Digitalis refers to a family of plants commonly called foxglove that contain digitalis glycosides, chemicals with actions and toxicities similar to the prescription drug **digoxin** (page 71).

Erythromycin can increase the serum level of digitalis glycosides, increasing the therapeutic effects and risk of side effects.[4] Erythromycin and digitalis-containing products should be used only under the direct supervision of a doctor trained in their use.

INTERACTIONS WITH FOODS AND OTHER COMPOUNDS

Food

Some forms of erythromycin are best absorbed when taken on an empty stomach, 1 hour before or 2 hours after food.[5] Individuals who experience stomach upset taking these forms of erythromycin on an empty stomach should use one of the other forms that can be taken with food.

Other forms of erythromycin may be taken with or without food.[6] People taking erythromycin should ask their pharmacist about the form of erythromycin they are taking and compatibility with or without food. Erythromycin is best taken with water, rather than other beverages, to prevent degradation of the drug before it reaches the intestines.[7] Erythromycin tablets should be swallowed whole, without cutting, chewing, or crushing.[8]

SUMMARY OF INTERACTIONS FOR ERYTHROMYCIN

Depletion or interference	*Multiple nutrients** *(Magnesium, Vitamin B_6, Vitamin B_{12})*
Adverse interaction	*None known*
Side effect reduction/prevention	*Bifidobacterium*
Supportive interaction	*Bromelain**
Reduced drug absorption/bioavailability	*None known*
Other (see text)	*Digitalis, Calcium, Folic Acid*

ESTRADIOL
(Estrace, Alora, Climara, Esclim, Estraderm, FemPatch, and Vivelle)

Estradiol is a semisynthetic human estrogenic hormone used to treat menopausal symptoms, to prevent osteoporosis in postmenopausal women, and as replacement therapy in other conditions of inadequate estrogen production. It is also used to treat some people with advanced breast or prostate cancers.

Estradiol is available as an oral drug (Estrace), as a transdermal (skin) patch (Alora, Climara, Esclim, Estraderm, FemPatch, and Vivelle), and as a vaginal cream (Estrace Vaginal Cream).

INTERACTIONS WITH DIETARY SUPPLEMENTS

Quercetin

Studies have shown that grapefruit juice significantly increases estradiol levels.[1][2] One of the flavonoids found in grapefruit juice is quercetin. In a test tube study, quercetin was found to change estrogen metabolism in human liver cells in a way that increases estradiol levels and reduces other forms of estrogen.[3] This effect is likely to increase estrogen activity in the body. However, the levels of quercetin used to alter estrogen metabolism in the test tube were much higher than levels found in the body after supplementing with quercetin. There is in vitro evidence that another flavonoid in grapefruit juice, naringenin, also has estrogenic activity.[4] It has yet to be shown that dietary or supplemental levels or quercetin (or naringenin) could create a significant problem.

Vitamin D

In a 2½-year, randomized study of 464 postmenopausal women without osteoporosis, hormone replacement with estradiol plus a progestin increased lumbar bone density and reduced femoral bone loss. Adding

300 IU of vitamin D_3 (cholecalciferol) per day did not improve the bone-sparing effects.[5] The outcome of this study therefore suggests against the common practice of nutritionally oriented doctors who frequently prescribe 400 IU vitamin D to women taking combination hormones.

INTERACTIONS WITH FOODS AND OTHER COMPOUNDS

Grapefruit Juice

In a randomized study of eight women with surgically removed ovaries, serum estradiol levels were significantly higher after estradiol was taken with grapefruit juice than when estradiol was taken alone.[6] These results have been independently confirmed,[7] suggesting that women taking oral estradiol should probably avoid grapefruit juice. The same effects might be seen from eating grapefruit as from drinking its juice.

SUMMARY OF INTERACTIONS FOR ESTRADIOL

Depletion or interference	*None known*
Adverse interaction	*Grapefruit juice,* Quercetin**
Side effect reduction/prevention	*None known*
Supportive interaction	*None known*
Reduced drug absorption/bioavailability	*None known*
Other (see text)	*Vitamin D*

ETODOLAC
(Lodine)

Etodolac is a member of the **nonsteroidal anti-inflammatory drug (NSAID** [page 157]**)** family. NSAIDs reduce inflammation (swelling), pain, and temperature. Etodolac is used to treat mild to moderate pain, arthritis, ankylosing spondylitis, tendinitis, bursistis, and other conditions.

INTERACTIONS WITH DIETARY SUPPLEMENTS

Copper

Supplementation may enhance the anti-inflammatory effects of NSAIDs while reducing their ulcerogenic effects. One study found that when various anti-inflammatory drugs were chelated with copper, the anti-inflammatory activity was increased.[1] Animal models of inflammation have found that the copper chelate of **aspirin** (page 18) was active at one-eighth the effective dose of aspirin. These copper complexes are less toxic than the parent compounds, as well.

Etodolac

Iron

NSAIDs cause gastrointestinal (GI) irritation, bleeding, and iron loss.[2] Iron supplements can cause GI irritation.[3] However, iron supplementation is sometimes needed in people taking NSAIDs if those drugs have caused enough blood loss to lead to iron deficiency. If both iron and etodolac are prescribed, they should be taken with food to reduce GI irritation and bleeding risk.

Potassium

NSAIDs have caused kidney dysfunction and increased blood potassium levels, especially in older people.[4] People taking NSAIDs, including etodolac, should not supplement potassium without consulting with their prescribing doctor or a nutritionally oriented doctor.

Sodium

Etodolac may cause sodium and water retention.[5] It is healthful to reduce dietary salt intake by eliminating table salt and heavily salted foods.

INTERACTIONS WITH HERBS

Licorice (Glycyrrhiza glabra)

The flavonoids found in the extract of licorice known as DGL (deglycyrrhizinated licorice) are helpful for avoiding the irritating actions **NSAIDs** (page 157) have on the stomach and intestines. One study found that 350 mg of chewable DGL taken together with each dose of aspirin reduced gastrointestinal bleeding caused by the aspirin.[6] DGL has been shown in controlled human research to be as effective as drug therapy (**cimetidine** [page 46]) in healing stomach ulcers.[7]

INTERACTIONS WITH FOODS AND OTHER COMPOUNDS

Food

Etodolac should be taken with food to prevent gastrointestinal upset.[8]

Alcohol

Etodolac may cause drowsiness, dizziness, or blurred vision.[9] Alcohol may intensify these effects and increase the risk of accidental injury. Use of alcohol during etodolac therapy increases the risk of stomach irritation and bleeding. People taking etodolac should avoid alcohol.

SUMMARY OF INTERACTIONS FOR ETODOLAC

Depletion or interference	*Iron*
Adverse interaction	*Sodium**

Side effect reduction/prevention	*Copper,* Licorice*
Supportive interaction	*Copper**
Reduced drug absorption/bioavailability	*None known*
Other (see text)	*Potassium*

FAMOTIDINE
(Pepcid, Pepcid AC)

Famotidine is a member of the H-2 blocker (histamine blocker) family of drugs that prevents the release of acid into the stomach. Famotidine is used to treat stomach and duodenal ulcers, reflux of stomach acid into the esophagus, and Zollinger-Ellison syndrome. Famotidine is available as the prescription drug Pepcid. It is also available as a nonprescription (OTC) product, Pepcid AC, for relief of heartburn, acid indigestion, and sour stomach.

INTERACTIONS WITH DIETARY SUPPLEMENTS

Iron

Stomach acid may increase absorption of iron from food. H-2 blocker drugs reduce stomach acid and are associated with decreased dietary iron absorption.[1] The iron found in supplements is available to the body without the need for stomach acid. People with ulcers may be iron deficient due to blood loss. If iron deficiency is present, iron supplementation may be beneficial. Iron levels in the blood can be checked with lab tests.

Magnesium-Containing Antacids

In healthy people, a **magnesium hydroxide** (page 135)/**aluminum hydroxide** (page 6) antacid, taken with famotidine, decreased famotidine absorption by 20 to 25%.[2] People can avoid this interaction by taking famotidine 2 hours before or after any aluminum/magnesium-containing antacids. Some magnesium supplements such as magnesium hydroxide are also antacids.

Vitamin B$_{12}$

Stomach acid is needed for vitamin B$_{12}$ in food to be absorbed. H-2 blocker drugs reduce stomach acid and may therefore inhibit absorption of the vitamin B$_{12}$ naturally present in food. However, the vitamin B$_{12}$ found in supplements does not depend on stomach acid for absorption.[3] Lab tests can determine vitamin B$_{12}$ levels in people.

Other Vitamins and Minerals

There is some evidence that other vitamins and minerals, such as folic acid[4] and copper,[5] require the presence of stomach acid for optimal absorption. Long-term use of H-2 blockers may therefore promote a deficiency of these nutrients. Individuals requiring long-term use of H-2 blockers may therefore benefit from a multiple vitamin/mineral supplement.

INTERACTIONS WITH FOODS AND OTHER COMPOUNDS

Food

Famotidine may be taken with or without food.[6] To prevent heartburn after meals, famotidine is best taken 1 hour before meals.[7]

Tobacco

In a study of eighteen healthy people, cigarette smoking was found to decrease the acid blocking effects of famotidine.[8] A double-blind, randomized study of 594 people with duodenal ulcers found that smoking inhibited the ulcer-healing effect of famotidine.[9]

SUMMARY OF INTERACTIONS FOR FAMOTIDINE

Depletion or interference	*Iron,* Vitamin B$_{12}$*
Adverse interaction	*Tobacco*
Side effect reduction/prevention	*None known*
Supportive interaction	*None known*
Reduced drug absorption/bioavailability	*None known*
Other (see text)	*Magnesium, Copper, Folic acid*

FEXOFENADINE
(Allegra)

Fexofenadine is a selective antihistamine used to relieve allergic rhinitis (seasonal allergy) symptoms including sneezing, runny nose, itching, and watery eyes.

INTERACTIONS WITH FOODS AND OTHER COMPOUNDS

Alcohol

Selective antihistamines, including fexofenadine, may cause drowsiness or dizziness, although it is less likely than with nonselective antihistamines.[1] Alcohol can intensify drowsiness and dizziness, increasing the risk of accidental injury. People taking fexofenadine should use alcohol only with caution.

SUMMARY OF INTERACTIONS FOR FEXOFENADINE

Depletion or interference	None known
Adverse interaction	None known
Side effect reduction/prevention	None known
Supportive interaction	None known
Reduced drug absorption/bioavailability	None known

FLUCONAZOLE
(Diflucan)

Fluconazole is an antifungal drug used to treat *Candida* infections. Fluconazole is also used to treat onychomycosis (fungal infection) of the toenails or fingernails and meningitis caused by *Cryptococcus*.

INTERACTIONS WITH FOODS AND OTHER COMPOUNDS

Food

Fluconazole may be taken with or without food.[1]

SUMMARY OF INTERACTIONS FOR FLUCONAZOLE

Depletion or interference	None known
Adverse interaction	None known
Side effect reduction/prevention	None known
Supportive interaction	None known
Reduced drug absorption/bioavailability	None known

FLUOROURACIL
(5-FU, Adrucil, Efudex, Fluoroplex)

Fluorouracil (Adrucil) is a **chemotherapy** (page 40) drug given intravenously (IV) to reduce symptoms of colon, rectum, breast, stomach, and pancreas cancers. Fluorouracil is also available in creams and solutions (Efudex and Fluoroplex) for topical treatment of some skin cancers and genital warts.

INTERACTIONS WITH DIETARY SUPPLEMENTS

Vitamin B$_6$

Fluorouracil occasionally causes problems on the skin of palms and soles. Preliminary reports have appeared showing that 100 mg per day of vitamin B$_6$ can sometimes eliminate the pain associated with this drug-induced condition.[1] [2]

SUMMARY OF INTERACTIONS FOR FLUOROURACIL

Depletion or interference	*None known*
Adverse interaction	*None known*
Side effect reduction/prevention	*Vitamin B$_6$*
Supportive interaction	*None known*
Reduced drug absorption/bioavailability	*None known*

FLUOXETINE
(Prozac)

Fluoxetine is a member of the selective serotonin reuptake inhibitor (SSRI) family of drugs. Fluoxetine is used to treat depression, bulimia (binge-eating and vomiting), obsessive-compulsive disorder, and others.

INTERACTIONS WITH DIETARY SUPPLEMENTS

Folic Acid

Low blood levels of folic acid have been correlated to poor response to fluoxetine.[1] It may be beneficial to supplement 200 mcg per day of folic acid in persons who have depression and are taking fluoxetine, though more study is required to determine if this is helpful.

Melatonin

Administration of fluoxetine for 6 weeks significantly lowered melatonin levels in people with seasonal affective disorder (SAD) and in healthy persons as well.[2] Further study is needed to determine if this might interfere with sleeping or whether melatonin supplementation might be appropriate.

L-Tryptophan

L-tryptophan is an amino acid found in protein-rich foods. Foods rich in L-tryptophan are not believed to cause any problems during fluoxetine use. However, dietary supplements of L-tryptophan taken during fluoxetine treatment have been reported to cause headache, sweating, dizziness, agitation, restlessness, nausea, vomiting, and other symptoms.[3]

5-Hydroxytryptophan (5-HTP)

Fluoxetine works by increasing serotonin activity in the brain. 5-HTP is converted to serotonin in the brain, and taking it with fluoxetine may increase fluoxetine-induced side effects. Until more is known, 5-HTP should not be taken with any SSRI drug, including fluoxetine.

INTERACTIONS WITH HERBS

Ginkgo (Ginkgo biloba)

In three men and two women treated with SSRI drugs (fluoxetine or **sertraline** [page 187]) for depression who experienced sexual dysfunction, addition of ginkgo biloba extract (GBE) in amounts up to 240 mg per day effectively reversed the sexual dysfunction.[4] In part this makes sense, because ginkgo, through its blood vessel–dilating action, has been reported to help men with some forms of impotence.[5]

St. John's Wort (Hypericum perforatum)

There have been no reports in the literature about negative consequences of combining St. John's wort and fluoxetine. There has been one reported case of an interaction between St. John's wort and a weak serotonin reuptake inhibitor drug known as **trazodone** (page 212) that is vaguely similar to fluoxetine.[6] Please refer to the section on trazodone for more information. In another case, a person experienced grogginess, lethargy, nausea, weakness, and fatigue after taking one dose of **paroxetine** (page 165) (Paxil, another SSRI drug) after 10 days of St. John's wort use.[7] Until more is known about interactions and adverse actions, people taking any SSRI drugs, including fluoxetine, should avoid St. John's wort.

INTERACTIONS WITH FOODS AND OTHER COMPOUNDS

Food

Fluoxetine may be taken with or without food.[8]

Alcohol

SSRI drugs, including fluoxetine, may cause dizziness or drowsiness.[9] Alcohol may intensify these actions and increase the risk of accidental injury. Alcohol should be avoided during fluoxetine therapy. Fluoxetine has been reported to decrease the desire to drink alcohol in a group of alcoholics.[10]

SUMMARY OF INTERACTIONS FOR FLUOXETINE

Depletion or interference	*Melatonin**
Adverse interaction	*5-HTP, L-tryptophan, St. John's wort*
Side effect reduction/prevention	*Ginkgo*
Supportive interaction	*Folic acid**
Reduced drug absorption/bioavailability	*None known*
Other (see text)	*Melatonin*

FLUVASTATIN
(Lescol)

Fluvastatin is a member of the HMG-CoA reductase inhibitor family of drugs that blocks the body's production of cholesterol. Fluvastatin is used to lower elevated cholesterol and to slow or prevent hardening of the arteries.

INTERACTIONS WITH DIETARY SUPPLEMENTS

Coenzyme Q_{10}

In a randomized, double-blind trial, blood levels of coenzyme Q_{10} (CoQ_{10}) were found in forty-five people with high cholesterol treated with **lovastatin** (page 133) or **pravastatin** (page 175) (drugs related to fluvastatin) for 18 weeks.[1] A significant decline in blood levels of CoQ_{10} occurred with either drug. One study found that supplementation with 100 mg of CoQ_{10} prevented declines in CoQ_{10} when taken with **simvastatin** (page 189) (another HMG-CoA reductase inhibitor drug).[2] Many nutritionally oriented doctors recommend that people taking HMG-CoA reductase inhibitor drugs such as fluvastatin also supplement with approximately 100 mg CoQ_{10} per day, although lower doses, such as 10 to 30 mg per day, might conceivably be effective in preventing the decline in CoQ_{10} levels.

Niacin

Niacin is the form of vitamin B_3 used to lower cholesterol. Fluvastatin and niacin used together have been shown to be more effective than either drug alone.[3] High-dose niacin taken with lovastatin (a drug closely related to fluvastatin) may cause muscle disorders (myopathy) that can become serious (rhabdomyolysis).[4][5] Such problems appear to be uncommon.[6][7] No interactions have yet been reported with fluvastatin and niacin. Nonetheless, people taking both fluvastatin and niacin should be monitored for muscle disorders by the prescribing physician until more is known.

Vitamin A

A study of thirty-seven people with high cholesterol treated with diet and HMG-CoA reductase inhibitors found blood vitamin A levels increased during 2 years of therapy.[8] Until more is known, people taking HMG-CoA reductase inhibitors, including fluvastatin, should have blood levels of vitamin A monitored if they intend to supplement vitamin A.

INTERACTIONS WITH FOODS AND OTHER COMPOUNDS

Food

Fluvastatin is equally effective taken with or without food in the evening.[9]

Alcohol

In a study of thirty-one people with primary hypercholesterolemia treated with fluvastatin, 6 weeks of daily, moderate alcohol consumption slowed the absorption and metabolism of fluvastatin but did not interfere with its effectiveness.[10]

SUMMARY OF INTERACTIONS FOR FLUVASTATIN

Depletion or interference	*Coenzyme Q_{10}*
Adverse interaction	*Vitamin A**
Side effect reduction/prevention	*None known*
Supportive interaction	*None known*
Reduced drug absorption/bioavailability	*None known*
Other (see text)	*Niacin*

FLUVOXAMINE
(Luvox)

Fluvoxamine is a selective serotonin reuptake inhibitor (SSRI) drug, related to **Fluoxetine** (Prozac) (page 94). It is used primarily to treat obsessive-compulsive disorder and is under investigation to treat depression.

INTERACTIONS WITH DIETARY SUPPLEMENTS

5-Hydroxytryptophan (5-HTP) and L-tryptophan

Fluvoxamine works by increasing serotonin activity in the brain. 5-HTP and L-tryptophan are converted to serotonin in the brain and taking them with fluvoxamine may increase fluvoxamine-induced side effects. Until more is known, 5-HTP and L-tryptophan should not be taken with any SSRI drug, including fluvoxamine.

INTERACTIONS WITH HERBS

Ginkgo (Ginkgo biloba)

In a clinical report of sixty-six men and women treated primarily with SSRI drugs (fluoxetine or **sertraline** [page 187]) for depression, ginkgo biloba extract (GBE) in amounts up to 240 mg per day effectively reversed the sexual dysfunction associated with these drugs.[1] In part this makes sense, because ginkgo, through its blood vessel–dilating action, has been reported to help men with some forms of impotence.[2]

St. John's Wort (Hypericum perforatum)

One report describes a case of serotonin syndrome in a person who took St. John's wort and **trazodone** (page 212), a weak SSRI drug.[3] The individual experienced mental confusion, muscle twitching, sweating, flushing, and ataxia. In another case, a person experienced grogginess, lethargy, nausea, weakness, and fatigue after taking one dose of **paroxeteine** (page 165) (Paxil, an SSRI drug related to fluvoxamine) after 10 days of St. John's wort.[4] Until more is known about interactions and adverse actions, people taking any SSRI drugs, including fluvoxamine, should avoid St. John's wort.

Yohimbe (Pausinystalia yohimbe)

The alkaloid yohimbine from the African yohimbe tree affects the nervous system in a way that may complement fluvoxamine. One report studied depressed people who had not responded to fluvoxamine. When 5 mg of yohimbine was added 3 times each day, there was significant improvement. Some people required higher doses of yohimbine before their depression improved. Because yohimbine can have side effects, it should only be taken under a doctor's supervision. Yohimbine is a prescription drug, but standardized extracts of yohimbe that contain yohimbine are available as a supplement.

INTERACTIONS WITH FOODS AND OTHER COMPOUNDS

Alcohol

SSRI drugs, including fluvoxamine, may cause dizziness or drowsiness.[5] Alcohol may intensify the drowsiness and increase the risk of accidental injury. People should avoid alcohol-containing products during fluvoxamine treatment.

Tobacco (Nicotiana species)

Smoking increases the metabolism of fluvoxamine, which may reduce effectiveness.[6] People should avoid smoking while taking fluvoxamine.

SUMMARY OF INTERACTIONS FOR FLUVOXAMINE

Depletion or interference	*None known*
Adverse interaction	*5-HTP, L-tryptophan, St. John's wort,* Tobacco*
Side effect reduction/prevention	*Ginkgo*
Supportive interaction	*Yohimbe**
Reduced drug absorption/bioavailability	*None known*

GABAPENTIN
(Neurontin)

Gabapentin is a drug used to treat or prevent seizures in people with seizure disorders.

INTERACTIONS WITH FOODS AND OTHER COMPOUNDS

Alcohol

Gabapentin may cause dizziness or sleepiness.[1] Alcohol may intensify these effects and increase the risk of accidental injury. To prevent problems, people taking gabapentin should avoid alcohol.

SUMMARY OF INTERACTIONS FOR GABAPENTIN

Depletion or interference	*None known*
Adverse interaction	*None known*
Side effect reduction/prevention	*None known*
Supportive interaction	*None known*
Reduced drug absorption/bioavailability	*None known*

GEMFIBROZIL
(Lopid, Apo-Gemfibrozil, Novo-Gemfibrozil, and Others)

Gemfibrozil is a drug used to lower cholesterol and triglycerides in people with high cholesterol. Other drugs, especially members of the HMG-CoA reductase inhibitor drug family, are more commonly used.

INTERACTIONS WITH DIETARY SUPPLEMENTS

Coenzyme Q_{10}

In a randomized study of twenty-one men with combined hyperlipidemia, 10 to 12 weeks of gemfibrozil therapy reduced coenzyme Q_{10} blood levels to the levels seen in healthy men.[1] The clinical significance of this finding is unknown.

Vitamin E

In a randomized study of twenty-one men with combined hyperlipidemia, 10 to 12 weeks of gemfibrozil therapy reduced alpha- and gamma-tocopherol blood levels to the levels seen in healthy men.[2] The clinical significance of this finding is unknown and may reflect a normal physiological response to a reduction in serum cholesterol levels.

Monascus Purpureus

Monascus purpureus, a form of red yeast, is fermented with rice to produce a dietary supplement, Cholestin, that contains low levels of **lovastatin** (page 133), a drug otherwise available only by prescription. Gemfibrozil taken with the prescription drug lovastatin has been reported to cause rhabdomyolysis, a potentially life-threatening muscle disease.[3] People taking gemfibrozil should avoid lovastatin-containing products, including Cholestin, until more is known. The levels of lovastatin in Cholestin are significantly lower than those given of the drug as a single agent. It also contains numerous other compounds that may alter the interaction of lovastatin and gemfibrozil.

INTERACTIONS WITH FOODS AND OTHER COMPOUNDS

Food

Gemfibrozil should be taken 30 minutes before meals.[4]

Alcohol

Gemfibrozil may cause dizziness or blurred vision.[5] Alcohol may intensify these effects, increasing the risk for accidental injury. People taking gemfibrozil should avoid alcohol.

SUMMARY OF INTERACTIONS FOR GEMFIBROZIL

Depletion or interference	*Coenzyme Q_{10},* Vitamin E*
Adverse interaction	Monascus purpureus
Side effect reduction/prevention	*None known*
Supportive interaction	*None known*
Reduced drug absorption/bioavailability	*None known*

GENTAMICIN
(Garamycin)

Gentamicin is an aminoglycoside **antibiotic** (page 14) used to treat infections caused by many different types of bacteria. Gentamicin is usually administered by intravenous (IV) infusion or intramuscular injection. There are special gentamicin-containing drug products to treat eye and skin infections.

INTERACTIONS WITH DIETARY SUPPLEMENTS

Calcium

Gentamicin has been associated with hypocalcemia (low calcium levels) in humans.[1] In a study using rats, authors reported oral calcium supplementation reduced gentamicin-induced kidney damage.[2] The implications of this report for humans are unclear. People receiving gentamicin should ask their prescribing doctor or a nutritionally oriented doctor about monitoring calcium levels and calcium supplementation.

Magnesium

Gentamicin has been associated with urinary loss of magnesium, resulting in hypomagnesemia (low magnesium levels) in humans.[3] [4]

Potassium

Gentamicin has been associated with hypokalemia (low potassium levels) in humans.[5]

Vitamin B$_6$

Gentamicin administration has been associated with vitamin B$_6$ depletion in rabbits.[6] The authors of this study mention early evidence that vitamin B$_6$ administration may protect against gentamicin-induced kidney damage.

SUMMARY OF INTERACTIONS FOR GENTAMICIN

Depletion or interference	*Calcium,* Magnesium, Potassium**
Adverse interaction	*None known*
Side effect reduction/prevention	*None known*
Supportive interaction	*None known*
Reduced drug absorption/bioavailability	*None known*
Other (see text)	*Vitamin B$_6$*

Glipizide

GLIPIZIDE
(Glucotrol)

Glipizide is a sulfonylurea drug used to lower blood sugar levels in people with non-insulin-dependent (type II) diabetes.

INTERACTIONS WITH DIETARY SUPPLEMENTS

Magnesium

In a study of people with poorly controlled type II diabetes and low blood levels of magnesium, treatment with glipizide was associated with a significant rise in magnesium levels.[1] In a randomized trial with eight healthy people, 850 mg **magnesium hydroxide** (page 135) increased glipizide absorption and activity.[2] In theory, such changes could be therapeutic or detrimental under varying circumstances. Therefore, people taking glipizide should consult with their prescribing doctor before taking magnesium supplements.

INTERACTIONS WITH HERBS

Fenugreek (Trigonella foenum-graecum)

In a randomized study of fifteen people with IDDM diabetes, fenugreek (100 grams per day for 10 days) was reported to reduce blood sugar, urinary sugar excretion, serum cholesterol, and triglycerides, with no change in insulin levels, compared with 10 days of placebo.[3] In a study of sixty people with NIDDM diabetes, fenugreek (25 grams per day for 24 weeks) was reported to significantly reduce blood glucose levels.[4] People using glipizide should talk with their prescribing doctor before making any therapy changes.

Gymnema sylvestre

Herbs such as *Gymnema sylvestre* will often improve blood-sugar control in diabetics.

INTERACTIONS WITH FOODS AND OTHER COMPOUNDS

Food

Glipizide works best when taken 30 minutes before meals.[5] Effective treatment of type II diabetes with glipizide includes adherence to recommended dietary guidelines.

SUMMARY OF INTERACTIONS FOR GLIPIZIDE

Depletion or interference	*None known*
Adverse interaction	*Fenugreek,** *Gymnema sylvestre**

Side effect reduction/prevention	*None known*
Supportive interaction	*None known*
Reduced drug absorption/bioavailability	*None known*
Other (see text)	*Magnesium*

GLYBURIDE
(Glibenclamide, Diabeta, Micronase, Pres Tab)

Glyburide is a sulfonylurea drug used to lower blood sugar levels in people with non-insulin-dependent diabetes (type II diabetes). Maintaining normal blood sugar levels helps reduce health problems associated with diabetes. People with diabetes should consult with their doctor before starting or stopping any form of treatment including drug therapy, herbal products, supplements, and others.

Consumption of a high-fiber diet and/or supplementation with nutrients such as chromium, biotin, vitamin E, and others or herbs such as *Gymnema sylvestre* will often improve blood-sugar control in diabetics. In such cases, the dose of blood sugar-lowering drugs may need to be reduced in order to avoid a hypoglycemic reaction. Anyone taking medication for diabetes should consult the prescribing physician before making dietary changes or taking nutrients or herbs that are designed to lower blood-sugar levels.

INTERACTIONS WITH HERBS

Aloe (*Aloe vera*)

One single-blind study in Thailand reported that combining 1 tablespoon of aloe juice twice daily with glyburide significantly improved blood sugar and lipid levels in people with diabetes, compared with placebo.[1] Previously, glyburide by itself had not effectively controlled the diabetes in the people in this study.

INTERACTIONS WITH FOODS AND OTHER COMPOUNDS

Food

Glyburide may be taken with food to avoid gastrointestinal (GI) upset.[2] Effective treatment of type II diabetes with glyburide includes adherence to recommended dietary guidelines.

Alcohol

Alcohol consumption may interfere with blood-sugar control during glyburide therapy.[3] Alcohol may interact with glyburide, causing facial flushing, headache, light-headedness, nausea, breathlessness, and other symptoms.[4] People taking glyburide should avoid alcohol.

SUMMARY OF INTERACTIONS FOR GLYBURIDE

Depletion or interference	*None known*
Adverse interaction	*None known*
Side effect reduction/prevention	*None known*
Supportive interaction	*Aloe vera**
Reduced drug absorption/bioavailability	*None known*
Other (see text)	*Biotin, Chromium, Gymnema, Vitamin E*

GRISEOFULVIN
(Fulvicin, Grifulvin, Gris-PEG, Gristatin)

Griseofulvin is an antifungal drug used to treat ringworm infections of the skin, hair, and nails caused by specific fungi.

INTERACTIONS WITH DIETARY SUPPLEMENTS

Vitamin E

Adding 50 IU of vitamin E per day was reported to increase blood levels of this drug within 4 weeks in children, allowing drug dose to be cut in half. Reducing the dose of griseofulvin should decrease the likelihood of side effects. This evidence is preliminary, so people taking griseofulvin should not supplement vitamin E on their own but may wish to discuss this matter with the prescribing doctor.[1]

INTERACTIONS WITH FOODS AND OTHER COMPOUNDS

Food

Food, especially with high fat content, increases griseofulvin absorption.[2] It is recommended that griseofulvin be taken with food to maximize absorption of the drug. People on lowfat diets who are taking griseofulvin should talk with their prescribing doctor or pharmacist.

Alcohol

Alcohol may interact with griseofulvin causing a reaction marked by facial flushing, headache, lightheadedness, nausea, and breathlessness.[3] To prevent unwanted reactions, people should avoid alcohol-containing products during griseofulvin therapy.

SUMMARY OF INTERACTIONS FOR GRISEOFULVIN

Depletion or interference	*None known*
Adverse interaction	*None known*
Side effect reduction/prevention	*None known*
Supportive interaction	*Vitamin E**
Reduced drug absorption/bioavailability	*None known*

GUAIFENESIN
(Guiatuss, Humibid, Robitussin, and Others)

Guaifenesin is a drug that reduces the thickness and stickiness of mucus. It is used for short-term relief of dry, nonproductive cough and mucus in the breathing passages. Guaifenesin is available in nonprescription products alone (Guiatuss, Robitussin, and others), in prescription products (Humibid and others), and in combination with other nonprescription drugs, to treat symptoms of allergy, colds, and upper respiratory infections, including:

- Guaifenesin/**phenylpropanolamine** (page 172) (Entex LA and others)
- Guaifenesin/**dextromethorphan** (page 70) (Robitussin DM and others)
- Guaifenesin/**dextromethorphan** (page 70)/**phenylpropanolamine** (page 172) (Robitussin CF and others)
- Guaifenesin/**ephedrine** (page 83)/**theophylline** (page 200) (Primatene Dual Action)

There are currently no reported nutrient or herb interactions involving guaifenesin.

HALOPERIDOL
(Haldol)

Haloperidol is a drug used to treat people with psychotic disorders, including schizophrenia.

INTERACTIONS WITH DIETARY SUPPLEMENTS

Glycine

Two double-blind studies have found that 0.4 to 0.8 mg/kg body weight per day of glycine combined with haloperidol and related drugs can reduce the so-called negative symptoms of schizophrenia.[1] [2] Negative symptoms include reduced emotional expression or general activity. The action of glycine in combination with the drugs was greater than the drugs alone, suggesting a synergistic action. Another double-blind study using approximately half the dose in the positive studies could not find any benefit from adding glycine to antipsychotic drug therapy.[3] People with low blood levels of glycine appeared to improve the most when given glycine in addition to their antipsychotic drugs.[4] No side effects were noticed in these studies, even when more than 30 grams of glycine were given daily.

Iron

Haloperidol may cause decreased blood levels of iron.[5] The importance of this interaction remains unclear. Iron should not be supplemented unless a deficiency is diagnosed.

Potassium

Haloperidol may cause hyperkalemia (high blood levels of potassium) or hypokalemia (low blood levels of potassium).[6] The incidence and severity of these changes remains unclear. Serum potassium can be measured by any doctor.

Vitamin E

Haloperidol and related antipsychotic drugs can cause a movement disorder called tardive dyskinesia. Several double-blind studies suggest that vitamin E may be beneficial for treatment of tardive dyskinesia.[7] Taking the large dose of 1,600 IU per day of vitamin E simultaneously with antipsychotic drugs has also been shown to lessen symptoms of tardive dyskinesia.[8] It is unknown if combining vitamin E with haloperidol could prevent tardive dyskinesia.

Sodium

Haloperidol may cause hyponatremia (low blood levels of sodium).[9] The incidence and severity of these changes remain unclear.

INTERACTIONS WITH HERBS

Milk Thistle (*Silybum marianum*)

Haloperidol may cause liver damage. A double-blind study in sixty women treated with drugs such as haloperidol were given 800 mg per day silymarin extract made from milk thistle.[10] There was a significant decrease in free radical levels of the test subjects who were given silymarin, unlike those given placebo.

INTERACTIONS WITH FOODS AND OTHER COMPOUNDS

Coffee and Tea

Coffee and tea are reported to cause precipitation of haloperidol in the test tube.[11] If this interaction happens in people, it would reduce the amount of haloperidol absorbed and the effectiveness of therapy. People taking haloperidol may avoid this possible interaction by taking haloperidol 1 hour before or 2 hours after drinking coffee or tea.

Alcohol

Haloperidol may cause drowsiness.[12] Alcohol may compound this drowsiness and increase the risk of accidents during activities requiring alertness. People should avoid alcohol-containing products during haloperidol therapy.

SUMMARY OF INTERACTIONS FOR HALOPERIDOL

Depletion or interference	Iron,* Sodium*
Adverse interaction	None known
Side effect reduction/prevention	Milk thistle,* Vitamin E
Supportive interaction	Glycine
Reduced drug absorption/bioavailability	Tea and coffee*
Other (see text)	Potassium

HEPARIN

Heparin, a natural product available by prescription, is used as an anticoagulant (slows the rate of blood clot formation). Blood clots can cause severe and life-threatening problems. Heparin is used to prevent formation of blood clots (after surgery and in other settings) and in circumstances to help dissolve blood clots already formed (deep vein thrombosis, pulmonary embolism, and other situations involving excessive blood clotting).

INTERACTIONS WITH DIETARY SUPPLEMENTS

Potassium

Heparin therapy may cause hyperkalemia (abnormally high potassium levels).[1]

Vitamin D

Heparin may interfere with activation of vitamin D in the body.[2] Osteoporosis (bone degeneration) has been reported in people who received high doses of heparin for several months.[3] Osteopenia (decreased bone density) has been reported in women who received heparin therapy during pregnancy.[4] [5]

INTERACTIONS WITH HERBS

Digitalis (Digitalis purpurea)

Digitalis refers to a group of plants commonly called foxglove, which contains chemicals related to the drug **digoxin** (page 71). Digitalis may interfere with the anticoagulant action of heparin, reducing its action.[6] People receiving heparin should avoid digitalis and digitalis-containing products. Digitalis should only be used under the direct supervision of a doctor trained in its use.

Ginger (Zingiber officinale)

Ginger has been shown to reduce platelet stickiness in test tubes. Although there are no reports of interactions with anticoagulant drugs, people should discuss it with a health-care professional if they are taking an anticoagulant and wish to use ginger.[7]

Ginkgo (Ginkgo biloba)

Ginkgo extracts may reduce the ability of platelets to stick together, possibly increasing the tendency toward bleeding.[8] Standardized extracts of ginkgo have been associated with two cases of spontaneous bleeding, although the ginkgo extracts were not definitively shown to be the cause of the problem.[9] [10] There is one case report of a person taking **warfarin** (page 224) in whom bleeding occurred after the addition of ginkgo.[11] People taking heparin should consult with a physician knowledgeable about botanical medicines if they are considering taking ginkgo.

Herbs Containing Coumarin Derivatives

Although there are no specific studies demonstrating interactions with anticoagulants, the following herbs contain coumarin-like substances that may interact with heparin and may cause bleeding.[12] These herbs include dong quai, fenugreek, horse chestnut, red clover, sweet clover, and sweet woodruff. People should consult their health-care professional if they are taking an anticoagulant and wish to use one of these herbs.

INTERACTIONS WITH FOODS AND OTHER COMPOUNDS

Alcohol

Alcohol consumption during heparin therapy may increase the risk of serious bleeding.[13] It is important for people receiving heparin to avoid alcohol during the entire course of heparin therapy.

SUMMARY OF INTERACTIONS FOR HEPARIN

Depletion or interference	*Vitamin D*
Adverse interaction	*Digitalis,* Dong quai,* Fenugreek,* Ginger, Ginkgo,* Horse chestnut,* Red clover,* Sweet clover,* Sweet woodruff**
Side effect reduction/prevention	*None known*
Supportive interaction	*None known*
Reduced drug absorption/bioavailability	*None known*
Other (see text)	*Potassium*

HYDRALAZINE
(Apresoline)

Hydralazine is a drug used to lower blood pressure in people with hypertension. Hydralazine relaxes the muscles that control the diameter of blood vessels. This relaxation allows the blood vessels to dilate (open wider), lowering blood pressure.

INTERACTIONS WITH DIETARY SUPPLEMENTS

Vitamin B$_6$

Vitamin B$_6$ can bind to hydralazine to form a complex that is excreted in the urine, increasing vitamin B$_6$ loss.[1] This may lead to vitamin B$_6$ deficiency.[2] People taking hydralazine should consult with their prescribing doctor and/or a nutritionally oriented doctor to discuss the possibility of vitamin B$_6$ supplementation.

INTERACTIONS WITH FOODS AND OTHER COMPOUNDS

Food

Taking hydralazine with food improves the absorption of the drug.[3] People with questions should ask their prescribing doctor or pharmacist.

Alcohol

Alcohol causes blood vessels to dilate, lowering blood pressure. This action may add to the blood pressure–lowering effect of hydralazine and increase the risk of dizziness, fainting, or accidental falls. People taking hydralazine should avoid alcohol and should read all product labels carefully for alcohol content.

SUMMARY OF INTERACTIONS FOR HYDRALAZINE

Depletion or interference	*Vitamin B6*
Adverse interaction	*None known*
Side effect reduction/prevention	*None known*
Supportive interaction	*None known*
Reduced drug absorption/bioavailability	*None known*

HYDROCODONE/ACETAMINOPHEN
(Vicodin, Lortab, and Others)

Hydrocodone is a narcotic analgesic used to relieve mild to moderate pain. Hydrocodone is available in the combination of hydrocodone/**acetaminophen** (page 2) (Vicodin, Lortab, and others).

INTERACTIONS WITH FOODS AND OTHER COMPOUNDS

Food

Hydrocodone may cause gastrointestinal (GI) upset. Hydrocodone-containing products may be taken with food to reduce or prevent GI upset.[1] A common side effect of narcotic analgesics is constipation.[2] Increasing dietary fiber (especially vegetables and whole-grain foods) and water intake can ease constipation.

Alcohol

Hydrocodone may cause drowsiness, dizziness, or blurred vision. Alcohol may intensify these effects and increase the risk of accidental injury.[3] To prevent problems, people taking hydrocodone should avoid alcohol.

SUMMARY OF INTERACTIONS FOR HYDROCODONE/ ACETAMINOPHEN

Depletion or interference	*None known*
Adverse interaction	*None known*
Side effect reduction/prevention	*None known*
Supportive interaction	*None known*
Reduced drug absorption/bioavailability	*None known*

IBUPROFEN
(Advil, Motrin, Motrin IB, Nuprin, and Others)

Ibuprofen is a member of the **nonsteroidal anti-inflammatory drug (NSAID** [page 157]**)** family. NSAIDs reduce inflammation (swelling), pain, and temperature. Ibuprofen is used to treat mild to moderate pain, fever, arthritis, primary dysmenorrhea, and other conditions. Ibuprofen is available in prescription strength (Motrin and others) and in nonprescription strength (Advil, Motrin IB, Nuprin, and others).

INTERACTIONS WITH DIETARY SUPPLEMENTS

Copper

Supplementation may enhance the anti-inflammatory effects of NSAIDs while reducing their ulcerogenic effects. One study found that when various anti-inflammatory drugs were chelated with copper, the anti-inflammatory activity was increased.[1] Animal models of inflammation have found that the copper chelate of **aspirin** (page 18) was active at one-eighth the effective dose of aspirin. These copper complexes are less toxic than the parent compounds as well.

Iron

NSAIDs cause gastrointestinal (GI) irritation, bleeding and iron loss.[2] Iron supplements can cause GI irritation.[3] However, iron supplementation is sometimes needed in people taking NSAIDs if those drugs have caused enough blood loss to lead to iron deficiency. If both iron and ibuprofen are prescribed, they should be taken with food to reduce GI irritation and bleeding risk.

Potassium

Ibuprofen has caused kidney dysfunction and increased blood potassium levels, especially in older people.[4] People taking ibuprofen should not supplement potassium without consulting with their prescribing doctor or a nutritionally oriented doctor.

Sodium

Ibuprofen may cause sodium and water retention.[5] It is healthful to reduce dietary salt intake by eliminating table salt and heavily salted foods.

INTERACTIONS WITH HERBS

Licorice (Glycyrrhiza glabra)

The flavonoids found in the extract of licorice known as DGL (deglycyrrhizinated licorice) are helpful for avoiding the irritating actions **NSAIDs** (page 157) have on the stomach and intestines. One study found that 350 mg of chewable DGL taken together with each dose of aspirin reduced gastrointestinal bleeding caused by the aspirin.[6] DGL has been shown in controlled human research to be as effective as drug therapy (**cimetidine** [page 46]) in healing stomach ulcers.[7]

INTERACTIONS WITH FOODS AND OTHER COMPOUNDS

Food

Ibuprofen should be taken with food to prevent gastrointestinal upset.[8]

Alcohol

Ibuprofen may cause drowsiness, dizziness, or blurred vision.[9] Alcohol may intensify these effects and increase the risk of accidental injury. Use of alcohol during ibuprofen therapy increases the risk of stomach irritation and bleeding. People taking ibuprofen should avoid alcohol.

SUMMARY OF INTERACTIONS FOR IBUPROFEN

Depletion or interference	Iron
Adverse interaction	Sodium*
Side effect reduction/prevention	Copper,* Licorice
Supportive interaction	Copper*
Reduced drug absorption/bioavailability	None known
Other (see text)	Potassium

INDOMETHACIN
(Indocin)

Indomethacin is a member of the **nonsteroidal anti-inflammatory drug (NSAID** [page 157]**)** family of drugs. NSAIDs reduce inflammation (swelling), pain, and temperature. Indomethacin is used to reduce pain/swelling involved in osteoarthritis, rheumatoid arthritis, bursitis, tendinitis, gout, ankylosing spondylitis, and headaches.

INTERACTIONS WITH DIETARY SUPPLEMENTS

Iron

Iron supplements can cause stomach irritation. Use of iron supplements with indomethacin increases the risk of stomach irritation and bleeding.[1] However, stomach bleeding causes iron loss. If both iron and indomethacin are prescribed, they should be taken with food to reduce stomach irritation and bleeding risk.

Potassium

Indomethacin may cause elevated blood potassium levels in people with normal and abnormal kidney function.[2] [3] [4] Until more is known, people taking indomethacin should not supplement potassium without medical supervision.

Vitamins and Minerals

Indomethacin has been reported to decrease absorption of folic acid and vitamin C.[5] Under certain circumstances, indomethacin may interfere with the actions of vitamin C.[6] Calcium and phosphate levels may also be reduced with indomethacin therapy.[7] It remains unclear whether people taking this drug need to supplement any of these nutrients.

Sodium

Indomethacin may cause sodium and water retention.[8] It is healthful to reduce dietary salt intake by eliminating table salt and heavily salted foods.

INTERACTIONS WITH FOODS AND OTHER COMPOUNDS

Food

Indomethacin should be taken with food to prevent stomach irritation.[9] However, applesauce, high-protein foods, and high-fat foods have been reported to interfere with indomethacin absorption and/or activity.[10]

Alcohol

Indomethacin may cause drowsiness or dizziness.[11] Alcohol may amplify these actions. Use of alcohol during indomethacin therapy increases the risk of stomach irritation and bleeding.[12] People taking indomethacin should avoid alcohol.

SUMMARY OF INTERACTIONS FOR INDOMETHACIN

Depletion or interference	*Calcium,[*] Folic acid, Vitamin C*
Adverse interaction	*Potassium, Sodium*
Side effect reduction/prevention	*None known*
Supportive interaction	*None known*
Reduced drug absorption/bioavailability	*None known*
Other (see text)	*Iron*

INFLUENZA VIRUS VACCINE
(Fluzone, FluShield, Fluvirin)

The influenza vaccine is given by injection to help prevent influenza (flu), particularly in people with compromised immune systems. The vaccine is altered yearly to correspond to mutations in the flu virus.

INTERACTIONS WITH HERBS

Asian Ginseng (Panax ginseng)

In a randomized, double-blind study, 227 people received influenza vaccine plus 100 mg of standardized extract of Asian ginseng or placebo 2 times per day for 4 weeks before and 8 weeks after influenza vaccination.[1] Compared with placebo, Asian ginseng extract was reported to prevent colds and flu, improve immune cell activity, and increase antibody levels after vaccination.

Eleuthero (Siberian ginseng)

Some Russian studies suggest that eleuthero (Siberian ginseng) may reduce the risk of postvaccination reactions.[2]

SUMMARY OF INTERACTIONS FOR INFLUENZA VACCINE

Depletion or interference	*None known*
Adverse interaction	*None known*
Side effect reduction/prevention	*Eleuthero[*]*

Supportive interaction	*Asian ginseng**
Reduced drug absorption/bioavailability	*None known*

INSULIN
(Animal-Source Insulin: Iletin; Human Analog Insulin: Humanlog; Human Insulin: Humulin, Novolin)

Insulin is a natural protein made by the pancreas that helps the body use sugar. Insulin is injected by all people with insulin-dependent diabetes mellitus (IDDM) and some people with non-insulin-dependent diabetes mellitus (NIDDM) to help control blood sugar levels.

Any substance (dietary, supplemental, herbal, and others) that affects blood sugar levels will directly or indirectly affect the amount of insulin required by a person with diabetes. For example, consumption of a high-fiber diet and/or supplementation with nutrients such as chromium, biotin, vitamin E, and others or herbs such as *Gymnema sylvestre* will often improve blood-sugar control in diabetics. In such cases, the dose of insulin may need to be reduced, in order to avoid a hypoglycemic reaction. Anyone taking insulin should consult the prescribing physician before making dietary changes or taking nutrients or herbs that are designed to lower blood-sugar levels. (For more information on diabetes, see *The Natural Pharmacy, 2nd Edition.*)

INTERACTIONS WITH HERBS

Fenugreek *(Trigonella foenum-graecum)*

In a randomized study of fifteen people with IDDM diabetes, fenugreek (100 grams per day for 10 days) was reported to reduce blood sugar, urinary sugar excretion, serum cholesterol, and triglycerides, with no change in insulin levels, compared with 10 days of placebo.[1] In a study of sixty people with NIDDM diabetes, fenugreek (25 grams per day for 24 weeks) was reported to significantly reduce blood glucose levels.[2] People using insulin should talk with their prescribing doctor before making any therapy changes.

Gymnema sylvestre

Although no interactions have been reported, gymnema may decrease the required daily dose of insulin.[3] Therefore, people currently using insulin for the treatment of diabetes should discuss the use of this herb with a health-care professional.

INTERACTIONS WITH FOODS AND OTHER COMPOUNDS

Food

Diet is an important factor in effective diabetes prevention and treatment. Diabetes is a serious disease. All treatment, including diet, requires the guidance and monitoring of a doctor. People using insulin should monitor their blood sugar carefully and consult with their prescribing doctor, a nutritionally oriented doctor, or clinical nutritionist to learn more about the role of diet in diabetes control.

Alcohol

Alcohol may increase the action of insulin, leading to hypoglycemia (low blood sugar).[4] People using insulin should avoid alcohol.

Tobacco (*Nicotiana* species)

Smoking may decrease insulin activity.[5] Smoking compounds the health problems associated with diabetes. People using insulin are cautioned to avoid smoking.

SUMMARY OF INTERACTIONS FOR INSULIN

Depletion or interference	*None known*
Adverse interaction	*Gymnema sylvestre,*[*] *Tobacco*
Side effect reduction/prevention	*None known*
Supportive interaction	*Fenugreek*
Reduced drug absorption/bioavailability	*None known*
Other (see text)	*Biotin, Chromium, Vitamin E*

INTERFERON

(Actimmune, Alferon N, Avonex, Betaseron, Intron A, Rebif, Roferon-A, Weferon)

Interferons are proteins made by the human immune system for fighting viral infections and regulating cell function. There are three types of interferons used as drugs: interferon alpha, interferon beta, and interferon gamma. They are used by injection to treat viral infections, hepatitis, multiple sclerosis, some cancers, and other diseases.

INTERACTIONS WITH DIETARY SUPPLEMENTS

N-Acetyl Cysteine (NAC)

An uncontrolled study found that adding 600 mg NAC 3 times per day to interferon therapy for people with chronic hepatitis C led to improvement in their conditions not seen with interferon alone.[1] Further study is needed to determine if NAC might benefit persons receiving interferon.

Thymus Peptides

Peptides (short proteins) from the immune organ known as the thymus gland have been investigated in combination with interferon therapy for people with hepatitis B and C. One study found that adding thymus humoral factor-gamma 2 to interferon therapy prevented decreases in white blood cell counts sometimes seen with interferon alone, and also seemed to improve the efficacy of interferon against hepatitis B.[2] Thymus humoral factor-gamma 2 has to be administered by injection, requiring consultation with a doctor familiar with natural medicine. More studies are necessary to determine if thymus peptides are of benefit in combination with interferon.

INTERACTIONS WITH HERBS

Bupleurum (Bupleurum chinense)

Bupleurum is the major constituent of a Japanese Kampo (herbal) medicine formula called sho-saiko-to. This formula has been used alone or with interferon to treat hepatitis. Eighty or more cases of drug-induced pneumonitis (inflammation of the lungs) have been associated with the use of sho-saiko-to alone or with interferon.[3,4,5,6] Until more is known, sho-saiko-to should not be combined with interferon.

Licorice (Glycyrrhiza glabra)

Injections of the licorice compound glycyrrhizin are commonly used to treat hepatitis in Japan. The combination of glycyrrhizin and interferon may be more effective than interferon alone.[7,8] Injectable glycyrrhizin is available from some nutritionally oriented physicians. So far, human studies have not used *orally* administered licorice extracts in conjunction with interferon.

SUMMARY OF INTERACTIONS FOR INTERFERON

Depletion or interference	*None known*
Adverse interaction	*Bupleurum*
Side effect reduction/prevention	*None known*

| Supportive interaction | Licorice,* N-acetyl cysteine (NAC),* Thymus peptides* |
| Reduced drug absorption/bioavailability | Thymus peptides* |

IPRATROPIUM BROMIDE
(Atrovent)

IPRATROPIUM BROMIDE/ALBUTEROL
(Combivent)

Ipratropium bromide is a drug used by oral inhalation to keep breathing passages open in chronic obstructive pulmonary diseases, including chronic bronchitis and emphysema. Ipratropium bromide for oral inhalation is available alone (Atrovent) and in the combination ipratropium bromide/**albuterol** (page 4) (Combivent). It is also available as a nasal spray to relieve runny nose associated with allergies and common colds.

INTERACTIONS WITH FOODS AND OTHER COMPOUNDS

Food

Atrovent and Combivent for oral inhalation contain soy lecithin. Rarely, people very sensitive to soy have reacted to these drugs,[1] and life-threatening anaphylactic reaction is possible, though extremely rare. Ipratropium bromide nasal spray and solution for inhalation contain no soy lecithin.

SUMMARY OF INTERACTIONS FOR IPRATROPIUM BROMIDE

Depletion or interference	None known
Adverse interaction	None known
Side effect reduction/prevention	None known
Supportive interaction	None known
Reduced drug absorption/bioavailability	None known
Other (see text)	Soy

ISONIAZID
(INH, Laniazid; Isoniazid/Rifampin, Rifamate, Rimactane)

Isoniazid is an **antibiotic** (page 14) used to prevent and treat tuberculosis. To prevent development of resistant tuberculosis bacteria, people with tuberculosis are treated with long courses of combination drug therapy, most commonly isoniazid, rifampin, and pyrazinamide.

INTERACTIONS WITH DIETARY SUPPLEMENTS

Vitamin B$_6$

Isoniazid can interfere with the activity of vitamin B$_6$.[1] Vitamin B$_6$ supplementation is recommended, especially in people with poor nutritional status, to prevent development of isoniazid-induced peripheral neuritis (inflamed nerves).[2] One case is reported in which injectable vitamin B$_6$ reversed isoniazid-induced coma.[3] Although the optimal amount remains unknown, some doctors suggest that adults taking isoniazid supplement vitamin B$_6$ 100 mg per day to prevent side effects.

Vitamin K

Many antibiotics taken by mouth, including isoniazid, may kill friendly bacteria in the large intestine that produce vitamin K.[4] Vitamin K$_1$ (phylloquinone) is now found in some multivitamins.

Other Nutrient Interactions

Isoniazid may interfere with the activity of other nutrients, including vitamins B$_3$ (niacin), B$_{12}$, D, and E, folic acid, calcium, and magnesium.[5][6] People should consider using a daily multivitamin/mineral supplement during isoniazid therapy.

INTERACTIONS WITH HERBS

Licorice (*Glycyrrhiza glabra*)

The potent anti-inflammatory substance known as glycyrrhizin from licorice has been combined with isoniazid for treatment of tuberculosis. An older study found a benefit from combining the two compared to using isoniazid alone.[7] Glycyrrhizin was given by injection, so it is not certain if licorice extracts containing glycyrrhizin would be as effective given by mouth. The treatment required at least 3 months of administration.

INTERACTIONS WITH FOODS AND OTHER COMPOUNDS

Food

Food decreases absorption of isoniazid. Isoniazid should be taken 1 hour before or 2 hours after eating. However, people may take isoniazid with food to decrease stomach upset.[8]

Isoniazid has some monoamine oxidase inhibitor (MAOI) activity.[9] Isoniazid can alter metabolism of tyramine-containing foods, leading to reactions associated with MAOI drugs (diarrhea, flushing, sweating, pounding chest, dangerous changes in blood pressure, and other symptoms).[10] People taking isoniazid should avoid tyramine-containing foods. Isoniazid can also alter metabolism of histamine-containing foods, leading to headaches, sweating, pounding chest, flushing, diarrhea, low blood pressure, and itching.[11] People taking isoniazid should avoid histamine-containing foods (for example, tuna, sauerkraut juice, or yeast extract).

Alcohol

Daily alcohol intake increases the risk of isoniazid-related hepatitis.[12] Alcohol may interact with isoniazid, causing facial flushing, headache, lightheadedness, nausea, breathlessness, and other symptoms.[13] To prevent unwanted reactions, people taking isoniazid should avoid alcohol-containing products.

SUMMARY OF INTERACTIONS FOR ISONIAZID

Depletion or interference	Calcium*, Folic acid,* Magnesium,* Vitamin B_3, Vitamin B_6, Vitamin B_{12}, Vitamin D,* Vitamin E,* Vitamin K
Adverse interaction	None known
Side effect reduction/prevention	None known
Supportive interaction	Licorice
Reduced drug absorption/bioavailability	None known

ISOSORBIDE MONONITRATE
(Imdur, ISMO, Monoket)

Isosorbide mononitrate is a member of the nitrate family of drugs used to prevent angina (chest pain). It is available in immediate-release (ISMO and Monoket) and extended-release (Imdur) products.

INTERACTIONS WITH DIETARY SUPPLEMENTS

N-Acetyl Cysteine (NAC)

In a double-blind trial, sustained-release isosorbide mononitrate (ISMN) plus oral NAC (2,400 mg twice per day) for 2 days led to significantly longer exercise time than ISMN plus placebo.[1] This outcome suggests that NAC may have increased the efficacy of ISMN. There were no differences in side effects between the two groups.

Vitamin C

Some persons taking **nitroglycerin** (page 154) or isosorbide mononitrate may find that it loses efficacy over time. This is because the body adapts to the drug, a process known as developing tolerance. One study found that taking 2 grams 3 times daily of vitamin C can decrease this effect when nitroglycerin patches are simultaneously used.[2] Similar benefits have been confirmed in another study.[3] However, it should be noted that it is also possible to avoid tolerance to these drugs by simply changing the dosing schedule. People taking ISMN or nitroglycerin should talk with their pharmacists about avoiding drug tolerance.

INTERACTIONS WITH FOODS AND OTHER COMPOUNDS

Food

Isosorbide mononitrate should be taken on an empty stomach with a glass of water.[4] Imdur may be taken with or without food[5] and should be swallowed whole, without chewing or crushing.[6]

Alcohol

Isosorbide mononitrate causes low blood pressure. Alcohol may increase this effect, leading to dangerously low blood pressure and other side effects.[7] To prevent problems, people taking isosorbide mononitrate should avoid alcohol.

SUMMARY OF INTERACTIONS FOR ISOSORBIDE MONONITRATE

Depletion or interference	*None known*
Adverse interaction	*None known*
Side effect reduction/prevention	*None known*
Supportive interaction	*N-acetyl cysteine*
Reduced drug absorption/bioavailability	*None known*
Other (see text)	*Vitamin C*

ISOTRETINOIN

(Accutane)

Isotretinoin is a modified vitamin A molecule used to treat severe acne.

INTERACTIONS WITH DIETARY SUPPLEMENTS

Vitamin A

Although little is known about how isotretinoin interacts with real vitamin A, the two are structurally similar and have similar toxicities. Therefore, it makes sense for people taking isotretinoin to avoid vitamin A supplements at levels higher than typically found in a multivitamin (10,000 IU per day).

SUMMARY OF INTERACTIONS FOR ISOTRETINOIN

Depletion or interference	*None known*
Adverse interaction	*Vitamin A*
Side effect reduction/prevention	*None known*
Supportive interaction	*None known*
Reduced drug absorption/bioavailability	*None known*

LACTASE
(Dairy Ease, LactAid, Lactrase, SureLac)

Lactase is a nonprescription enzyme used by people who have an impaired ability to digest lactose (milk sugar) because their bodies make insufficient lactase.

INTERACTIONS WITH DIETARY SUPPLEMENTS

Calcium

Dairy products are rich in calcium. Lactase-deficient people may not consume milk and therefore have fewer dietary sources of calcium available to them. Lactase products allow lactase-deficient people to digest milk products, increasing their sources and intake of dietary calcium.

SUMMARY OF INTERACTIONS FOR LACTASE

Depletion or interference	*None known*
Adverse interaction	*None known*
Side effect reduction/prevention	*None known*
Supportive interaction	*None known*
Reduced drug absorption/bioavailability	*None known*
Other (see text)	*Calcium*

LANSOPRAZOLE
(Prevacid)

Lansoprazole is a "proton pump inhibitor" drug that blocks production of stomach acid. Lansoprazole is used to treat diseases in which stomach acid causes damage, including stomach and duodenal ulcers, esophagitis, and Zollinger-Ellison syndrome.

INTERACTIONS WITH DIETARY SUPPLEMENTS

Beta-Carotene

Omeprazole (page 159), a closely related drug, taken for 7 days led to a near-total loss of stomach acid in healthy people and interfered with the absorption of a single 120 mg dose of beta-carotene.[1] It is unknown if repeated beta-carotene doses would overcome this problem or if absorption of carotenes from food would be imparied. Persons taking omeprazole and related acid-blocking drugs for long periods may want to have carotenoid blood levels checked, eat plenty of fruits and vegetables, and consider supplementing with carotenoids.

Vitamin B_{12}

Omeprazole, a drug closely related to lansoprazole, has interfered with the absorption of vitamin B_{12} from food (though not supplements) in some,[2][3] but not all, studies.[4][5] This interaction has not yet been reported with lansoprazole. However, a fall in vitamin B_{12} status may result from decreased stomach acid caused by acid blocking drugs, including lansoprazole.[6] Unlike dietary vitamin B_{12} (which is bound to protein), supplemental B_{12} does not require stomach acid for absorption.

INTERACTIONS WITH HERBS

Cranberry (Vaccinium macrocarpon)

Omeprazole (page 159) was shown to reduce protein-bound vitamin B_{12} absorption and cranberry juice was shown to increase protein-bound vitamin B_{12} absorption in eight people treated with omeprazole (a drug closely related to lansoprazole).[7] While this effect has not been studied with lansoprazole, people taking lansoprazole may choose to drink cranberry juice or other acidic liquids with vitamin B_{12}–containing foods. Unlike vitamin B_{12} found in food, vitamin B_{12} found in supplements is not bound to peptides (pieces of protein).

Levodopa

The absorption of B_{12} supplements therefore does not require acid and is unlikely to be improved by drinking cranberry juice.

INTERACTIONS WITH FOODS AND OTHER COMPOUNDS

Food

The initial dose of lansoprazole should be taken thirty minutes before a meal.[8] Subsequent doses are equally effective taken with or without food but should be taken at the same time every day.[9] Capsules and granule contents should not be chewed or crushed. However, lansoprazole capsules may be opened, the granule contents sprinkled on one tablespoon of applesauce, then immediately swallowed.

SUMMARY OF INTERACTIONS FOR LANSOPRAZOLE

Depletion or interference	*Beta-carotene,* * *Vitamin B$_{12}$* * *(dietary, not supplemental B$_{12}$)*
Adverse interaction	*None known*
Side effect reduction/prevention	*None known*
Supportive interaction	*Cranberry* *
Reduced drug absorption/bioavailability	*None known*

LEVODOPA
(L-dopa, Dopar, Larodapa)

CARBIDOPA/LEVODOPA
(Sinemet)

Levodopa is the precursor required by the brain to produce dopamine, a neurotransmitter (chemical messenger in the nervous system). People with Parkinson's disease have depleted levels of dopamine. Levodopa is used to increase dopamine in the brain, which reduces the symptoms of Parkinson's disease. Levodopa is broken down by the body before it reaches the brain. To avoid this, levodopa is used with **carbidopa** (page 36), a drug that protects levodopa from breakdown. Levodopa is available alone (L-dopa, Dopar, Larodapa) or in the combination **carbidopa/levodopa** (page 36) (Sinemet).

INTERACTIONS WITH DIETARY SUPPLEMENTS

Vitamin B$_6$

Levodopa is broken down in the body by a process requiring vitamin B$_6$. Breakdown may deplete available vitamin B$_6$. **Carbidopa** (page 36) blocks levodopa breakdown and prevents vitamin B$_6$ depletion. People taking **Sinemet** (page 36) (levodopa/carbidopa), or levodopa plus carbidopa (Lodosyn), have no risk for levodopa-induced vitamin B$_6$ deficiency; it is not a problem for people to supplement vitamin B$_6$ while taking Sinemet. For people taking levodopa alone, small amounts of vitamin B$_6$ (5 to 10 mg per day) may prevent levodopa-induced vitamin B$_6$ deficiency.[1] Amounts of vitamin B$_6$, slightly higher than required to replace depleted levels, may reduce the effectiveness of levodopa therapy and should not be taken.[2]

INTERACTIONS WITH FOODS AND OTHER COMPOUNDS

Food

Foods, especially those high in protein, compete with levodopa for absorption. However, levodopa may be taken with food to avoid stomach upset.[3] It is important to take levodopa at the same time every day, always with or always without food. People with questions about levodopa and food should ask their prescribing doctor or pharmacist. Taking sustained-release **Sinemet CR** (page 36) with food may increase blood levels of levodopa.[4] It is important to take Sinemet CR at the same time every day, always with or always without food. People with questions about Sinemet CR and food should ask their prescribing doctor or pharmacist.

SUMMARY OF INTERACTIONS FOR LEVODOPA

Depletion or interference	*Vitamin B$_6$*
Adverse interaction	*None known*
Side effect reduction/prevention	*None known*
Supportive interaction	*None known*
Reduced drug absorption/bioavailability	*None known*

LISINOPRIL
(Prinivil, Zestril)

Lisinopril is an **angiotensin-converting enzyme (ACE) inhibitor** (page 1), a family of drugs used to treat high blood pressure and some types of heart failure. Lisinopril is also used in some cases to improve survival after a heart attack.

INTERACTIONS WITH DIETARY SUPPLEMENTS

Potassium

ACE inhibitors may increase blood potassium levels.[1] This problem is more likely to occur with advanced kidney disease. Potassium supplements, potassium-containing salt substitutes (No Salt, Morton Salt Substitute, and others), and even foods uncommonly high in potassium (primarily fruit), will increase the chances of potentially dangerous elevations in blood potassium. People taking ACE inhibitors should avoid unnecessary potassium supplementation.

Zinc

In a study of thirty-four people with hypertension, 6 months of **captopril** (page 35) or **enalapril** (page 82) (ACE inhibitors related to lisinopril) treatment led to decreased zinc levels in certain white blood cells,[2] raising concerns about possible ACE inhibitor–induced zinc depletion. While zinc depletion has not been reported with lisinopril, until more is known, it makes sense for people taking lisinopril long term to consider, as a precaution, taking a zinc supplement or a multimineral tablet containing zinc. (Such multiminerals usually contain no more than 99 mg of potassium, probably not enough to trigger the above-mentioned interaction.) Supplements containing zinc should also contain copper, to protect against a zinc-induced copper deficiency.

INTERACTIONS WITH FOODS AND OTHER COMPOUNDS

Food

Lisinopril may be taken with or without food.[3]

SUMMARY OF INTERACTIONS FOR LISINOPRIL

Depletion or interference	*Zinc*[*]
Adverse interaction	*Potassium*[*]
Side effect reduction/prevention	*None known*
Supportive interaction	*None known*

Reduced drug absorption/bioavailability *None known*

LITHIUM
(Eskalith, Lithobid, Lithonate, Lithotabs)

The prescription drug lithium is a mineral with antidepressant and antimanic actions. It is used to treat bipolar disorder (manic-depression) and severe depression.

INTERACTIONS WITH DIETARY SUPPLEMENTS

Essential Fatty Acids

In one report, supplementation with essential fatty acids in the form of safflower oil (3 to 5 grams per day) reversed symptoms of lithium toxicity such as tremor and ataxia (an abnormality of gait).[1] Controlled studies are needed to confirm the benefit of combination of lithium and essential fatty acids.

Folic Acid

Some studies have found that people taking lithium long-term who have high blood levels of folic acid respond better to lithium.[2][3] Not all studies have confirmed these findings, however.[4]

A double-blind study was conducted combining 200 mcg folic acid per day with lithium therapy.[5] Even though the volunteers in this study were doing well on lithium alone before the study, addition of folic acid further improved their condition, whereas placebo did not. There is no evidence that folic acid reduces side effects of lithium. Based on the available evidence, it is suggested people taking lithium also take at least 200 mcg of folic acid per day.

L-Tryptophan

A small double-blind study found that combining 2 to 4 grams 3 times per day of L-tryptophan with lithium significantly improved symptoms in people with bipolar disorder or a mild form of schizophrenia.[6] L-tryptophan is only available from doctors of natural medicine. It should be taken several hours before or after meals.

Sodium

Lithium may cause sodium depletion, especially during initial therapy until consistent blood levels are achieved.[7] A low-sodium (salt-restricted) diet can decrease lithium elimination, leading to increased lithium levels and risk of toxicity.[8] People starting lithium therapy should maintain adequate water intake as well as a normal diet and salt intake. Sodium loss due to diarrhea, illness, extreme sweating, or other causes may alter lithium levels.

INTERACTIONS WITH HERBS

Psyllium (Plantago ovata)

Addition of psyllium husk 2 times per day to the regimen of a woman treated with lithium was associated with decreased lithium blood levels and lithium levels increased after psyllium was stopped.[9]

INTERACTIONS WITH FOODS AND OTHER COMPOUNDS

Food

Lithium should be taken with food to avoid stomach upset.[10]

Foods that alkalinize the urine may increase elimination of lithium from the body, potentially decreasing the actions of the drug.[11] Urine-alkalinizing foods include dairy products, nuts, fruits, vegetables (except corn and lentils), and others.

Coffee

Mild hand tremor is a common side effect of lithium therapy. Two cases of women treated with lithium who experienced increased tremor when they stopped drinking coffee have been reported.[12] Lithium levels increased almost 50% in one of the women, who had been drinking 17 cups of coffee per day, requiring a 20% reduction in her lithium dose. In eleven people treated with lithium who drank 4 to 6 cups of coffee per day, 2 weeks without coffee resulted in increased lithium blood levels, anxiety, and depression.[13] Lithium levels, anxiety, and depression ratings returned to base line 2 weeks after resuming coffee consumption. Until more is known, people taking lithium should avoid abrupt changes in their coffee consumption.

SUMMARY OF INTERACTIONS FOR LITHIUM

Depletion or interference	*None known*
Adverse interaction	*None known*
Side effect reduction/prevention	*Essential fatty acids**
Supportive interaction	*Folic acid, L-tryptophan**
Reduced drug absorption/bioavailability	*None known*
Other (see text)	*Coffee, Psyllium, Sodium*

LOOP DIURETICS

Loop diuretics are a family of drugs that include bumetanide (Bumex), ethacrynic acid (Edecrin), furosemide (Lasix), and torsemide (Demadex).

Loop diuretics constitute a family of drugs that remove water from the body. They are referred to as potassium-depleting, as they cause the body to lose potassium as well as water. Potassium-depleting diuretics also cause the body to lose magnesium. Loop diuretics are more potent than **thiazide diuretics** (page 202). They are used to lower blood pressure in people with hypertension and to reduce the amount of work the heart has to do, allowing it to pump better in people with congestive heart failure. Loop diuretics are also used to reduce water accumulation caused by other diseases.

INTERACTIONS WITH DIETARY SUPPLEMENTS

Magnesium and Potassium

Potassium-depleting diuretics, including loop diuretics, cause the body to lose potassium. Loop diuretics may also cause cellular magnesium depletion,[1] although this deficiency may not be reflected by a subnormal blood level of magnesium.[2] Magnesium loss induced by potassium-depleting diuretics can cause additional potassium loss. Evaluating whether potassium loss is increased by magnesium depletion can be difficult. Until more is known, it has been suggested that people taking potassium-depleting diuretics, including **thiazide diuretics** (page 202), should supplement both potassium and magnesium.[3]

People taking loop diuretics should be monitored by their prescribing doctor, who will prescribe potassium supplements if needed. Fruit is high in potassium, and increasing fruit intake is another way of supplementing potassium. Nutritionally oriented doctors often suggest 300 to 400 mg of magnesium per day.

Vitamin B$_1$

People with congestive heart failure (CHF) treated with the loop diuretic furosemide may be at risk for vitamin B$_1$ deficiency due to: 1) the disease, 2) treatment with furosemide, and/or 3) inadequate dietary vitamin B$_1$ intake.[4] In a study of people with CHF, long-term furosemide therapy was associated with clinically significant vitamin B$_1$ deficiency due to urinary loss.[5] This furosemide-induced vitamin B$_1$ deficiency may worsen heart function in people with CHF and may be prevented or corrected with vitamin B$_1$ supplementation.[6]

Sodium

Diuretics, including loop diuretics, cause increased loss of sodium in the urine. By removing sodium from the body, diuretics also cause water to leave the body. This reduction of body water is the purpose of taking diuretics. Therefore, there is usually no reason to replace lost sodium, although strict limitation of salt intake in combination with the actions of diuretics can sometimes cause excessive sodium depletion. On the other hand, people who restrict sodium intake and in the process reduce blood pressure may need to have their dose of diuretics lowered.

INTERACTIONS WITH HERBS

Herbs that have a diuretic effect should be avoided when taking diuretic medications, as they may potentiate the effect of these drugs and lead to possible cardiovascular side effects. These herbs include dandelion, uva ursi, juniper, buchu, cleavers, horsetail, and gravel root.[7]

Digitalis *(Digitalis purpurea)*

Digitalis refers to a family of plants commonly called foxglove that contain digitalis glycosides, chemicals with actions and toxicities similar to the prescription drug **digoxin** (page 71). Loop diuretics can increase the risk of digitalis-induced heart disturbances.[8] Loop diuretics and digitalis-containing products should only be used under the direct supervision of a doctor trained in their use.

Licorice *(Glycyrrhiza glabra)*

Licorice may potentiate the side effects of potassium-depleting diuretics, including loop diuretics.[9] Loop diuretics and licorice should be used together only under careful medical supervision. Deglycyrrhizinated licorice (DGL) may be used safely with all diuretics.

INTERACTIONS WITH FOODS AND OTHER COMPOUNDS

Food

Furosemide (Lasix) is most effective taken on an empty stomach, 1 hour before eating.[10] However, furosemide may be taken with food to prevent gastrointestinal (GI) upset.[11] Torsemide (Demadex) may be taken with or without food.[12]

SUMMARY OF INTERACTIONS FOR LOOP DIURETICS

Depletion or interference	*Magnesium, Potassium, Vitamin B$_1$*

Adverse interaction	*Buchu, Cleavers, Dandelion, Digitalis, Gravel root, Horsetail, Juniper, Licorice, Uva ursi*
Side effect reduction/prevention	*None known*
Supportive interaction	*None known*
Reduced drug absorption/bioavailability	*None known*
Other (see text)	*Sodium*

LOPERAMIDE
(Imodium)

Loperamide is a drug used to treat diarrhea. It is available as a prescription drug (Imodium and others) and as a nonprescription drug product (Imodium AD and others).

INTERACTIONS WITH FOODS AND OTHER COMPOUNDS

Alcohol

Loperamide may cause drowsiness or dizziness.[1] Alcohol may intensify these effects and increase the risk of accidental injury. To prevent problems, people taking loperamide should avoid alcohol.

SUMMARY OF INTERACTIONS FOR LOPERAMIDE

Depletion or interference	*None known*
Adverse interaction	*None known*
Side effect reduction/prevention	*None known*
Supportive interaction	*None known*
Reduced drug absorption/bioavailability	*None known*

LORATADINE
(Claritin)

LORATADINE/PSEUDOEPHEDRINE
(Claritin-D)

Loratadine is a selective antihistamine used to relieve allergic rhinitis (seasonal allergy) symptoms, including sneezing, runny nose, itching, and watery eyes. It is also used to treat people with idiopathic urticaria. Loratadine is available alone (Claritin) and in the combination loratadine/**pseudoephedrine** (page 83) (Claritin-D).

INTERACTIONS WITH FOODS AND OTHER COMPOUNDS

Food

Food slows the absorption of loratadine and also increases the total amount of the drug absorbed.[1] It is recommended that loratadine be taken on an empty stomach.[2]

Alcohol

Selective antihistamines, including loratadine, may cause drowsiness or dizziness, although it is less likely than with nonselective antihistamines.[3] Alcohol can intensify drowsiness and dizziness, increasing the risk of accidental injury. People taking loratadine should use alcohol only with caution.

SUMMARY OF INTERACTIONS FOR LORATADINE

Depletion or interference	*None known*
Adverse interaction	*None known*
Side effect reduction/prevention	*None known*
Supportive interaction	*None known*
Reduced drug absorption/bioavailability	*None known*

LOSARTAN
(Cozaar)

Losartan is a member of the angiotensin II receptor antagonist family of drugs used to lower blood pressure in people with hypertension.

INTERACTIONS WITH DIETARY SUPPLEMENTS

Minerals

In a randomized, double-blind study of twenty-three healthy people on a low-sodium diet, a single oral dose of losartan increased urinary excretion of calcium, magnesium, potassium, sodium, chloride, and phosphate.[1] The clinical significance of these findings is not known.

INTERACTIONS WITH FOODS AND OTHER COMPOUNDS

Food

Food slows the rate of losartan absorption but has little impact on the total amount of the dose absorbed.[2] Losartan should be taken at the same time every day.

SUMMARY OF INTERACTIONS FOR LOSARTAN

Depletion or interference	*Calcium,* Chloride, Magnesium,* Potassium,* Sodium,* Phosphate*
Adverse interaction	*None known*
Side effect reduction/prevention	*None known*
Supportive interaction	*None known*
Reduced drug absorption/bioavailability	*None known*

LOVASTATIN
(Mevacor)

Lovastatin is a member of the HMG-CoA reductase inhibitor family of drugs, which blocks the body's production of cholesterol. Lovastatin is used to lower elevated cholesterol levels. Cholestin, a dietary supplement advertised to help maintain healthy cholesterol, but not to lower high cholesterol, contains several HMG-CoA reductase inhibitor chemicals, including lovastatin.

INTERACTIONS WITH DIETARY SUPPLEMENTS

Coenzyme Q_{10}

In a randomized, double-blind trial, blood levels of coenzyme Q_{10} (CoQ_{10}) were measured in forty-five people with high cholesterol treated with lovastatin (20 to 80 mg per day) or **pravastatin** (page 175) (10 to 40 mg per day) for 18 weeks.[1] A significant decline in blood levels of CoQ_{10} occurred with both drugs. Supplementation with 100 mg CoQ_{10} has been shown to prevent reductions in blood levels of CoQ_{10} due to **simvastatin** (page 189).[2] Combining 180 mg CoQ_{10} daily with lovastatin therapy in a double-blind study did not show that adding CoQ_{10} provided significant benefits.[3] In other words, although taking CoQ_{10} may prevent decreased blood levels of CoQ_{10}, it may not otherwise benefit the person taking the supplement. If no adverse effects of lowered blood levels of CoQ_{10} can be demonstrated, then merely bringing the levels back up may not be justified. Most nutritionally oriented doctors recommend that people taking lovastatin supplement with 30 to 100 mg CoQ_{10} per day.

Fiber (Soluble)

Soluble fiber is found primarily in fruit, beans, and oats, but it is also available separately as pectin, oat bran, and glucomannan. Two sources of soluble fiber, pectin (found in fruit) and oat bran (a component of oatmeal also available by itself), have been reported to interact with lovastatin.[4] It appears that the fiber binds the drug in the gastrointestinal tract and reduces absorption of the drug as a consequence. People taking this drug should avoid concentrated intake of soluble fiber, as taking lovastatin with a high soluble-fiber diet leads to reduced drug effectiveness.

Niacin (Vitamin B₃, Nicotinic Acid)

Niacin is a vitamin used to lower cholesterol. High-dose niacin taken with lovastatin has been reported to cause potentially serious muscle disorders (myopathy or rhabdomyolysis).[5] However, most research reports that lovastatin and niacin have complementary, supportive actions.[6] Taking as little as 500 mg 3 times per day of niacin with lovastatin has been shown to have these complementary, supportive actions with almost none of the side effects seen when higher amounts of niacin are taken.[7]

Vitamin A

A study of thirty-seven people with high cholesterol treated with diet and HMG-CoA reductase inhibitors found serum vitamin A levels increased over 2 years of therapy.[8] It remains unclear whether this moderate increase should suggest that people taking lovastatin have a particular need to restrict vitamin A supplementation.

Red Yeast Rice

A supplement containing red yeast *(Monascus purpureus)* rice (cholestin) has been shown to effectively lower cholesterol and triglycerides in people with moderately elevated levels of these blood lipids.[9] This extract contains small amounts of naturally occurring HMG-CoA reductase inhibitors such as lovastatin and should not be used if you are currently taking lovastatin or pravastatin.

INTERACTIONS WITH HERBS

Milk Thistle *(Silybum marianum)*

One of the possible side effects of lovastatin is liver toxicity. Although there are no clinical studies to substantiate its use with lovastatin, a milk thistle extract standardized to 70 to 80% silymarin may reduce the potential liver toxicity of lovastatin. The suggested use is 200 mg of the extract 3 times daily.

INTERACTIONS WITH FOODS AND OTHER COMPOUNDS

Food

Food increases blood levels of lovastatin.[10] Lovastatin should be taken with a meal, at the same time every day.[11] Due to the possibility of reduced lovastatin absorption in the presence of soluble fiber (see soluble fiber, above), it makes sense to avoid eating fruit or oatmeal within 2 hours before or after taking lovastatin.

Grapefruit Juice

In a small, single-dose trial with healthy volunteers, grapefruit juice was found to significantly increase lovastatin blood levels compared with placebo.[12] The same effect might be seen from eating grapefruit as from drinking its juice. Using grapefruit juice to reduce the dose of lovastatin has not been sufficiently studied.

SUMMARY OF INTERACTIONS FOR LOVASTATIN

Depletion or interference	*Coenzyme Q$_{10}$*
Adverse interaction	*Red yeast rice*
Side effect reduction/prevention	*Milk thistle**
Supportive interaction	*None known*
Reduced drug absorption/bioavailability	*Fiber (soluble)*
Other (see text)	*Grapefruit juice, Niacin, Vitamin A*

MAGNESIUM HYDROXIDE
(MOM, Milk of Magnesia)

Magnesium hydroxide is used as an **antacid** (page 13) for short-term relief of stomach upset and as a laxative for short-term treatment of constipation. Magnesium hydroxide is available in nonprescription products alone (Milk of Magnesia and others) and in combination with other nonprescription ingredients, to relieve stomach upset, including:

- Magnesium hydroxide/**aluminum hydroxide** (page 6) (Maalox, Mylanta, and others)

- Magnesium hydroxide/calcium carbonate (Calcium Rich Rolaids)
- Magnesium hydroxide/calcium carbonate/**simethicone** (page 189) (Advanced Formula Di-Gel Tablets)
- Magnesium hydroxide/**aluminum hydroxide** (page 6)/calcium carbonate/**simethicone** (page 189) (Tempo tablets)

INTERACTIONS WITH DIETARY SUPPLEMENTS

Iron

Antacids (page 13), including magnesium hydroxide, may reduce the absorption of dietary iron. Iron supplements do not require stomach acid for absorption and one human study found that a magnesium hydroxide/aluminum hydroxide antacid did not decrease supplemental iron absorption.[1]

Potassium

Individuals taking **potassium-depleting diuretics** (page 129) and those who are otherwise at risk of developing potassium deficiency (such as people with chronic diarrhea or vomiting) may experience a fall in serum potassium levels if they take magnesium without taking additional potassium.[2] This could lead to muscle cramps or, in individuals taking **digoxin** (page 71) or digitalis, more serious problems such as cardiac arrhythmias. Individuals who have a history of potassium deficiency and those who are at risk of developing potassium deficiency, as well as people taking digoxin or digitalis, should consult a physician before taking magnesium-containing products.

SUMMARY OF INTERACTIONS FOR MAGNESIUM HYDROXIDE

Depletion or interference	*Iron**
Adverse interaction	*None known*
Side effect reduction/prevention	*None known*
Supportive interaction	*None known*
Reduced drug absorption/bioavailability	*None known*
Other (see text)	*Potassium*

MEDROXYPROGESTERONE
(Cycrin, Provera, Depo-Provera)

MEDROXYPROGESTERONE/CONJUGATED ESTROGENS
(Prempro)

Medroxyprogesterone is a semisynthetic compound that differs in structure from the naturally occurring human hormone progesterone. It is added to estrogen replacement therapy to prevent uterine cancer caused by unopposed estrogen. It is also used to treat absence of menstrual bleeding (amenorrhea) and abnormal menstrual bleeding. Medroxyprogesterone is available alone (Cycrin and Provera) and in the combination medroxyprogesterone/**conjugated estrogens** (page 57) (Prempro). An injection product, Depo-Provera, is used for contraception.

INTERACTIONS WITH DIETARY SUPPLEMENTS

Minerals

In a group of thirty-seven postmenopausal women treated with conjugated estrogens and medroxyprogesterone for 12 months, urinary zinc and magnesium loss was reduced in those women who began the study with signs of osteoporosis and elevated zinc and magnesium excretion.[1] The clinical significance of this interaction remains unclear.

Vitamin A

In a 1-year study of predominantly malnourished women in India and Thailand, medroxyprogesterone used for contraception was associated with increased blood levels of vitamin A and folic acid.[2] The clinical meaning of these changes remains unclear.

Vitamin D

In a study of postmenopausal women, treatment with estrogen alone increased vitamin D blood levels, whereas estrogen plus medroxyprogesterone lowered vitamin D back to the level seen without estrogen use.[3] This outcome might suggest that medroxyprogesterone interferes with beneficial effects estrogen may have on vitamin D metabolism and vitamin D supplementation would be called for. However, some research has not found the addition of vitamin D to estrogen/progestin combinations to be helpful.[4] Therefore, while many nutritionally oriented doctors recommend 400 IU vitamin D to women taking estrogen/progestin combination hormone products, the efficacy of such supplementation has not been proven.

SUMMARY OF INTERACTIONS FOR MEDROXYPROGESTERONE

Depletion or interference	*None known*
Adverse interaction	*None known*
Side effect reduction/prevention	*None known*
Supportive interaction	*None known*
Reduced drug absorption/bioavailability	*None known*
Other (see text)	*Calcium, Folic acid, Magnesium, Vitamin A, Vitamin D, Zinc*

MENTHOL

Menthol is a compound obtained from peppermint oil or other mint oils or made synthetically. Menthol has local anesthetic and counterirritant qualities. It is contained in nonprescription products for short-term relief of minor sore throat and minor mouth or throat irritation. Menthol is also contained in combination products used for relief of muscle aches, sprains, and similar conditions.

There are currently no reported nutrient or herb interactions involving menthol. People using combination products that include menthol are advised to review the other ingredients for possible herb and/or nutrient interactions.

METFORMIN
(Glucophage)

Metformin is a drug used to lower blood sugar levels in people with non-insulin-dependent diabetes (type II diabetes).

INTERACTIONS WITH DIETARY SUPPLEMENTS

Folic Acid and Vitamin B$_{12}$

In a study of seventy people with diabetes, serum vitamin B$_{12}$ levels, but not folic acid levels, were significantly lower in those treated with metformin compared with **insulin** (page 115) or sulfonylurea drugs.[1] In a study of sixty nondiabetic men with cardiovascular disease treated with **lovastatin** (page 133), 40 weeks of metformin treatment reduced vitamin

B_{12} and folic acid serum levels and increased blood levels of homocysteine, compared to placebo.[2] Until more is known, people taking metformin should supplement vitamin B_{12} and folic acid or ask their prescribing doctor or a nutritionally oriented doctor to monitor folic acid and vitamin B_{12} levels.

Magnesium

In a study of people with poorly controlled type II diabetes, low blood levels of magnesium, and high urine magnesium loss, metformin therapy was associated with reduced urinary magnesium excretion but no change in low blood levels of magnesium.[3] It remains unclear whether this interaction has clinical importance.

Guar Gum

In a study with six healthy people, guar gum plus metformin slowed the rate of metformin absorption.[4] In people with diabetes, this interaction could reduce the blood sugar–lowering effectiveness of metformin. Until more is known, metformin should be taken 2 hours before or 2 hours after guar gum–containing supplements. It remains unclear whether the small amounts of guar gum found in many processed foods is enough to significantly affect metformin absorption.

INTERACTIONS WITH FOODS AND OTHER COMPOUNDS

Food

Food interferes with metformin absorption.[5][6] Metformin should be taken on an empty stomach.

Alcohol

Lactic acidosis is a rare but serious side effect of metformin. Alcohol increases the production of lactic acid caused by metformin, increasing the risk of lactic acidosis.[7] People taking metformin should avoid alcohol or consult with their prescribing doctor before consuming alcohol.

SUMMARY OF INTERACTIONS FOR METFORMIN

Depletion or interference	*Folic acid,* Vitamin B₁₂*
Adverse interaction	*None known*
Side effect reduction/prevention	*None known*
Supportive interaction	*None known*
Reduced drug absorption/bioavailability	*Guar gum**
Other (see text)	*Magnesium*

METHOTREXATE
(Folex, Rheumatrex)

Methotrexate (MTX) is a **chemotherapy** (page 40) drug that interferes with folic acid activation, preventing cell reproduction. Methotrexate is used to treat some forms of cancer; severe, disabling psoriasis; and severe, active rheumatoid arthritis.

INTERACTIONS WITH DIETARY SUPPLEMENTS

Folic Acid

In cancer treatment, methotrexate works by blocking activation of folic acid. Folic acid-containing supplements may interfere with methotrexate therapy in people with cancer.[1] Methotrexate therapy can lead to folic acid deficiency. People using methotrexate for cancer treatment should ask their prescribing doctor before using any folic acid–containing supplements. There is no concern about folic acid supplementation for people with cancer using **chemotherapy drugs** (page 40) other than methotrexate.

Until recently, it was believed that methotrexate helped people with rheumatoid arthritis also by interfering with folic acid metabolism. However, recent research has shown that this is not so. In fact, it now appears that people with rheumatoid arthritis taking methotrexate should supplement large amounts of folic acid. In separate double-blind studies, 5,000 mcg per day of folic acid and 2.5 to 5 mg per day of folinic acid (an activated form of folic acid) have substantially reduced side effects of methotrexate without interfering with the therapeutic action in people with rheumatoid arthritis.[2] [3] Folic or folinic acid were taken at a different time from methotrexate and sometimes only 5 days per week. Similarly, recent evidence suggests that people who are prescribed methotrexate to treat severe psoriasis experience fewer side effects if they also supplement high amounts (5 mg per day) of folic acid.[4] As is the case with methotrexate and rheumatoid arthritis, supplementing folic acid did not interfere with the activity of methotrexate. Such high levels of folic acid should not be taken without clinical supervision.

PABA (Para-Aminobenzoic Acid)

PABA can increase methotrexate levels, activity, and side effects.[5] The incidence and severity of this interaction remains unclear.

INTERACTIONS WITH FOODS AND OTHER COMPOUNDS

Food

Food can interfere with methotrexate absorption, and methotrexate causes stomach upset.[6]

Alcohol

Alcohol should be avoided during methotrexate therapy, due to concerns of increased risk of liver damage.[7]

SUMMARY OF INTERACTIONS FOR METHOTREXATE

Depletion or interference	*None known*
Adverse interaction	*Folic acid (for people with cancer), PABA**
Side effect reduction/prevention	*Folic acid (for people with rheumatoid arthritis), Folic acid* (for people with psoriasis)*
Supportive interaction	*None known*
Reduced drug absorption/bioavailability	*None known*

METHYLCELLULOSE
(Citrucel)

Methylcellulose is a semisynthetic, bulk laxative used for short-term treatment of constipation. It is available as a nonprescription drug.

There are currently no reported nutrient or herb interactions involving methylcellulose.

METHYLDOPA
(Aldomet)

Methyldopa is a drug used to lower blood pressure in people with hypertension (high blood pressure).

INTERACTIONS WITH DIETARY SUPPLEMENTS

Iron

Iron supplements have been found to decrease methyldopa absorption.[1][2] Taking melthyldopa 2 hours before or after iron-containing products can help avoid this interaction.

Vitamin B$_{12}$

Methyldopa can decrease vitamin B$_{12}$ levels, thus increasing the risk of vitamin B$_{12}$ deficiency.[3]

Sodium

Excess dietary sodium (salt) intake can cause fluid retention and interfere with the blood pressure lowering action of methyldopa.[4] Reducing the use of table salt and heavily salted foods during methyldopa therapy reduces the likelihood of this interference.

INTERACTIONS WITH FOODS AND OTHER COMPOUNDS

Food

Food can interfere with methyldopa absorption.[5] Taking methyldopa 1 hour before or 2 hours after eating can prevent this interference.

SUMMARY OF INTERACTIONS FOR METHYLDOPA

Depletion or interference	*Vitamin B$_{12}$*[*]
Adverse interaction	*Sodium*
Side effect reduction/prevention	*None known*
Supportive interaction	*None known*
Reduced drug absorption/bioavailability	*Iron*

METHYLPHENIDATE
(Ritalin and Others)

Methylphenidate is a stimulant drug with actions similar to amphetamines. It is used as an adjunct to a complete program to treat children with attention deficit hyperactivity disorders. Methylphenidate is also used to treat people with narcolepsy.

INTERACTIONS WITH FOODS AND OTHER COMPOUNDS

Food

Some researchers have recommended that methylphenidate be taken 30 to 45 minutes before meals,[1] although it has been reported that methylphenidate was absorbed faster[2] and was equally effective[3] taken with food. Sustained-release methylphenidate (Ritalin-SR) tablets should be swallowed whole, without crushing or chewing.[4]

Alcohol

Methylphenidate may impair physical coordination and cause dizziness or drowsiness.[5] Alcohol may intensify these effects, increasing the risk of accidental injury. To prevent problems, people taking methylphenidate should avoid alcohol.

SUMMARY OF INTERACTIONS FOR METHYLPHENIDATE

Depletion or interference	*None known*
Adverse interaction	*None known*
Side effect reduction/prevention	*None known*
Supportive interaction	*None known*
Reduced drug absorption/bioavailability	*None known*

METOPROLOL
(Lopressor, Toprol XL)

METOPROLOL/HYDROCHLOROTHIAZIDE
(Lopressor HCT)

Metoprolol is a beta-blocker drug used to reduce the symptoms of angina pectoris (chest pain), lower blood pressure in people with hypertension, and treat people after heart attacks. Metoprolol is available alone (Lopressor and Toprol XL) and in the combination metoprolol/**hydrochlorothiazide** (page 202) (Lopressor HCT) used to lower blood pressure.

INTERACTIONS WITH FOODS AND OTHER COMPOUNDS

Food

Food increases the absorption of metoprolol.[1] Metoprolol should be taken at the same time every day,[2] always with or always without food.

Alcohol

Metoprolol may cause drowsiness, dizziness, lightheadedness, or blurred vision.[3] Alcohol may intensify these effects and increase the risk of accidental injury. To prevent problems, people taking metoprolol should avoid alcohol.

SUMMARY OF INTERACTIONS FOR METOPROLOL

Depletion or interference	*None known*
Adverse interaction	*None known*
Side effect reduction/prevention	*None known*
Supportive interaction	*None known*
Reduced drug absorption/bioavailability	*None known*

METRONIDAZOLE
(Flagyl, Protostat)

METRONIDAZOLE/BISMUTH SUBSALICYLATE/TETRACYCLINE
(Helidac)

Metronidazole is an **antibiotic** (page 14) used to treat a variety of bacterial and parasitic infections, such as amebiasis, trichomoniasis, and giardiasis. It is also used as a component of multidrug antibiotic combinations to heal stomach and duodenal ulcers caused by *Helicobacter pylori* infections. Metronidazole is available alone (Flagyl, Protostat) and in the combination metronidazole/**bismuth subsalicylate** (page 30)/**tetracycline** (page 199) (Helidac).

INTERACTIONS WITH HERBS

Milk Thistle *(Silybum marianum)*

Milk thistle has been reported to protect the liver from harm caused by some prescription drugs.[1] While milk thistle has not yet been studied directly for protecting people against the known potentially liver-damaging actions of metronidazole, it is often used for this purpose by doctors of natural medicine.

INTERACTIONS WITH FOODS AND OTHER COMPOUNDS

Food

Metronidazole should be taken with food to avoid stomach upset.

Alcohol

Alcohol may interact with metronidazole, causing facial flushing, headache, lightheadedness, nausea, breathlessness, and other symptoms.[2] Vinegar typically contains small amounts of alcohol and should be avoided during metronidazole therapy. People should read all product labels carefully for alcohol content and should avoid alcohol-containing products during metronidazole therapy.

SUMMARY OF INTERACTIONS FOR METRONIDAZOLE

Depletion or interference	*None known*
Adverse interaction	*None known*
Side effect reduction/prevention	*None known*
Supportive interaction	*None known*
Reduced drug absorption/bioavailability	*None known*
Other (see text)	*Milk thistle*

MINERAL OIL

Mineral oil is a laxative used to soften stools in people with constipation. Mineral oil is also used as a vehicle to carry other ingredients in some topical skin products.

INTERACTIONS WITH DIETARY SUPPLEMENTS

Vitamins and Minerals

Mineral oil has interfered with the absorption of many nutrients, including beta-carotene, calcium, phosphorus, potassium, and vitamins A, D, K, and E in some[1] but not all[2] research. Taking mineral oil on an empty stomach may reduce this interference. It makes sense to take a daily multivitamin/mineral supplement 2 hours before or after mineral oil. It is important to read labels; because many multivitamins do not contain vitamin K or contain inadequate (less than 100 mcg per daily dose) amounts.

SUMMARY OF INTERACTIONS FOR MINERAL OIL

Depletion or interference	*Beta-carotene,* Calcium,* Phosphorus,* Potassium,* Vitamin A,* Vitamin D,* Vitamin E,* Vitamin K**
Adverse interaction	*None known*
Side effect reduction/prevention	*None known*
Supportive interaction	*None known*
Reduced drug absorption/bioavailability	*None known*

MUPIROCIN
(Bactroban, Bactroban Nasal)

Mupirocin is an **antibiotic** (page 14) applied to the skin to treat bacterial skin infections. It is also used to prevent hospital outbreaks of dangerous antibiotic-resistant *Staph aureus* infections.

There are currently no reported nutrient or herb interactions involving mupirocin.

NABUMETONE
(Relafen)

Nabumetone is a member of the **nonsteroidal anti-inflammatory drug (NSAID** [page 157]**)** family. NSAIDs reduce inflammation (swelling), pain, and temperature. Nabumetone is used to treat arthritis.

INTERACTIONS WITH DIETARY SUPPLEMENTS

Copper

Supplementation may enhance the anti-inflammatory effects of NSAIDs while reducing their ulcerogenic effects. One study found that when various anti-inflammatory drugs were chelated with copper, the anti-inflammatory activity was increased.[1] Animal models of inflammation have found that the copper chelate of **aspirin** (page 18) was active at one-eighth the effective dose of aspirin. These copper complexes are less toxic than the parent compounds, as well.

Iron

NSAIDs cause gastrointestinal (GI) irritation, bleeding and iron loss.[2] Iron supplements can cause GI irritation.[3] However, iron supplementation is sometimes needed in people taking NSAIDs if those drugs have caused enough blood loss to lead to iron deficiency. If both iron and nabumetone are prescribed, they should be taken with food to reduce GI irritation and bleeding risk.

Potassium

NSAIDs have caused kidney dysfunction and increased blood potassium levels, especially in older people.[4] People taking NSAIDs, including nabumetone, should not supplement potassium without consulting with their prescribing doctor or a nutritionally oriented doctor.

Sodium

Nabumetone may cause sodium and water retention.[5] It is healthful to reduce dietary salt intake by eliminating table salt and heavily salted foods.

INTERACTIONS WITH HERBS

Licorice (Glycyrrhiza glabra)

The flavonoids found in the extract of licorice known as DGL (deglycyrrhizinated licorice) are helpful for avoiding the irritating actions **NSAIDs** (page 157) have on the stomach and intestines. One study found that 350 mg of chewable DGL taken together with each dose of **aspirin** (page 18) reduced gastrointestinal bleeding caused by the aspirin.[6] DGL has been shown in controlled human research to be as effective as drug therapy (**cimetidine** [page 46]) in healing stomach ulcers.[7]

INTERACTIONS WITH FOODS AND OTHER COMPOUNDS

Food

Nabumetone should be taken with food to prevent gastrointestinal upset.[8]

Alcohol

Nabumetone may cause drowsiness, dizziness, or blurred vision.[9] Alcohol may intensify these effects and increase the risk of accidental injury. Use of alcohol during nabumetone therapy increases the risk of stomach irritation and bleeding. People taking nabumetone should avoid alcohol.

SUMMARY OF INTERACTIONS FOR NABUMETONE

Depletion or interference	Iron
Adverse interaction	Sodium*
Side effect reduction/prevention	Copper,* Licorice
Supportive interaction	Copper*
Reduced drug absorption/bioavailability	None known
Other (see text)	Potassium

NAPROXEN
(Napralen, Naprosyn, and Others)

NAPROXEN SODIUM
(Aleve, Anaprox, and Others)

Naproxen/naproxen sodium are members of the nonsteroidal anti-inflammatory drug (**NSAID** [page 157]) family. NSAIDs reduce inflammation (swelling), pain, and temperature. Naproxen is used to treat mild to moderate pain, arthritis, ankylosing spondylitis, primary dysmenorrhea, tendinitis, bursitis, and other conditions. Naproxen is available in prescription strength (naproxen: Napralen, Naprosyn, and others; naproxen sodium: Anaprox and others). Naproxen sodium is also available in nonprescription strength (Aleve).

INTERACTIONS WITH DIETARY SUPPLEMENTS

Copper

Supplementation may enhance the anti-inflammatory effects of NSAIDs while reducing their ulcerogenic effects. One study found that when various anti-inflammatory drugs were chelated with copper, the anti-inflammatory activity was increased.[1] Animal models of inflammation have found that the copper chelate of **aspirin** (page 18) was active at one-eighth the effective dose of aspirin. These copper complexes are less toxic than the parent compounds, as well.

Iron

NSAIDs cause gastrointestinal (GI) irritation, bleeding, and iron loss.[2] Iron supplements can cause GI irritation.[3] However, iron supplementation is sometimes needed in people taking NSAIDs if those drugs have caused enough blood loss to lead to iron deficiency. If both iron and naproxen are prescribed, they should be taken with food to reduce GI irritation and bleeding risk.

Potassium

Naproxen has caused kidney dysfunction and increased blood potassium levels, especially in older people.[4] People taking naproxen should not supplement potassium without consulting with their prescribing doctor or a nutritionally oriented doctor.

Sodium

Naproxen may cause sodium and water retention.[5] It is healthful to reduce dietary salt intake by eliminating table salt and heavily salted foods.

INTERACTIONS WITH HERBS

Licorice (Glycyrrhiza glabra)

The flavonoids found in the extract of licorice known as DGL (deglycyrrhizinated licorice) are helpful for avoiding the irritating actions **NSAIDs** (page 157) have on the stomach and intestines. One study found that 350 mg of chewable DGL taken together with each dose of **aspirin** (page 18) reduced gastrointestinal bleeding caused by the aspirin.[6] DGL has been shown in controlled human research to be as effective as drug therapy (**cimetidine** [page 46]) in healing stomach ulcers.[7]

INTERACTIONS WITH FOODS AND OTHER COMPOUNDS

Food

Naproxen should be taken with food to prevent gastrointestinal upset.[8]

Alcohol

Naproxen may cause drowsiness, dizziness, or blurred vision.[9] Alcohol may intensify these effects and increase the risk of accidental injury. Use of alcohol during naproxen therapy increases the risk of stomach irritation and bleeding. People taking naproxen should avoid alcohol.

SUMMARY OF INTERACTIONS FOR NAPROXEN

Depletion or interference	Iron
Adverse interaction	Sodium*
Side effect reduction/prevention	Copper,* Licorice
Supportive interaction	Copper*
Reduced drug absorption/bioavailability	None known
Other (see text)	Potassium

NEFAZODONE
(Serzone)

Nefazodone is a drug used to treat people with depression.

INTERACTIONS WITH HERBS

Digitalis (Digitalis lanata, Digitalis purpurea)

Digitalis refers to a family of plants commonly called foxglove that contain digitalis glycosides, chemicals with actions and toxicities similar to the prescription drug **digoxin** (page 71).

Nefazodone increased serum digoxin levels in a three-way crossover study of eighteen healthy men.[1] No interactions between nefazodone and digitalis have been reported. Until more is known, nefazodone and digitalis-containing products should be used only under the direct supervision of a doctor trained in their use.

St. John's Wort (*Hypericum perforatum*)

Although there have been no interactions reported in the medical literature, it is best to avoid using nefazodone with St. John's wort unless you are under the supervision of a qualified health-care professional.

INTERACTIONS WITH FOODS AND OTHER COMPOUNDS

Food

Nefazodone may be taken with or without food.[2]

Alcohol

People taking nefazodone are advised to avoid alcohol.[3]

SUMMARY OF INTERACTIONS FOR NEFAZODONE

Depletion or interference	*None known*
Adverse interaction	*St. John's wort*[*]
Side effect reduction/prevention	*None known*
Supportive interaction	*None known*
Reduced drug absorption/bioavailability	*None known*
Other (see text)	*Digitalis*

NEOMYCIN

Neomycin is an **antibacterial** (page 14) drug that is poorly absorbed when taken by mouth. It is combined with enteric coated **erythromycin** (page 86) to suppress gastrointestinal (GI) bacteria before surgery to avoid infection. Neomycin is used to treat hepatic coma in cases of liver failure and is included in some antibiotic products used to treat infections of the eyes, ears, or skin.

INTERACTIONS WITH DIETARY SUPPLEMENTS

Vitamins and Minerals

Neomycin can decrease absorption or increase elimination of many nutrients, including calcium, carbohydrates, beta-carotene, fats, folic acid, iron, magnesium, potassium, sodium, and vitamins A, B_{12}, D, and K.[1] [2] Surgery preparation with oral neomycin is unlikely to lead to deficiencies. It makes sense for people taking neomycin for more than a few days to also take a multivitamin/mineral supplement.

Vitamin B_6

Neomycin may inactivate vitamin B_6.[3] Surgery preparation with oral neomycin is unlikely to lead to vitamin B_6 deficiency. People taking oral neomycin for more than a few days should ask their prescribing doctor or a nutritionally oriented doctor about vitamin B_6 supplementation to prevent deficiency.

SUMMARY OF INTERACTIONS FOR NEOMYCIN

Depletion or interference	*Calcium, Carbohydrates, Beta-carotene, Fats, Folic acid, Iron, Magnesium, Potassium, Sodium, Vitamin A, Vitamin B_6, Vitamin B_{12}, Vitamin D, Vitamin K*
Adverse interaction	*None known*
Side effect reduction/prevention	*None known*
Supportive interaction	*None known*
Reduced drug absorption/bioavailability	*None known*

NICOTINE GUM
(Nicorette)

NICOTINE NASAL SPRAY
(Nicotrol NS)

NICOTINE ORAL INHALER
(Nicotrol Inhaler)

NICOTINE SKIN PATCH
(Habitrol, Nicoderm, Nicotrol)

Nicotine is available in various forms as an aid to quitting smoking. Nicotine skin patches are available in nonprescription (Nicoderm CQ, Nicotrol) and prescription (Habitrol) strengths. Nicotine gum is available without prescription

(Nicorette). Nicotine nasal spray (Nicotrol NS) and oral inhaler (Nicotrol Inhaler) are available by prescription.

INTERACTIONS WITH HERBS

Lobelia (Lobelia inflata)

Lobelia is the plant from which the drug lobeline was isolated. Lobeline produces effects similar to nicotine.[1] Combined use of nicotine and lobeline may increase the risk of nicotine side effects. No interactions have been reported with nicotine and lobelia, and in fact research has suggested lobeline may be useful as an aid to stopping smoking.[2]

INTERACTIONS WITH FOODS AND OTHER COMPOUNDS

Food

Absorption of nicotine from nicotine gum requires mildly alkaline saliva.[3] Acidic foods and beverages (coffee, colas, fruit/fruit juices, and others) may reduce nicotine absorption. This potential interaction may be avoided by chewing nicotine gum 1 hour before or after consuming acidic food and beverages.

SUMMARY OF INTERACTIONS FOR NICOTINE ALTERNATIVES

Depletion or interference	*None known*
Adverse interaction	*None known*
Side effect reduction/prevention	*None known*
Supportive interaction	*None known*
Reduced drug absorption/bioavailability	*None known*
Other (see text)	*Lobelia*

NIFEDIPINE
(Procardia, Adalat, and Others)

Nifedipine is a calcium channel blocker used to treat angina pectoris and high blood pressure.

INTERACTIONS WITH FOODS AND OTHER COMPOUNDS

Grapefruit Juice

Ingestion of grapefruit juice has been shown to increase the absorption of felodipine (a drug similar in structure and action to that of nifedipine) and to increase the adverse effects of the medication in people with hypertension. Until more is known, it seems that grapefruit juice should not be ingested at the same time as nifedipine or similar drugs.[1] The same effects might be seen from eating grapefruit as from drinking its juice.

Food

Nifedipine may be taken with or without food.[2] Nifedipine products should be swallowed whole, without crushing or chewing.[3]

Tobacco

In a double-blind study of ten cigarette smokers with angina treated with nifedipine for 1 week, angina episodes were significantly reduced during the nonsmoking phase compared to the smoking phase.[4] People with angina taking nifedipine should not smoke tobacco.

SUMMARY OF INTERACTIONS FOR NIFEDIPINE

Depletion or interference	*None known*
Adverse interaction	*Tobacco**
Side effect reduction/prevention	*None known*
Supportive interaction	*None known*
Reduced drug absorption/bioavailability	*None known*
Other (see text)	*Grapefruit juice*

NITROFURANTOIN
(Macrobid, Macrodantin, and Others)

Nitrofurantoin is an **antibiotic** (page 14) used to treat urinary tract bacterial infections.

INTERACTIONS WITH DIETARY SUPPLEMENTS

Magnesium

In six healthy men, nitrofurantoin absorption was reduced by also taking magnesium trisilicate.[1] Another magnesium compound, magnesium oxide (commonly found in supplements) was shown to bind with nitrofurantoin in a test tube.[2]

In a study of eleven people, the rate of nitrofurantoin absorption was delayed despite the fact that the amount of nitrofurantoin ultimately absorbed remained the same when the drug was administered in a colloidal magnesium aluminum silicate suspension.[3] It remains unclear whether this interaction is clinically important or if typical magnesium supplements would have the same effect.

INTERACTIONS WITH FOODS AND OTHER COMPOUNDS

Food

Taking nitrofurantoin with food improves absorption[4] and reduces gastrointestinal (GI) upset.[5]

SUMMARY OF INTERACTIONS FOR NITROFURANTOIN

Depletion or interference	None known
Adverse interaction	None known
Side effect reduction/prevention	None known
Supportive interaction	None known
Reduced drug absorption/bioavailability	Magnesium*

NITROGLYCERIN

(Deponit, Nitro-Bid, Nitrodisc, Nitro-Dur, Nitrogard, Nitrolingual, Nitrostat, Transderm-Nitro, Minitran)

Nitroglycerin dilates blood vessels by relaxing the smooth muscles surrounding them, increasing blood flow. Nitroglycerin is used to treat or prevent chest pain in people with angina pectoris and to treat instances of congestive heart failure.

INTERACTIONS WITH DIETARY SUPPLEMENTS

N-Acetyl Cysteine (NAC)

Continuous nitroglycerin use leads to development of nitroglycerin tolerance and loss of effectiveness. Intravenous (IV) N-acetyl cysteine (NAC), during short-term studies of people receiving continuous nitroglycerin, was reported to reverse nitroglycerin tolerance.[1] [2] In a double-blind placebo-controlled trial, transdermal nitroglycerin plus oral NAC (600 mg 3 times per day) was associated with fewer failures of medical treatment than placebo, NAC, or nitroglycerin alone. However, when combined with nitroglycerin use, NAC has led to intolerable headaches.[3] [4] In two double-blind, randomized trials of people with angina treated with transdermal nitroglycerin, oral NAC 200 mg or 400 mg 3 times per day failed to prevent nitroglycerin tolerance.[5] [6]

People using long-acting nitroglycerin can avoid tolerance with a 10- to 12-hour nitroglycerin-free period every day. People taking long-acting nitroglycerin should ask their prescribing doctor or pharmacist about preventing nitroglycerin tolerance.

INTERACTIONS WITH FOODS AND OTHER COMPOUNDS

Alcohol

Alcohol, when consumed during nitroglycerin therapy, may cause low blood pressure and circulatory collapse in extreme cases.[7] People using nitroglycerin should avoid alcohol.

SUMMARY OF INTERACTIONS FOR NITROGLYCERIN

Depletion or interference	*None known*
Adverse interaction	*N-acetyl cysteine*[*]
Side effect reduction/prevention	*None known*
Supportive interaction	*None known*
Reduced drug absorption/bioavailability	*None known*

NITROUS OXIDE

Nitrous oxide is an anesthetic gas. It is used during dental work and with people who are not candidates for more commonly used **anesthetics** (page 12) during surgery.

INTERACTIONS WITH DIETARY SUPPLEMENTS

Folic Acid and Vitamin B_{12}

Nitrous oxide interferes with activity of vitamin B_{12}, which further interferes with the activity of folic acid, causing adverse actions.[1] [2] Administration of folic acid or folinic acid (activated folic acid) has reversed nitrous oxide–induced bone marrow changes.[3] [4] People with vitamin B_{12} deficiency may be especially susceptible.[5] People who will undergo nitrous oxide anesthesia for several hours may benefit from vitamin B_{12} and folic acid supplementation.[6] Some doctors of natural medicine recommend 100 mcg of vitamin B_{12} and 1,000 mcg folic acid, starting 1 week before through 1 week after prolonged exposure to nitrous oxide. People with normal vitamin B_{12} levels who undergo short-duration nitrous oxide anesthesia (less than 2 hours) do not require supplementation.

SUMMARY OF INTERACTIONS FOR NITROUS OXIDE

Depletion or interference	*Folic acid, Vitamin B$_{12}$*
Adverse interaction	*None known*
Side effect reduction/prevention	*None known*
Supportive interaction	*None known*
Reduced drug absorption/bioavailability	*None known*

NIZATIDINE
(Axid, Axid AR)

Nizatidine is a member of the H-2 blocker (histamine blocker) family of drugs that prevents the release of acid into the stomach. Nizatidine is used to treat stomach and duodenal ulcers and reflux of stomach acid into the esophagus. Nizatidine is available as the prescription drug Axid. It is also available as a nonprescription product, Axid AR, for relief of heartburn, acid indigestion, and sour stomach.

INTERACTIONS WITH DIETARY SUPPLEMENTS

Iron

Stomach acid may increase absorption of iron from food. H-2 blocker drugs reduce stomach acid and are associated with decreased dietary iron absorption.[1] The iron found in supplements is available to the body without the need for stomach acid. People with ulcers may be iron deficient due to blood loss. If iron deficiency is present, iron supplementation may be beneficial. Iron levels in the blood can be checked with lab tests.

Magnesium-Containing Antacids

In healthy people, a **magnesium hydroxide** (page 135)/**aluminum hydroxide** (page 6) antacid, taken with nizatidine, decreased nizatidine absorption by 12%.[2] People can avoid this interaction by taking nizatidine 2 hours before or after any aluminum/magnesium-containing antacids. Some magnesium supplements such as magnesium hydroxide are also **antacids** (page 13).

Vitamin B$_{12}$

Stomach acid is needed for vitamin B$_{12}$ in food to be absorbed by the body. H-2 blocker drugs reduce stomach acid and may therefore inhibit absorption of the vitamin B$_{12}$ naturally present in food. However, the vitamin B$_{12}$ found in supplements does not depend on stomach acid for absorption.[3] Lab tests can determine vitamin B_{12} levels in people.

Other Vitamins and Minerals

There is some evidence that other vitamins and minerals, such as folic acid[4] and copper,[5] require the presence of stomach acid for optimal absorption. Long-term use of H-2 blockers may therefore promote a deficiency of these nutrients. Individuals requiring long-term use of H-2 blockers may therefore benefit from a multiple vitamin/mineral supplement.

INTERACTIONS WITH FOODS AND OTHER COMPOUNDS

Food

To prevent heartburn after meals, nizatidine is best taken 30 minutes before meals.[6] For other conditions, nizatidine works best taken with an early evening meal.[7]

Tobacco

In a randomized, double-blind, 1-year study of 513 people with recently healed duodenal ulcers, smokers were found to have a significantly higher recurrence rate than nonsmokers during maintenance therapy with nizatidine.[8]

SUMMARY OF INTERACTIONS FOR NIZATIDINE

Depletion or interference	*Iron,* Vitamin B_{12}*
Adverse interaction	*Tobacco*
Side effect reduction/prevention	*None known*
Supportive interaction	*None known*
Reduced drug absorption/bioavailability	*None known*
Other (see text)	*Copper, Folic acid, Magnesium*

NONSTEROIDAL ANTI-INFLAMMATORY DRUGS
(NSAIDs)

NSAIDs are drugs that reduce swelling, pain, and fever. They are used to treat mild to moderate pain, arthritis, ankylosing spondylitis, bursitis, headaches, tendinitis, and other conditions. Although **aspirin** (page 18) reduces swelling, pain, and fever just like NSAIDs, it is classed as a member of the salicylate

Ofloxacin

family of drugs. **Acetaminophen** (page 2) reduces pain and fever but not swelling and is not an NSAID.

A variety of prescription and over-the-counter NSAIDs are available, including:

- **Etodolac** (page 89) (Lodine)
- **Ibuprofen** (page 111) (Motrin and others)
- **Indomethacin** (page 113) (Indocin)
- **Nabumetone** (page 146) (Relafen)
- **Naproxen** (page 148) (Napralen and others)
- **Oxaprozin** (page 162) (Daypro)

For detailed interaction information, see the individual NSAID.

OFLOXACIN
(Floxin, Oculflox)

Ofloxacin is a "fluoroquinolone" **antibiotic** (page 14) used to treat bacterial infections. Ofloxacin is available in special preparations to treat eye infections and ear infections.

INTERACTIONS WITH DIETARY SUPPLEMENTS

Minerals

Minerals including calcium, iron, magnesium, and zinc can bind to fluoroquinolones, including ofloxacin, greatly reducing drug absorption.[1] Ofloxacin should be taken 4 hours before or 2 hours after consuming **antacids** (page 13) (Maalox, Mylanta, Tums, Rolaids, and others) that may contain these minerals and mineral-containing supplements.[2]

Vitamin K

Unlike with most other antibiotics, preliminary research suggests that people taking ofloxacin do not need to supplement vitamin K to protect against possible drug-induced depletion.[3]

INTERACTIONS WITH FOODS AND OTHER COMPOUNDS

Food

Ofloxacin may be taken with or without food. Food slows the absorption but not the total amount of ofloxacin absorbed from each dose.[4] [5] Milk does not alter ofloxacin absorption.[6]

SUMMARY OF INTERACTIONS FOR OFLOXACIN

Depletion or interference	*None known*
Adverse interaction	*None known*
Side effect reduction/prevention	*None known*
Supportive interaction	*None known*
Reduced drug absorption/bioavailability	*Calcium, Iron, Magnesium, Zinc*
Other (see text)	*Vitamin K*

OMEPRAZOLE
(Prilosec)

Omeprazole is a member of the proton pump inhibitor family of drugs, which blocks production of stomach acid. Omeprazole is used to treat diseases in which stomach acid causes damage, including gastric and duodenal ulcers, gastroesophageal reflux disease, erosive esophagitis, and Zollinger-Ellison syndrome.

INTERACTIONS WITH DIETARY SUPPLEMENTS

Vitamin B_{12}

Omeprazole interferes with the absorption of vitamin B_{12} from food (though not from supplements) in some[1][2] but not all[3][4] studies. The fall in vitamin B_{12} status may result from the decrease in stomach acid caused by the drug.[5] Unlike dietary vitamin B_{12} (which is bound to protein), supplemental B_{12} does not require stomach acid for absorption.

INTERACTIONS WITH HERBS

Cranberry (Vaccinium marocarpon)

People taking omeprazole may increase absorption of dietary vitamin B_{12} by drinking cranberry juice or other acidic liquids with vitamin B_{12}-containing foods.[6]

SUMMARY OF INTERACTIONS FOR OMEPRAZOLE

Depletion or interference	*Vitamin B_{12}*[*]
Adverse interaction	*None known*
Side effect reduction/prevention	*Cranberry*[*]

Supportive interaction   *None known*

Reduced drug absorption/bioavailability   *None known*

ORAL CONTRACEPTIVES

Oral contraceptives (OCs) are a family of drugs that include Brevicon, Demulen, Genora, Levlen, Loestrin, Micronor, Modicon, Nordette, Norinyl, Ortho-Novum, Ovcon, Ovral, Ovrette, Triphasil, and others.

OCs contain combinations of estrogens and progestins (female hormones) or only progestins. They are used primarily to prevent human pregnancy. Oral contraceptives are also used to treat women with menstrual irregularities and endometriosis. Oral contraceptives should not be confused with hormone replacement therapy, which uses different estrogen and/or progestin-containing products.

INTERACTIONS WITH DIETARY SUPPLEMENTS

Folic Acid

OCs use can cause folic acid depletion.[1] In a 3-month, double-blind placebo-controlled trial of OC users with cervical dysplasia, supplementation with very large doses (10,000 mcg) of folic acid improved cervical health. Women with cervical dyplasia diagnosed while they are taking OCs should consult a nutritionally oriented doctor. Mega-folate supplementation should not be attempted without a doctor's supervision, nor is there any reason to believe that folic acid supplementation would help people with cervical cancer.

Iron

Menstrual blood loss is typically reduced with use of OCs. This can lead to increased iron stores and, presumably, a decreased need for iron in premenopausal women.[2] Premenopausal women taking oral contraceptives should have their iron levels monitored and talk with their prescribing doctor before using iron-containing supplements.

Magnesium

Ninety-three women using OCs were found to have significantly lower serum magnesium levels compared with a control group.[3] In a study of thirty-two women, serum magnesium decreased after 6 months of taking an OC containing ethinyl estradiol and levonorgestrel.[4] Although the importance of this interaction remains somewhat unclear, supplementation with 250 to 350 mg of magnesium per day is a safe and reasonable supplemental level for most adults.

Vitamin B$_6$

Oral contraceptives have been associated with vitamin B$_6$ depletion and clinical depression. In a small, double-blind study of women with depression taking OCs, vitamin B$_6$ (20 mg twice per day) improved depression.[5] Half of the women in the study showed laboratory evidence of vitamin B$_6$ deficiency.

Other Nutrients

A review of literature suggests that women who use OCs may experience decreased vitamin B$_1$, B$_2$, B$_3$, B$_{12}$, C, and zinc levels.[6][7][8] OC use has been associated with increased absorption of calcium and copper and with increased serum vitamin A levels.[9][10] OCs may interfere with manganese absorption.[11] The clinical importance of these actions remains unclear.

INTERACTIONS WITH FOODS AND OTHER COMPOUNDS

Tobacco (*Nicotiana* species)

Women who smoke and use OCs have a five-times greater risk of dying from a heart attack than OC users who do not smoke.[12] Women over the age of thirty-five who smoke and use OCs have a greatly increased risk of death related to circulatory disease.[13] Avoiding or quitting smoking is good for health.

SUMMARY OF INTERACTIONS FOR ORAL CONTRACEPTIVES

Depletion or interference	*Magnesium,* * *Vitamin B$_1$,* * *Vitamin B$_2$,* * *Vitamin B$_3$,* * *Vitamin B$_6$,* * *Vitamin B$_{12}$,* * *Vitamin C,* * *Zinc* *
Adverse interaction	*Tobacco*
Side effect reduction/prevention	*Vitamin B$_6$*
Supportive interaction	*None known*
Reduced drug absorption/bioavailability	*None known*
Other (see text)	*Calcium, Copper, Folic acid, Iron, Manganese, Vitamin A*

OXAPROZIN
(Daypro)

Oxaprozin is a member of the **nonsteroidal anti-inflammatory drug (NSAID** [page 157]**)** family. NSAIDs reduce inflammation (swelling), pain, and temperature. Oxaprozin is used to treat arthritis.

INTERACTIONS WITH DIETARY SUPPLEMENTS

Copper

Supplementation may enhance the anti-inflammatory effects of NSAIDs while reducing their ulcerogenic effects. One study found that when various anti-inflammatory drugs were chelated with copper, the anti-inflammatory activity was increased.[1] Animal models of inflammation have found that the copper chelate of **aspirin** (page 18) was active at one-eighth the effective dose of aspirin. These copper complexes are less toxic than the parent compounds, as well.

Iron

NSAIDs cause gastrointestinal (GI) irritation, bleeding, and iron loss.[2] Iron supplements can cause GI irritation.[3] However, iron supplementation is sometimes needed in people taking NSAIDs if those drugs have caused enough blood loss to lead to iron deficiency. If both iron and oxaprozin are prescribed, they should be taken with food to reduce GI irritation and bleeding risk.

Potassium

NSAIDs have caused kidney dysfunction and increased blood potassium levels, especially in older people.[4] People taking NSAIDs, including oxaprozin, should not supplement potassium without consulting with their prescribing doctor or a nutritionally oriented doctor.

Sodium

Oxaprozin may cause sodium and water retention.[5] It is healthful to reduce dietary salt intake by eliminating table salt and heavily salted foods.

INTERACTIONS WITH HERBS

Licorice (Glycyrrhiza glabra)

The flavonoids found in the extract of licorice known as DGL (deglycyrrhizinated licorice) are helpful for avoiding the irritating actions **NSAIDs** (page 157) have on the stomach and intestines. One study found that 350 mg of chewable DGL taken together with each dose of aspirin reduced gastrointestinal bleeding caused by the aspirin.[6] DGL has been shown in controlled human research to be as effective as drug therapy (**cimetidine** [page 46]) in healing stomach ulcers.[7]

INTERACTIONS WITH FOODS AND OTHER COMPOUNDS

Food

Oxaprozin should be taken with food to prevent gastrointestinal upset.[8]

Alcohol

Oxaprozin may cause drowsiness, dizziness, or blurred vision.[9] Alcohol may intensify these effects and increase the risk of accidental injury. Use of alcohol during oxaprozin therapy increases the risk of stomach irritation and bleeding. People taking oxaprozin should avoid alcohol.

SUMMARY OF INTERACTIONS FOR OXAPROZIN

Depletion or interference	*Iron*
Adverse interaction	*Sodium**
Side effect reduction/prevention	*Copper,* Licorice*
Supportive interaction	*Copper**
Reduced drug absorption/bioavailability	*None known*
Other (see text)	*Potassium*

OXYCODONE/ACETAMINOPHEN
(Percocet, Roxicet, and Others)

OXYCODONE/ASPIRIN
(Percodan, Roxiprin, and Others)

Oxycodone is a narcotic analgesic used to relieve moderate to severe pain. Oxycodone is available in combination with other drugs, including oxycodone/**acetaminophen** (page 2) (Percocet, Roxicet, and others) and oxycodone/**aspirin** (page 18) (Percodan, Roxiprin, and others).

INTERACTIONS WITH FOODS AND OTHER COMPOUNDS

Food

Oxycodone may cause gastrointestinal (GI) upset. Oxycodone-containing products may be taken with food to reduce or prevent GI upset.[1] A common side effect of narcotic analgesics is constipation.[2]

Increasing dietary fiber (especially vegetables and whole-grain foods) and water intake can ease constipation.

Alcohol

Oxycodone may cause drowsiness, dizziness, or blurred vision. Alcohol may intensify these effects and increase the risk of accidental injury.[3] To prevent problems, people taking oxycodone should avoid alcohol.

SUMMARY OF INTERACTIONS FOR OXYCODONE

Depletion or interference	*None known*
Adverse interaction	*None known*
Side effect reduction/prevention	*None known*
Supportive interaction	*None known*
Reduced drug absorption/bioavailability	*None known*

PACLITAXEL
(Taxol)

Paclitaxel is a natural (though quite toxic) substance derived from the yew tree by taking a naturally present substance from the tree and chemically altering it to form the drug; it is used as a **chemotherapy** (page 40) drug to treat people with a wide variety of cancers. The resultant drug is administered intravenously.

INTERACTIONS WITH DIETARY SUPPLEMENTS

Glutamine

Paclitaxel commonly causes muscle and joint pain. Five cases of people experiencing these symptoms who responded to the amino acid glutamine have been reported.[1] All five were given 10 grams glutamine by mouth 3 times per day beginning 24 hours after the paclitaxel treatment. Although the report does not state how many days glutamine supplements were taken, it may have been for 10 days or less—the typical time it takes for these symptoms to subside following paclitaxel administration. Whereas all five had experienced moderate to severe symptoms from the drug when taken previously without glutamine, none of the five experienced these symptoms when glutamine was added. Glutamate, an amino acid structurally related to glutamine, had previously been reported to reduce paclitaxel-induced nerve damage in animals.[2]

SUMMARY OF INTERACTIONS FOR PACLITAXEL

Depletion or interference	*None known*
Adverse interaction	*None known*
Side effect reduction/prevention	*Glutamine*
Supportive interaction	*None known*
Reduced drug absorption/bioavailability	*None known*

PAROXETINE
(Paxil)

Paroxetine is a member of the selective serotonin reuptake inhibitor (SSRI) family of drugs used to treat people with depression.

INTERACTIONS WITH DIETARY SUPPLEMENTS

5-Hydroxytryptophan (5-HTP)

Paroxetine increases serotonin activity in the brain. 5-HTP and L-tryptophan are converted to serotonin in the brain, and taking them with paroxetine may increase paroxetine-induced side effects. While no interactions with paroxetine and 5-HTP or L-tryptophan have been reported, until more is known, 5-HTP or L-tryptophan should not be taken with any SSRI drug, including paroxetine.

L-Tryptophan

L-tryptophan is an amino acid found in protein-rich foods. Foods rich in L-tryptophan do not cause problems during paroxetine use. However, dietary supplements of L-tryptophan (available only by prescriptions from special compounding pharmacies) taken with paroxetine have been reported to cause headache, sweating, dizziness, agitation, restlessness, nausea, vomiting, and other symptoms.[1] The combination of 45 mg DL-tryptophan per pound of body weight (high dose) with zimelidine, a drug with a similar action to paroxetine, did not cause these side effects in another trial.[2] These contradictory findings show that it remains unclear whether tryptophan causes side effects in people taking paroxetine.

Sodium

SSRI drugs, including paroxetine, have been reported to cause sodium depletion.[3][4][5] The risk for SSRI-induced sodium depletion appears to be increased during the first few weeks of treatment in women, the elderly, and people also using **diuretics** (page 76). Doctors prescribing SSRI drugs, including paroxetine, should monitor their patients for signs of sodium depletion.

INTERACTIONS WITH HERBS

Ginkgo (Ginkgo biloba)

In three men and two women treated with **fluoxetine** (page 94) or **sertraline** (page 187) (SSRI drugs closely related to paroxetine) for depression who experienced sexual dysfunction, addition of ginkgo biloba extract (GBE) in the amount of 240 mg per day effectively reversed the sexual dysfunction.[6] In part, this makes sense because ginkgo has been reported to help men with some forms of impotence.[7]

St. John's Wort (Hypericum perforatum)

One report described a case of serotonin syndrome in an individual who took St. John's wort and **trazodone** (page 212), a weak SSRI drug.[8] The person reportedly experienced mental confusion, muscle twitching, sweating, flushing, and ataxia. In another case, a person experienced grogginess, lethargy, nausea, weakness, and fatigue after taking one dose of paroxetine after 10 days of St. John's wort use.[9]

INTERACTIONS WITH FOODS AND OTHER COMPOUNDS

Food

Paroxetine may be taken with or without food.[10]

Alcohol

SSRI drugs, including paroxetine, may cause dizziness or drowsiness.[11] Alcohol may intensify these effects and increase the risk of accidental injury. Alcohol should be avoided during paroxetine therapy.

SUMMARY OF INTERACTIONS FOR PAROXETINE

Depletion or interference	*Sodium*
Adverse interaction	*5-Hydroxytryptophan (5-HTP),* * *L-tryptophan,* * *St. John's wort* *
Side effect reduction/prevention	*Ginkgo* *
Supportive interaction	*None known*
Reduced drug absorption/bioavailability	*None known*

PENICILLAMINE
(Cuprimine, Depen)

Penicillamine is a chelating agent (binds metals and carries them out of the body). Penicillamine is used to treat people with Wilson's disease, cystinuria, and severe rheumatoid arthritis.

INTERACTIONS WITH DIETARY SUPPLEMENTS

Copper

One of the main uses of penicillamine is to reduce toxic copper deposits in people with Wilson's disease. People with Wilson's disease taking penicillamine should not take copper supplements, including the small amounts found in multivitamin/mineral supplements.

Iron

Penicillamine binds iron. When taken with iron, penicillamine absorption and activity are reduced.[1] Four cases of penicillamine-induced kidney damage were reported when concomitant iron therapy was stopped, which presumably led to the increased penicillamine absorption and toxicity.[2]

Vitamin B$_6$

Penicillamine may increase vitamin B$_6$ excretion, reduce activity, and increase the risk for vitamin B$_6$ deficiency.[3] It makes sense for people taking penicillamine to supplement with small (5 to 20 mg per day) amounts of vitamin B$_6$. Others have suggested that as much as 50 mg per day of vitamin B$_6$ may be necessary.[4]

Zinc

Penicillamine can bind zinc, interfering with the absorption of both agents.[5] People taking penicillamine should avoid zinc-containing supplements, unless otherwise directed by their prescribing doctor. However, with proper medical supervision, people with Wilson's disease can often supplement zinc instead of taking penicillamine.

Sodium

Penicillamine therapy has been associated with sodium depletion.[6] The frequency of this association remains unclear.

INTERACTIONS WITH FOODS AND OTHER COMPOUNDS

Food

Food decreases penicillamine absorption.[7] Penicillamine should be taken 1 hour before or 2 hours after any food to avoid this interaction.

SUMMARY OF INTERACTIONS FOR PENICILLAMINE

Depletion or interference	*Sodium,* *Vitamin B$_6$*
Adverse interaction	*None known*
Side effect reduction/prevention	*None known*
Supportive interaction	*None known*
Reduced drug absorption/bioavailability	*Iron*
Other (see text)	*Copper, Zinc*

PENICILLIN V
(Pen-Vee K, Veetids, and Others)

Penicillin V is an **antibiotic** (page 14) used to treat bacterial infections.

INTERACTIONS WITH DIETARY SUPPLEMENTS

Bromelain

One report found bromelain improved the action of antibiotic drugs, including penicillin and **erythromycin** (page 86), in treating a variety of infections. In that trial, twenty-two out of twenty-three people who had previously not responded to the antibiotics did so after adding bromelain 4 times per day.[1] Doctors of natural medicine will sometimes prescribe enough bromelain to equal 2,400 gelatin dissolving units (listed as GDU on labels) per day. This amount would equal approximately 3,600 MCU (milk clotting units), another common measure of bromelain activity.

Guar Gum

In a double-blind study with ten healthy people, guar gum reduced penicillin absorption.[2] Until more is known, to avoid this interaction, people taking penicillin should take it 2 hours before or after any guar gum–containing supplements. It remains unclear whether the smaller amounts of guar gum found in many processed foods would have a significant effect.

INTERACTIONS WITH FOODS AND OTHER COMPOUNDS

Food

Penicillin V should be taken at least 1 hour before or 2 hours after eating.[3] [4]

SUMMARY OF INTERACTIONS FOR PENICILLIN V

Depletion or interference	*None known*
Adverse interaction	*None known*
Side effect reduction/prevention	*None known*
Supportive interaction	*Bromelain**
Reduced drug absorption/bioavailability	*Guar gum**

PENTOXIFYLLINE
(Trental)

Pentoxifylline decreases blood thickness and improves red blood cell flexibility. Pentoxifylline is used to improve symptoms of intermittent claudication and in the treatment of other circulatory disorders.

INTERACTIONS WITH FOODS AND OTHER COMPOUNDS

Food

Pentoxifylline should be taken with meals.[1]

SUMMARY OF INTERACTIONS FOR PENTOXIFYLLINE

Depletion or interference	*None known*
Adverse interaction	*None known*
Side effect reduction/prevention	*None known*
Supportive interaction	*None known*
Reduced drug absorption/bioavailability	*None known*

PHENELZINE
(Nardil)

Phenelzine is a member of a group of drugs called monoamine oxidase (MAO) inhibitors (also called MAOIs). Phenelzine is sometimes used to treat people with depression who do not respond to other antidepressant drug therapy.

INTERACTIONS WITH DIETARY SUPPLEMENTS

Vitamin B$_6$

Phenelzine has a chemical structure similar to other drugs (**isoniazid** [page 118] and **hydralazine** [page 109]) that can cause vitamin B$_6$ deficiency. One case of phenelzine-induced vitamin B$_6$ deficiency has been reported.[1] Little is known about this interaction. People taking phenelzine should ask their prescribing doctor or a nutritionally oriented doctor about monitoring vitamin B$_6$ levels and supplementation.

INTERACTIONS WITH HERBS

Ephedra sinica (Ma huang)

Ephedra contains the chemical **ephedrine** (page 83), which may interact with phenelzine, causing unwanted actions.[2] People should read product labels for ephedra/ephedrine content. Ephedra and ephedrine-containing products should be avoided during phenelzine therapy. People with questions about phenelzine and ephedra/ephedrine should ask their prescribing doctor, pharmacist, or an herbally oriented doctor.

Ginseng (Species Not Specified)

In a case report of a woman treated with phenelzine, addition of a ginseng-containing tea was associated with insomnia, headache, and tremor.[3] Other contents of the tea were not reported. In a case report of a woman treated with phenelzine for depression, addition of ginseng (not further identified) was associated with hypomania, which the woman had not previously experienced.[4] Until more is known, people should combine ginseng and phenelzine with caution and consult an herbally oriented doctor.

St. John's Wort *(Hypericum perforatum)*

Although St. John's wort contains low-level chemicals that bind MAOI in test tubes, it is believed that the action of St. John's wort is not due to MAOI activity.[5] However, because St. John's wort may have serotonin reuptake inhibiting action, it is best to avoid concomitant use with MAOI drugs.

Scotch Broom *(Cytisus scoparius)*

Scotch broom contains high levels of tyramine. Combining phenelzine and Scotch broom may cause MAOI-type reactions (diarrhea, flushing, sweating, pounding chest, dangerous changes in blood pressure, and other symptoms).[6] It is important for people taking phenelzine to avoid Scotch broom. People with questions about phenelzine and Scotch broom should ask their prescribing doctor or an herbally oriented doctor.

INTERACTIONS WITH FOODS AND OTHER COMPOUNDS

Tyramine-Containing Foods

Phenelzine can alter metabolism of tyramine-containing foods, leading to diarrhea, flushing, sweating, pounding chest, dangerous changes in blood pressure, and other symptoms.[7] It is important for people taking phenelzine to avoid tyramine-containing foods. People with questions about phenelzine and tyramine-containing foods should ask their prescribing doctor, pharmacist, a nutritionally oriented doctor, or clinical nutritionist.

Aspartame

Two cases were reported involving men treated with phenelzine who experienced restlessness, agitation, tremor, and insomnia after drinking large quantities of cola beverages containing aspartame.[8]

SUMMARY OF INTERACTIONS FOR PHENELZINE

Depletion or interference	*Vitamin B$_6$*
Adverse interaction	*Aspartame,* Ephedra,* Ginseng,* Scotch broom, St. John's wort,* Tyramine-containing foods*
Side effect reduction/prevention	*None known*
Supportive interaction	*None known*
Reduced drug absorption/bioavailability	*None known*

PHENTERMINE
(Fastin, Ionamin, and Others)

Phentermine is a nonamphetamine drug used as a short-term adjunct to calorie restriction for weight loss. Phentermine is available in two forms, phentermine hydrochloride (Fastin and others) and phentermine resin (Ionamin and others).

INTERACTIONS WITH FOODS AND OTHER COMPOUNDS

Food

Phentermine should be taken on an empty stomach.[1]

Alcohol

Phentermine may cause dizziness or blurred vision.[2] Alcohol may intensify these effects, increasing the risk for accidental injury. People taking phentermine should avoid alcohol.

SUMMARY OF INTERACTIONS FOR PHENTERMINE

Depletion or interference	*None known*
Adverse interaction	*None known*
Side effect reduction/prevention	*None known*
Supportive interaction	*None known*
Reduced drug absorption/bioavailability	*None known*

PHENYLPROPANOLAMINE
(PPA, Propagest, Rhindecon, Acutrim, Dexatrim, Dex-A-Diet, Unitrol, and Others)

Phenylpropanolamine is a drug used to relieve nasal congestion due to colds, hay fever, upper respiratory allergies, and sinusitis. It is available in nonprescription products alone (Propagest, Rhindecon, and others) and in combination with other nonprescription drugs, to treat symptoms of allergy, colds, and upper respiratory infections, including:

- Phenylpropanolamine/**brompheniramine** (page 31) (Dimetapp, DayQuil Allergy Relief, and others)
- Phenylpropanolamine/**chlorpheniramine** (page 45) (Contac 12 Hour, Triaminic-12, and others)
- Phenylpropanolamine/**clemastine** (page 52) (Tavist D)
- Phenylpropanolamine/**guaifenesin** (page 105) (Entex LA and others)
- Phenylpropanolamine/**guaifenesin** (page 105)/**dextromethorphan** (page 70) (Robitussin CF and others)

Phenylpropanolamine is also used as an adjunct to calorie restriction in short-term weight loss. It is available in nonprescription products alone (Acutrim, Dexatrim, Dex-A-Diet, Unitrol, and others) and in combination with other ingredients for weight loss, including:

- Phenylpropanolamine/multiple vitamins and minerals (Appedrine)

- Phenylpropanolamine/vitamin C (Dex-A-Diet Plus Vitamin C, Dexatrim Plus Vitamin C)
- Phenylpropanolamine/grapefruit extract (Diadex Grapefruit Diet Plan)

INTERACTIONS WITH HERBS

Ephedra sinica (Ma huang)

Ephedra is the plant from which the drug **ephedrine** (page 83) was originally isolated. Phenylpropanolamine and ephedrine have similar effects and side effects.[1] Ephedra, also called ma huang, is used in many herbal products including supplements promoted for weight loss. While interactions between phenylpropanolamine and ephedra have not been reported, it seems likely that such interactions could occur. To prevent potential problems, people taking phenylpropanolamine-containing products should avoid using ephedra/ephedrine-containing products.

INTERACTIONS WITH FOODS AND OTHER COMPOUNDS

Caffeine

Phenylpropanolamine can increase blood pressure,[2] a danger especially in people with high blood pressure.[3] In a double-blind study of six healthy people, administration of caffeine and phenylpropanolamine produced an additive increase in blood pressure.[4] Additionally, in a study of sixteen healthy people, phenylpropanolamine plus caffeine resulted in higher serum caffeine levels than when caffeine was given alone.[5]

Caffeine (page 33) is found in coffee, tea, soft drinks, chocolate, guaraná *(Paullinia cupana)*, nonprescription drugs, and supplement products containing caffeine or guaraná. People taking phenyl-propanolamine-containing products can minimize the interaction with caffeine by limiting or avoiding caffeine.

SUMMARY OF INTERACTIONS FOR PHENYL-PROPANOLAMINE

Depletion or interference	*None known*
Adverse interaction	***Caffeine*** *(page 33), Ephedra sinica* (Ma huang)*
Side effect reduction/prevention	*None known*
Supportive interaction	*None known*
Reduced drug absorption/bioavailability	*None known*

POTASSIUM CHLORIDE
(Kaochlor, K-Dur, Klorvess, Slow-K, and Others)

Potassium chloride is a prescription drug used to replace potassium in people with low blood levels of potassium, to prevent potassium depletion in specific diseases or resulting from specific drug therapies, and to help lower mild high blood pressure in some people. Potassium chloride is also available without prescription in some supplements and in salt substitutes found in grocery stores. While potassium depletion is a health risk, high levels of potassium are also associated with health risks. Potassium-containing drugs should be used only under medical supervision. The potassium found in fruit is both safe and healthful for most people, except those taking potassium-sparing **diuretic drugs** (page 76) and individuals with kidney failure.

INTERACTIONS WITH DIETARY SUPPLEMENTS

Salt Substitutes

Salt substitutes (No Salt, Morton Salt Substitute, Lite Salt, and others) contain potassium chloride in place of sodium chloride. They are used by people on sodium-restricted diets. When used in moderation, they are a more healthful choice for many people compared with using regular table salt. However, people taking potassium chloride drug products should consult with their prescribing doctor before using salt substitutes[1] or even eating large amounts of high-potassium foods (primarily fruit).

INTERACTIONS WITH HERBS

Digitalis (Digitalis lanata, Digitalis purpurea)

Digitalis refers to a family of plants commonly called foxglove that contain digitalis glycosides, chemicals with actions and toxicities similar to the prescription drug **digoxin** (page 71). Low serum potassium increases the risk of digitalis toxicity.[2] People using digitalis-containing products should have their potassium status monitored by the health-care professional overseeing the digitalis therapy.

INTERACTIONS WITH FOODS AND OTHER COMPOUNDS

Food

Potassium chloride drugs should be taken after meals to avoid stomach upset.[3] Potassium-containing salt substitutes, however, are meant to be taken with food. Tablets should be swallowed whole and chewing or crushing should be avoided.[4] Liquid, powder, and effervescent potassium chloride products may be dissolved in a glass of cold water or juice to mask the unpleasant flavor.[5]

SUMMARY OF INTERACTIONS FOR POTASSIUM CHLORIDE

Depletion or interference	*None known*
Adverse interaction	*None known*
Side effect reduction/prevention	*None known*
Supportive interaction	*None known*
Reduced drug absorption/bioavailability	*None known*
Other (see text)	*Digitalis, Salt substitutes*

PRAVASTATIN
(Pravachol)

Pravastatin is a member of the HMG-CoA reductase inhibitor family of drugs, also called "statins," such as **lovastatin** (page 133) and **simvastatin** (page 189). Pravastatin blocks a key step in the body's production of cholesterol and is used to lower cholesterol levels in people with hypercholesterolemia (high cholesterol).

INTERACTIONS WITH DIETARY SUPPLEMENTS

Coenzyme Q_{10}

In a randomized, double-blind trial, blood levels of coenzyme Q_{10} (CoQ_{10}) were measured in forty-five people with high cholesterol treated with **lovastatin** (page 133) (20 to 80 mg per day) or pravastatin (10 to 40 mg per day) for 18 weeks.[1] A significant decline in blood levels of CoQ_{10} levels was reported with both drugs. Supplementation with 100 mg CoQ_{10} has been shown to prevent reductions in blood levels of CoQ_{10} due to **simvastatin** (page 189).[2] Combining 180 mg CoQ_{10} daily with lovastatin therapy in a double-blind study did not show that adding CoQ_{10} provided significant benefits.[3] In other words, although taking CoQ_{10} may prevent decreased blood levels of CoQ_{10}, it may not otherwise benefit the person taking the supplement. If no adverse effects of lowered blood levels of CoQ_{10} can be demonstrated, then merely bringing the levels back up may not be justified. Until more is known, people taking pravastatin should ask a nutritionally oriented doctor about supplementation with 30 to 100 mg CoQ_{10} per day.

Niacin (Vitamin B₃, Nicotinic Acid)

Niacin is a vitamin used to lower cholesterol. Sixteen people with diabetes and high cholesterol were given pravastatin plus low-dose niacin to lower cholesterol.[4] Niacin was added to a maximum dose of 500 mg 3 times per day for 2 weeks, and the combination of pravastatin plus niacin continued for 4 weeks. Compared with pravastatin, low-dose niacin plus pravastatin resulted in significantly reduced cholesterol. Others have also shown that the combination of pravastatin and niacin is more effective in lowering cholesterol levels.[5] However, high-dose niacin taken with pravastatin might cause serious muscle disorders (myopathy or rhabdomyolysis).[6]

Red Yeast Rice

A supplement containing red yeast *(Monascus purpureus)* rice (cholestin) has been shown to effectively lower cholesterol and triglycerides in people with moderately elevated levels of these blood lipids.[7] This extract contains small amounts of naturally occurring HMG-CoA reductase inhibitors such as **lovastatin** (page 133) and should not be used if you are currently taking lovastatin or pravastatin.

Vitamin A

A study of thirty-seven people with high cholesterol treated with diet and HMG-CoA reductase inhibitors found serum vitamin A levels increased over 2 years of therapy.[8] It remains unclear whether this moderate increase should suggest that people taking lovastatin have a particular need to restrict vitamin A supplementation.

INTERACTIONS WITH HERBS

Milk Thistle *(Silybum marianum)*

One of the possible side effects of pravastatin is liver toxicity. Although there are no clinical studies to substantiate its use with pravastatin, a milk thistle extract standardized to 70 to 80% silymarin may reduce the potential liver toxicity of pravastatin. The suggested use is 200 mg of the extract 3 times daily.

INTERACTIONS WITH FOODS AND OTHER COMPOUNDS

Food

Pravastatin may be taken with or without food.[9]

Grapefruit Juice

A study of grapefruit juice and lovastatin (a drug closely related to pravastatin) reported significantly increased **lovastatin** (page 133) levels in people who drank grapefruit juice compared with water.[10]

This interaction has not yet been reported with pravastatin. Until more is known, it is prudent to avoid grapefruit juice during pravastatin therapy or discuss grapefruit juice intake (before consuming any) with the prescribing doctor. Anyone taking pravastatin and drinking grapefruit juice would require very careful monitoring. The idea of using grapefruit juice to reduce the needed drug dose remains theoretical. The same effects might be seen from eating grapefruit as from drinking its juice.

SUMMARY OF INTERACTIONS FOR PRAVASTATIN

Depletion or interference	Coenzyme Q_{10}
Adverse interaction	Niacin,* Red yeast rice
Side effect reduction/prevention	Milk thistle*
Supportive interaction	Niacin
Reduced drug absorption/bioavailability	None known
Other (see text)	Grapefruit juice, Vitamin A

PRAZOSIN
(Minipress)

Prazosin is a member of the alpha blocker family of drugs used to lower blood pressure in people with hypertension. Prazosin is also used to treat some instances of heart failure.

INTERACTIONS WITH FOODS AND OTHER COMPOUNDS

Food

Prazosin may be taken with or without food.[1]

SUMMARY OF INTERACTIONS FOR PRAZOSIN

Depletion or interference	None known
Adverse interaction	None known
Side effect reduction/prevention	None known
Supportive interaction	None known
Reduced drug absorption/bioavailability	None known

PROMETHAZINE
(Phenergan and Others)

Promethazine is an antihistamine used to relieve allergic rhinitis (seasonal allergy) symptoms including sneezing, runny nose, itching, and watery eyes and itching and swelling associated with uncomplicated allergic skin reactions. It is also used as a sleep aid for surgical procedures and to prevent/treat motion sickness, nausea, and vomiting. Promethazine is available in nonprescription products alone (Phenergan and others) and in the combination promethazine/phenylephrine (Phenergan VC and others) to treat symptoms of allergy, colds, and upper respiratory infections.

Promethazine is also available in prescription products with **codeine** (page 54), to treat coughs associated with colds and upper respiratory infections, including:

- Promethazine/**codeine** (page 54) (Phenergan with Codeine and others)
- Promethazine/phenylephrine/**codeine** (page 54) (Phenergan VC with Codeine and others)

INTERACTIONS WITH HERBS

Henbane *(Hyoscyamus niger)*

Antihistamines, including promethazine, can cause "anticholinergic" side effects such as dryness of mouth and heart palpitations. Henbane also has anticholinergic activity and side effects. Therefore, use with promethazine could increase the risk of anticholinergic side effects,[1] though apparently no interactions have yet been reported with promethazine and henbane. Henbane should not be taken except by prescription from a physician trained in herbal medicine, as it is extremely toxic.

INTERACTIONS WITH FOODS AND OTHER COMPOUNDS

Alcohol

Promethazine causes drowsiness.[2] Alcohol may intensify this effect and increase the risk of accidental injury.[3] To prevent problems, people taking promethazine or promethazine-containing products should avoid alcohol.

SUMMARY OF INTERACTIONS FOR PROMETHAZINE

Depletion or interference	*None known*
Adverse interaction	*Henbane*[*]

Side effect reduction/prevention	None known
Supportive interaction	None known
Reduced drug absorption/bioavailability	None known

PROPOXYPHENE
(Darvon, Darvon-N, and Others)

PROPOXYPHENE-N/ACETAMINOPHEN
(Darvocet N and Others)

PROPOXYPHENE/ASPIRIN/CAFFEINE
(Darvon Compound)

Propoxyphene is a narcotic analgesic used to relieve mild to moderate pain. Propoxyphene is available alone (propoxyphene hydrochloride, Darvon; propoxyphene napsylate, Darvon-N) and in combination with other drugs, including propoxyphene-N/**acetaminophen** (page 2) (Darvocet N and others) and propoxyphene/**aspirin** (page 18)/**caffeine** (page 33) (Darvon Compound).

INTERACTIONS WITH FOODS AND OTHER COMPOUNDS

Food

Propoxyphene may cause gastrointestinal (GI) upset. Propoxyphene-containing products may be taken with food to reduce or prevent GI upset.[1] A common side effect of narcotic analgesics is constipation.[2] Increasing dietary fiber (especially vegetables and whole-grain foods) and water intake can ease constipation.

Alcohol

Propoxyphene may cause drowsiness, dizziness, or blurred vision. Alcohol may intensify these effects and increase the risk of accidental injury.[3] To prevent problems, people taking propoxyphene should avoid alcohol.

SUMMARY OF INTERACTIONS FOR PROPOXYPHENE

Depletion or interference	None known
Adverse interaction	None known

Side effect reduction/prevention	*None known*
Supportive interaction	*None known*
Reduced drug absorption/bioavailability	*None known*
Other (see text)	*Fiber*

PROPRANOLOL
(Inderal)

Propranolol is a beta-blocker drug. Propranolol is used to treat or prevent some heart conditions, reduce the symptoms of angina pectoris (chest pain), lower blood presssure in people with hypertension, and improve survival after a heart attack. Propranolol is sometimes used to prevent migraine headaches, to reduce movement associated with essential tremor, and to reduce performance anxiety.

INTERACTIONS WITH DIETARY SUPPLEMENTS

Coenzyme Q$_{10}$

Propranolol inhibits enzymes dependent on coenzyme Q$_{10}$ (CoQ$_{10}$). In one trial, propranolol-induced symptoms were reduced in people given 60 mg of CoQ$_{10}$ per day.[1]

INTERACTIONS WITH HERBS

Pepper (Piper nigrum, Piper longum)

In a single-dose human study, piperine, a chemical found in black pepper and long pepper, was reported to increase blood levels of propranolol,[2] which could increase the activity and risk of side effects of the drug.

INTERACTIONS WITH FOODS AND OTHER COMPOUNDS

Food

Food increases the absorption of propranolol.[3] Propranolol should be taken at the same time every day, always with or always without food. High-protein foods may interfere with propranolol metabolism, increasing propranolol blood levels and activity.[4]

Alcohol

Propranolol may cause drowsiness or dizziness.[5] Alcohol may intensify this action. To prevent accidental injury, people taking propranolol should avoid alcohol.

Tobacco

In a double-blind study of ten cigarette smokers with angina treated with propranolol for 1 week, angina episodes were significantly reduced during the nonsmoking phase compared with the smoking phase.[6] People with angina taking propranolol who do not smoke should avoid starting. Those who smoke should consult with their prescribing doctor about quitting.

SUMMARY OF INTERACTIONS FOR PROPRANOLOL

Depletion or interference	*Coenzyme Q$_{10}$*[*]
Adverse interaction	*Tobacco*
Side effect reduction/prevention	*Coenzyme Q$_{10}$*[*]
Supportive interaction	*None known*
Reduced drug absorption/bioavailability	*None known*
Other (see text)	*Pepper*

PSYLLIUM

(Effer-syllium, Fiberall, Hydrocil Instant, Konsyl, Metamucil, Modane Bulk, Perdiem Fiber, Reguloid, Serutan, Siblin, Syllact, V-Lax, and Others)

Psyllium is a bulk laxative used for short-term treatment of constipation. It is also used to treat people with irritable bowel syndrome, diverticular disease, and hemorrhoids and to lower cholesterol in people with high cholesterol. Psyllium is available as nonprescription drug products and as herbal dietary supplement products.

There are currently no reported nutrient or herb interactions involving psyllium.

QUINAPRIL

(Accupril)

Quinapril is an **angiotensin-converting enzyme (ACE) inhibitor** (page 1), a family of drugs used to treat high blood pressure and some types of heart failure.

Quinapril

INTERACTIONS WITH DIETARY SUPPLEMENTS

Potassium

ACE inhibitors may increase blood potassium levels.[1] This problem is more likely to occur with advanced kidney disease. Potassium supplements, potassium-containing salt substitutes (No Salt, Morton Salt Substitute, and others), and even foods that are uncommonly high in potassium (primarily fruit) will increase the chances of potentially dangerous elevations in blood potassium. People taking ACE inhibitors should avoid unnecessary potassium supplementation.

Zinc

In a study of thirty-four people with hypertension, 6 months of **captopril** (page 35) or **enalapril** (page 82) (ACE inhibitors related to quinapril) treatment led to decreased zinc levels in certain white blood cells,[2] raising concerns about possible ACE inhibitor–induced zinc depletion. While zinc depletion has not been reported with quinapril, until more is known, it makes sense for people taking quinapril long term to consider, as a precaution, taking a zinc supplement or a multimineral tablet containing zinc. (Such multiminerals usually contain no more than 99 mg of potassium, probably not enough to trigger the above-mentioned interaction.) Supplements containing zinc should also contain copper, to protect against a zinc-induced copper deficiency.

INTERACTIONS WITH FOODS AND OTHER COMPOUNDS

Food

High-fat meals may reduce quinapril absorption;[3] otherwise quinapril may be taken with or without food.[4]

SUMMARY OF INTERACTIONS FOR QUINAPRIL

Depletion or interference	Zinc*
Adverse interaction	Potassium*
Side effect reduction/prevention	None known
Supportive interaction	None known
Reduced drug absorption/bioavailability	None known

RAMIPRIL
(Altace)

Ramipril is an **angiotensin-converting enzyme (ACE) inhibitor** (page 1), a family of drugs used to treat high blood pressure and some types of heart failure.

INTERACTIONS WITH DIETARY SUPPLEMENTS

Potassium

ACE inhibitors may increase blood potassium levels.[1] This problem is more likely to occur with advanced kidney disease. Potassium supplements, potassium-containing salt substitutes (No Salt, Morton Salt Substitute, and others), and even foods that are uncommonly high in potassium (primarily fruit) will increase the chances of potentially dangerous elevations in blood potassium. People taking ACE inhibitors should avoid unnecessary potassium supplementation.

Zinc

In a study of thirty-four people with hypertension, 6 months of **captopril** (page 35) or **enalapril** (page 82) (ACE inhibitors related to ramipril) treatment led to decreased zinc levels in certain white blood cells,[2] raising concerns about possible ACE inhibitor–induced zinc depletion. While zinc depletion has not been reported with ramipril, until more is known, it makes sense for people taking ramipril long term to consider, as a precaution, taking a zinc supplement or a multimineral tablet containing zinc. (Such multiminerals usually contain no more than 99 mg of potassium, probably not enough to trigger the above-mentioned interaction.) Supplements containing zinc should also contain copper, to protect against a zinc-induced copper deficiency.

INTERACTIONS WITH FOODS AND OTHER COMPOUNDS

Food

Food slows the rate of ramipril absorption but not the total amount of drug absorbed.[3]

SUMMARY OF INTERACTIONS FOR RAMIPRIL

Depletion or interference	Zinc*
Adverse interaction	Potassium*
Side effect reduction/prevention	None known
Supportive interaction	None known
Reduced drug absorption/bioavailability	None known

RANITIDINE
(Zantac)

Ranitidine is a member of the H-2 (histamine blocker) family of drugs, which prevents the release of acid into the stomach. Ranitidine is used to treat stomach and duodenal ulcers, gastroesophageal reflux disease, erosive esophagitis, and Zollinger-Ellison syndrome. Ranitidine is available as the prescription drug Zantac and also as a nonprescription over-the-counter product for relief of heartburn.

INTERACTIONS WITH DIETARY SUPPLEMENTS

Iron

Stomach acid may facilitate iron absorption. H-2 blocker drugs reduce stomach acid and are associated with decreased dietary iron absorption.[1] People with ulcers may also be iron deficient due to blood loss and benefit from iron supplementation. Iron levels in the blood can be checked with lab tests.

Magnesium

In healthy volunteers, a **magnesium hydroxide** (page 135)/**aluminum hydroxide** (page 6) antacid, taken with ranitidine, decreased ranitidine absorption by 20 to 25%.[2] It was unclear from this study if magnesium or the specific form of magnesium as magnesium hydroxide was part of the problem. It is not known if other forms of magnesium would cause this problem. People can avoid this interaction by taking ranitidine 2 hours before or after any aluminum/magnesium-containing **antacids** (page 13), including magnesium hydroxide found in some vitamin/mineral supplements.

Vitamin B$_{12}$

Stomach acid is needed to release vitamin B$_{12}$ from food so it can be absorbed by the body. H-2 blocker drugs reduce stomach acid and are associated with decreased dietary vitamin B$_{12}$ absorption.[3]

The vitamin B_{12} found in supplements is available to the body without the need for stomach acid. Lab tests can determine vitamin B_{12} levels.

INTERACTIONS WITH FOODS AND OTHER COMPOUNDS

Food

Ranitidine may be taken with or without food.[4]

Tobacco (*Nicotiana* species)

A study of eighteen healthy people found that smoking decreased the acid blocking effects of ranitidine.[5]

SUMMARY OF INTERACTIONS FOR RANITIDINE

Depletion or interference	*Iron, Vitamin B_{12}*[*]
Adverse interaction	*None known*
Side effect reduction/prevention	*None known*
Supportive interaction	*None known*
Reduced drug absorption/bioavailability	***Magnesium hydroxide** (page 135), Tobacco*

RISPERIDONE
(Risperdal)

Risperidone is a drug used in the management of psychosis disorders.

INTERACTIONS WITH FOODS AND OTHER COMPOUNDS

Food

Risperidone oral solution should be mixed in half a glass of water, coffee, orange juice, or lowfat milk and immediately consumed.[1] It should not be mixed with cola or tea.[2]

Alcohol

Risperidone may cause drowsiness.[3] Alcohol may intensify this effect, increasing the risk of accidental injury. People taking risperidone should avoid alcohol.

SUMMARY OF INTERACTIONS FOR RISPERIDONE

Depletion or interference	*None known*
Adverse interaction	*None known*

Side effect reduction/prevention	*None known*
Supportive interaction	*None known*
Reduced drug absorption/bioavailability	*None known*

SALMETEROL
(Serevent)

Salmeterol is a long-acting, beta-adrenergic bronchodilator drug. It is inhaled by mouth, into the lungs, to treat asthma and prevent bronchospasm. Salmeterol is also used to prevent exercise-induced bronchospasm.

There are currently no reported nutrient or herb interactions involving salmeterol.

SENNA
(Black-Draught, Fletcher's Castoria, Gentlax, Senexon, Senolax, Senokot, Senna-Gen, and Others)

Senna is a laxative used for short-term treatment of constipation. It is available as nonprescription drugs and as herbal products.

INTERACTIONS WITH DIETARY SUPPLEMENTS

Sodium and Potassium

Overuse or misuse of laxatives, including senna, can cause water, sodium, and potassium depletion.[1] To avoid depletion problems, people should limit laxative use, including senna, to 1 week or less.[2]

INTERACTIONS WITH HERBS

Digitalis *(Digitalis lanata, Digitalis purpurea)*

Digitalis refers to a family of plants commonly called foxglove that contain digitalis glycosides, chemicals with actions and toxicities similar to the prescription drug **digoxin** (page 71). While the interaction has not been reported, overuse or misuse of senna (leading to potassium loss) may increase digitalis effects and risk of side effects.[3] Senna and digitalis-containing products should be used only under the direct supervision of a doctor trained in their use.

SUMMARY OF INTERACTIONS FOR SENNA

Depletion or interference	*None known*
Adverse interaction	*None known*
Side effect reduction/prevention	*None known*
Supportive interaction	*None known*
Reduced drug absorption/bioavailability	*None known*
Other (see text)	*Digitalis, Potassium, Sodium*

SERTRALINE
(Zoloft)

Sertraline is a member of the selective serotonin reuptake inhibitor (SSRI) family of drugs used to treat people with depression.

INTERACTIONS WITH DIETARY SUPPLEMENTS

5-Hydroxytryptophan (5-HTP) and L-Tryptophan

L-tryptophan is an amino acid found in protein-rich foods. Foods rich in L-tryptophan do not cause problems during sertraline use. However, dietary supplements of L-tryptophan (available only by prescriptions from special compounding pharmacies) taken with **fluoxetine** (page 94) (a drug closely related to sertraline) have been reported to cause headache, sweating, dizziness, agitation, restlessness, nausea, vomiting, and other symptoms.[1] The combination of 45 mg DL-tryptophan (a synthetic variation of L-tryptophan) per pound of body weight (high dose) with zimelidine, a drug with a similar action to sertraline, did not cause these side effects in another trial.[2] These contradictory findings show that it remains unclear whether tryptophan causes side effects in people taking sertraline.

Sertraline increases serotonin activity in the brain. 5-HTP and L-tryptophan are converted to serotonin in the brain, and taking one with sertraline may increase sertraline-induced side effects. While no interactions with sertraline and 5-HTP or L-tryptophan have been reported, until more is known, 5-HTP and L-tryptophan should not be taken with any SSRI drug, including sertraline.

Sodium

SSRI drugs, including sertraline, have been reported to cause sodium depletion.[3] [4] [5] The risk for SSRI-induced sodium depletion appears to be increased during the first few weeks of treatment in women, the elderly, and people also using **diuretics** (page 76). Doctors prescribing SSRI drugs, including sertraline, should monitor their patients for signs of sodium depletion.

INTERACTIONS WITH HERBS

Ginkgo (Ginkgo biloba)

In three men and two women treated with SSRI drugs (**fluoxetine** [page 94] or sertraline) for depression who experienced sexual dysfunction, addition of ginkgo biloba extract (GBE) in the amount of 240 mg per day effectively reversed the sexual dysfunction.[6] In part, this makes sense because ginkgo has been reported to help men with some forms of impotence.[7]

St. John's Wort (Hypericum perforatum)

One report described a case of serotonin syndrome in an individual who took St. John's wort and **trazodone** (page 212), a weak SSRI drug.[8] The person reportedly experienced mental confusion, muscle twitching, sweating, flushing, and ataxia. In another case, a person experienced grogginess, lethargy, nausea, weakness, and fatigue after taking one dose of **paroxetine** (page 165) (Paxil, another SSRI drug) after 10 days of St. John's wort use.[9]

INTERACTIONS WITH FOODS AND OTHER COMPOUNDS

Food

Results of two nonblinded randomized studies in healthy people suggest sertraline may be taken with or without food.[10]

Alcohol

SSRI drugs, including sertraline, may cause dizziness or drowsiness.[11] Alcohol may intensify these effects and increase the risk of accidental injury. Alcohol should be avoided during sertraline therapy.

SUMMARY OF INTERACTIONS FOR SERTRALINE

Depletion or interference	Sodium
Adverse interaction	5-Hydroxytryptophan (5-HTP), L-tryptophan, St. John's wort
Side effect reduction/prevention	Ginkgo
Supportive interaction	None known
Reduced drug absorption/bioavailability	None known

SIMETHICONE
(Gas-X, Mylicon, and Others)

Simethicone is a nonprescription drug used for short-term relief of excess gas in the gastrointestinal (GI) tract. It is also used to relieve symptoms of infant colic. Simethicone is available as a nonprescription product alone (Gas-X, Mylicon, and others) and in combination with nonprescription **antacids** (page 13), for relief of stomach upset, including:

- Simethicone/calcium carbonate/**magnesium hydroxide** (page 135) (Advanced Formula Di-Gel Tablets)
- Simethicone/**aluminum hydroxide** (page 6)/calcium carbonate/**magnesium hydroxide** (page 135) (Tempo tablets)

There are currently no reported nutrient or herb interactions involving simethicone.

SIMVASTATIN
(Zocor)

Simvastatin is a member of the HMG-CoA reductase inhibitor family of drugs that blocks the body's production of cholesterol. Simvastatin is used to lower elevated cholesterol and to reduce the risk of heart attack and death.

INTERACTIONS WITH DIETARY SUPPLEMENTS

Coenzyme Q_{10}

In people with hypercholesterolemia, simvastatin therapy results in decreased serum coenzyme Q_{10} (CoQ_{10}) levels.[1][2] One study found that supplementation with 100 mg of CoQ_{10} prevented declines in CoQ_{10} when taken with simvastatin.[3] Many nutritionally oriented doctors recommend that people taking HMG-CoA reductase inhibitor drugs such as simvastatin also supplement with approximately 100 mg CoQ_{10} per day, although lower doses, such as 10 to 30 mg per day might conceivably be effective in preventing the decline in CoQ_{10} levels.

Niacin

Niacin is the form of vitamin B_3 used to lower cholesterol. High-dose niacin taken with **lovastatin** (page 133) (a drug closely related to sim-

Sodium Bicarbonate

vastatin) or with simvastatin itself may cause muscle disorders (myopathy) that can become serious (rhabdomyolysis).[4] [5] Such problems appear to be uncommon.[6] [7] Moreover, niacin has been successfully combined with statin drugs to reduce cholesterol more effectively than using these drugs without niacin.[8] [9] People taking both simvastatin and niacin should be monitored for muscle disorders by the prescribing physician.

Vitamin A

A study of thirty-seven people with high cholesterol treated with diet and HMG-CoA reductase inhibitors found blood vitamin A levels increased over 2 years of therapy.[10] Until more is known, people taking HMG-CoA reductase inhibitors, including simvastatin, should have blood levels of vitamin A monitored if they intend to supplement vitamin A.

Vitamin E

In a study of seven people with hypercholesterolemia, 8 weeks of simvastatin plus vitamin E 300 IU improved markers of blood vessel elasticity more than simvastatin alone.[11]

INTERACTIONS WITH FOODS AND OTHER COMPOUNDS

Food

Simvastatin may be taken with or without food.[12]

SUMMARY OF INTERACTIONS FOR SIMVASTATIN

Depletion or interference	Coenzyme Q_{10}
Adverse interaction	Vitamin A*
Side effect reduction/prevention	None known
Supportive interaction	Vitamin E*
Reduced drug absorption/bioavailability	None known
Other (see text)	Niacin

SODIUM BICARBONATE

Sodium bicarbonate (baking soda) is used as an **antacid** (page 13) for short-term relief of stomach upset, to correct acidosis in kidney disorders, to make the urine alkaline during bladder infections, and to minimize uric acid crystallization during gout treatment. A prescription sodium bicarbonate product is given by injection to treat metabolic acidosis and some drug intoxications. Sodium bicarbonate is available as a nonprescription drug alone (sodium bicarbonate tablets) or in combination with other nonprescription drugs for short-term treatment of various conditions, including sodium bicarbonate/**aspirin** (page 18)/citric acid (Alka-Seltzer) to treat fever and mild to moderate pain.

INTERACTIONS WITH DIETARY SUPPLEMENTS

Iron

In a study of nine healthy people, sodium bicarbonate administered with 10 mg of iron led to lower iron levels compared to iron administered alone.[1] This interaction may be avoided by taking sodium bicarbonate-containing products 2 hours before or after iron-containing supplements.

SUMMARY OF INTERACTIONS FOR SODIUM BICARBONATE

Depletion or interference	*Iron**
Adverse interaction	*None known*
Side effect reduction/prevention	*None known*
Supportive interaction	*None known*
Reduced drug absorption/bioavailability	*None known*

SPIRONOLACTONE
(Aldactone)

SPIRONOLACTONE/HYDROCHLOROTHIAZIDE
(Aldactazide)

Spironolactone is a potassium-sparing diuretic. **Diuretics** (page 76) cause water loss and are used to treat a variety of conditions, including high blood pressure, heart failure, and diseases of the kidneys and liver. Spironolactone is available as a single agent and in the combination drug product spironolactone/**hydrochlorothiazide** (page 202) (Aldactazide).

INTERACTIONS WITH DIETARY SUPPLEMENTS

Magnesium

Preliminary research in animals suggests that **amiloride** (page 8), a drug similar to spironolactone, may prevent excess magnesium loss.[1] It is unknown if this same effect would occur in humans or with spironolactone. Persons taking more than 300 mg of magnesium per day and spironolactone should consult with a nutritionally oriented doctor as this may lead to potentially dangerous levels of magnesium in the body. The combination of spironolactone and **hydrochlorothiazide** (page 110) would likely eliminate this problem, as hydrochlorothiazide may deplete magnesium.

INTERACTIONS WITH HERBS

Herbs that have a diuretic effect should be avoided when taking diuretic medications, as they may potentiate the effect of these drugs and lead to possible cardiovascular side effects. These herbs include dandelion, uva ursi, juniper, buchu, cleavers, horsetail, and gravel root.[2]

Potassium

As a potassium-sparing diuretic, spironolactone reduces urinary loss of potassium, which can lead to elevated potassium levels. People taking spironolactone should avoid potassium supplements, potassium-containing salt substitutes (Morton Salt Substitute, No Salt, Lite Salt, and others), and even high-potassium foods (primarily fruit). Doctors should monitor potassium blood levels in people taking spironolactone to prevent problems associated with elevated potassium levels.

Sodium

Diuretics (page 76), including spironolactone, cause increased loss of sodium in the urine. By removing sodium from the body, diuretics also cause water to leave the body. This reduction of body water is the purpose of taking diuretics. Therefore, there is usually no reason to replace lost sodium, although strict limitation of salt intake in combination with the actions of diuretics can sometimes cause excessive sodium depletion. On the other hand, people who restrict sodium intake and in the process reduce blood pressure may need to have their dose of diuretics lowered. People taking spironolactone should talk with their prescribing doctor before severely restricting salt.

INTERACTIONS WITH FOODS AND OTHER COMPOUNDS

Food

Food can increase absorption of spironolactone.[3] Spironolactone should be taken at the same time and always with food or always without food, every day for best results. People with questions about spironolactone and food should ask their prescribing doctor or pharmacist.

SUMMARY OF INTERACTIONS FOR SPIRONOLACTONE

Depletion or interference	*None known*
Adverse interaction	*Buchu, Cleavers, Dandelion, Gravel root, Horsetail, Juniper, Magnesium,* Potassium, Uva ursi*
Side effect reduction/prevention	*None known*
Supportive interaction	*None known*
Reduced drug absorption/bioavailability	*None known*
Other (see text)	*Sodium*

STANOZOLOL
(Winstrol)

Stanozolol is a synthetic anabolic steroid related to the natural hormone testosterone. Stanozolol is used to treat hereditary angioedema (episodic swelling of areas of the body).

INTERACTIONS WITH DIETARY SUPPLEMENTS

Iron

Stanozolol was associated with iron depletion in a group of sixteen people.[1] The results suggest that people taking this drug on a regular basis have their iron status monitored by the prescribing doctor. There is insufficient information to recommend routine iron supplementation during stanozolol treatment.

SUMMARY OF INTERACTIONS FOR STANOZOLOL

Depletion or interference	*Iron**
Adverse interaction	*None known*
Side effect reduction/prevention	*None known*
Supportive interaction	*None known*
Reduced drug absorption/bioavailability	*None known*

SULFAMETHOXAZOLE
(Gantanol)

TRIMETHOPRIM/SULFAMETHOXAZOLE
(TMP/SMX, Bactrim, Cotrim, Septra, Uroplus, and Others)

Sulfamethoxazole is a member of the sulfonamide family of **antibiotics** (page 14). It is used for people with infections caused by a variety of bacteria and protozoa. The combination drug product **trimethoprim/sulfamethoxazole (TMP/SMX)** (page 219) is used to treat a wide variety of bacterial infections and some infections due to parasites.

INTERACTIONS WITH DIETARY SUPPLEMENTS

Calcium, Magnesium, Vitamin B_{12}

Sulfonamides, including sulfamethoxazole, can decrease absorption of calcium, magnesium, and vitamin B_{12}.[1] This is generally not a problem when taking sulfamethoxazole for 2 weeks or less. People taking sulfamethoxazole for longer than 2 weeks should ask their prescribing doctor or a nutritionally oriented doctor about nutrient monitoring and supplementation.

Folic Acid, Vitamin B_6, Vitamin K

Sulfonamides, including sulfamethoxazole, can interfere with the activity of folic acid, vitamin B_6, and vitamin K.[2] This is generally not a problem when taking sulfamethoxazole for 2 weeks or less. People taking sulfamethoxazole for longer than 2 weeks should ask their prescribing doctor or a nutritionally oriented doctor about nutrient monitoring and supplementation.

PABA (Para-Aminobenzoic Acid)

PABA may interfere with the activity of sulfamethoxazole. PABA should not be taken with this drug until more is known.

Potassium

TMP/SMX (page 219) has been reported to elevate potassium and other constituents of blood (creatine and BUN).[3] In particular, people with impaired kidney function should be closely monitored by their prescribing doctor for these changes. People taking sulfamethoxazole or TMP/ SMX should talk with their prescribing doctor before taking any potassium supplements or potassium-containing products, such as No Salt, Morton Salt Substitute, Lite Salt, and even high-potassium foods (primarily fruit).

INTERACTIONS WITH FOODS AND OTHER COMPOUNDS

Food

Food may interfere with the absorption of sulfonamides, including sulfamethoxazole. It is best to take sulfamethoxazole on an empty stomach with a full glass of water.[4] [5]

SUMMARY OF INTERACTIONS FOR SULFAMETHOXAZOLE

Depletion or interference	*Calcium,*[*] *Folic acid,*[*] *Magnesium,*[*] *Vitamin B$_6$,*[*] *Vitamin B$_{12}$,*[*] *Vitamin K*[*]
Adverse interaction	*PABA,*[*] *Potassium*
Side effect reduction/prevention	*None known*
Supportive interaction	*None known*
Reduced drug absorption/bioavailability	*None known*

SULFASALAZINE
(Azulfidine)

Sulfasalazine is a member of the sulfonamide drug family. It is used to treat people with ulcerative colitis, Crohn's disease, and rheumatoid arthritis.

INTERACTIONS WITH DIETARY SUPPLEMENTS

Folic Acid

Sulfasalazine decreases the absorption of folic acid.[1] Biochemical evidence of depletion of folic acid has been reported in people taking this drug,[2] although available evidence remains mixed.[3] [4]

Folic acid is needed for the normal healthy replication of cells. Perhaps as a result, there is evidence that folic acid can reverse precancerous changes in humans.[5] Ulcerative colitis, a disease commonly treated with sulfasalazine, is associated with an increased risk of colon cancer. Folate deficiency has also been linked to an increased risk for colon cancer.[6] It is plausible that some of the increased risk for colon cancer in people with ulcerative colitis may be related to folate depletion caused by sulfasalazine.

Folic acid supplementation may help protect against colon cancer specifically.[7] One study found that people who have ulcerative colitis *and* who supplement folic acid had a 55% lower risk of getting colon cancer, compared with people with ulcerative colitis who do not supplement folate (although this dramatic association with protection did not quite reach statistical significance).[8] Researchers at the University of Chicago Medical Center reported a 62% lower risk of colon cancer in folic acid supplementers.[9] They suggest that the link between folic acid supplementation and protection from colon cancer may well be linked with overcoming the folic acid deficiency induced by sulfasalazine.

Until more is known, many nutritionally oriented doctors believe that it is important for all people taking sulfasalazine to supplement folic acid. Folic acid in the amount of 800 mcg can be found in many multivitamins and B-complex vitamins. People wishing to supplement more—typically 1,000 mcg—should consult their nutritionally oriented doctor beforehand.

Iron

Iron can bind with sulfasalazine, decreasing sulfasalazine absorption and possibly decreasing iron absorption.[10] This interaction can be minimized by taking iron-containing products 2 hours before or after sulfasalazine.

PABA (Para-Aminobenzoic Acid)

PABA may interfere with the activity of sulfasalazine. PABA should not be taken with this drug until more is known.

INTERACTIONS WITH FOODS AND OTHER COMPOUNDS

Food

Sulfasalazine is best taken after meals, and it is important to swallow the tablets whole to avoid inactivation by stomach acid.[11]

SUMMARY OF INTERACTIONS FOR SULFASALAZINE

Depletion or interference	Folic acid
Adverse interaction	PABA*
Side effect reduction/prevention	Folic acid*
Supportive interaction	None known
Reduced drug absorption/bioavailability	Iron

SUMATRIPTAN
(Imitrex)

Sumatriptan is a member of the selective serotonin receptor agonist family of drugs used to treat, but not prevent, migraine headaches. Sumatriptan is available in injection, nasal spray, and oral tablet forms.

INTERACTIONS WITH DIETARY SUPPLEMENTS

5-Hydroxytryptophan (5-HTP) and L-Tryptophan

Sumatriptan works by stimulating serotonin receptors in the brain. 5-HTP and L-tryptophan are converted to serotonin in the brain, and taking it with sumatriptan could increase sumatriptan-induced side effects. However, no interactions have yet been reported with sumatriptan and 5-HTP or L-tryptophan.

INTERACTIONS WITH FOODS AND OTHER COMPOUNDS

Food

Sumatriptan tablets may begin to work faster when taken with fluid on an empty stomach at the first sign of migraine.[1] [2]

SUMMARY OF INTERACTIONS FOR SUMATRIPTAN

Depletion or interference	*None known*
Adverse interaction	*5-Hydroxytryptophan (5-HTP), L-tryptophan*
Side effect reduction/prevention	*None known*
Supportive interaction	*None known*
Reduced drug absorption/bioavailability	*None known*

TAMOXIFEN
(Nolvadex and Others)

Tamoxifen is an anti-estrogen drug primarily used to treat women with breast cancer or possibly help prevent breast cancer in women at high risk. It is also used to treat mastalgia and gynecomastia.

INTERACTIONS WITH DIETARY SUPPLEMENTS

Melatonin

In preliminary research, high-dose melatonin was used successfully in combination with tamoxifen in a few people with breast cancer for whom tamoxifen had previously failed.[1] The amounts used in this study should be taken only under the supervision of a doctor of natural medicine.

SUMMARY OF INTERACTIONS FOR TAMOXIFEN

Depletion or interference	*None known*
Adverse interaction	*None known*
Side effect reduction/prevention	*None known*
Supportive interaction	*Melatonin**
Reduced drug absorption/bioavailability	*None known*

TERAZOSIN
(Hytrin)

Terazosin is a member of the alpha blocker family of drugs used to lower blood pressure in people with hypertension. Terazosin is also used to treat some instances of heart failure and symptoms of benign prostatic hyperplasia (BPH).

There are currently no reported nutrient or herb interactions involving terazosin.

TERBINAFINE
(Lamisil)

Terbinafine is an antifungal drug used to treat onychomycosis (fungal infection) of the toenails and fingernails.

INTERACTIONS WITH FOODS AND OTHER COMPOUNDS

Food

Food increases absorption of terbinafine.[1] People taking terbinafine should take it at the same time every day, always with or always without food.

SUMMARY OF INTERACTIONS FOR TERBINAFINE

Depletion or interference	*None known*
Adverse interaction	*None known*
Side effect reduction/prevention	*None known*
Supportive interaction	*None known*
Reduced drug absorption/bioavailability	*None known*

TETRACYCLINE
(Achromycin, Sumycin, and Others)

Tetracycline is a member of the tetracycline family of **antibiotics** (page 14). Tetracycline is used to treat a wide variety of infections and severe acne.

INTERACTIONS WITH DIETARY SUPPLEMENTS

Probiotics

Though there have not been studies specifically showing that taking *Lactobacillus acidophilus* or similar normal gut bacteria or yeasts can prevent diarrhea or nausea due to tetracycline, it is theoretically likely. Most doctors of natural medicine recommend persons taking tetracycline supplement probiotics.

Minerals

Many minerals can decrease the absorption of tetracycline, reducing effectiveness, including aluminum (in **antacids** [page 13]), calcium (in antacids, dairy products, and supplements), magnesium (in antacids and supplements), iron (in food and supplements), zinc (in food and supplements), and others.

Vitamins

Tetracycline can interfere with the activity of folic acid, potassium, and vitamins B_2, B_6, B_{12}, C, and K.[1] This is generally not a problem when taking tetracycline for 2 weeks or less. People taking tetracycline for longer than 2 weeks should ask their prescribing doctor or a nutritionally oriented doctor about supplementation. Taking 500 mg vitamin C simultaneously with tetracycline was shown to increase blood levels of tetracycline in one study.[2]

Berberine-Containing Herbs

Berberine is a chemical extracted from goldenseal *(Hydrastis canadensis)*, barberry *(Berberis vulgaris)*, and Oregon grape *(Berberis aquifolium)*, which has been shown to have antibacterial activity. One double-blind study found that giving 100 mg of berberine at the same time as 500 mg of tetracycline 4 times daily led to a reduction of the efficacy of tetracycline in people with cholera.[3] Berberine may have decreased absorption of tetracycline. Another double-blind trial did not find that berberine interfered with tetracycline in people with cholera.[4] Until more studies are completed to clarify this issue, berberine-containing herbs should not be taken simultaneously with tetracycline.

INTERACTIONS WITH FOODS AND OTHER COMPOUNDS

Food

Tetracycline should be taken on an empty stomach, 1 hour before or 2 hours after any other food, drugs, or supplements, with a full glass of water.[5]

SUMMARY OF INTERACTIONS FOR TETRACYCLINE

Depletion or interference	*Folic acid, Potassium, Vitamin B_2, Vitamin B_6, Vitamin B_{12}, Vitamin C, Vitamin K*
Adverse interaction	*Berberine-containing herbs such as goldenseal, barberry, and Oregon grape*
Side effect reduction/prevention	*None known*
Supportive interaction	*Probiotics,* Vitamin C**
Reduced drug absorption/bioavailability	*Minerals (Aluminum, Calcium, Iron, Magnesium, Zinc)*

THEOPHYLLINE
(Slo-Bid, Slo-Phyllin, Theolair, Theo-Dur, Uniphyl)

AMINOPHYLLINE
(Phyllocontin, Truphylline)

Theophylline and aminophylline are bronchodilator (open lung passages) drugs used to treat people with asthma. Aminophylline is a modified form of theophylline. Theophylline and aminophylline are used systemically (carried in the bloodstream through the body) and have side effects throughout the body. Other drugs, which are inhaled by mouth, are more commonly used to treat asthma because they go directly to the lungs and have fewer side effects.

INTERACTIONS WITH DIETARY SUPPLEMENTS

Potassium and Magnesium

There is preliminary evidence that theophylline can promote potassium and magnesium deficiency.[1] [2] Some doctors of natural medicine have noted a tendency for persons on theophylline to become deficient in these minerals. Therefore it may be necessary to supplement these minerals during theophylline therapy. Consult with a nutritionally oriented doctor to make this determination.

Theophylline

Vitamin B$_6$

Theophylline has been associated with depressed serum vitamin B$_6$ levels in children with asthma[3] and adults with chronic obstructive pulmonary disease.[4] In a short-term study of healthy adults, theophylline reduced serum vitamin B$_6$ levels and supplementation with vitamin B$_6$ (10 mg per day) normalized vitamin B$_6$ levels.[5] Until more is known, some nutritionally oriented doctors believe that it makes sense for people taking this drug to accompany it with 10 mg of vitamin B$_6$.

INTERACTIONS WITH HERBS

Pepper (Piper nigrum, Piper longum)

Piperine is a chemical found in black peppers. A human study found that single doses of piperine could increase blood levels of theophylline.[6] Such an elevation could lead to increased theophylline side effects hypothetically or for dose reductions without loss of drug efficacy. However, further study is required before such conclusions are made. People should not change their theophylline dose without consulting an herbally oriented physician.

Tannin-Containing Herbs

Herbs high in tannins can impair the absorption of theophylline.[7] High-tannin herbs include green tea, black tea, uva ursi (*Arctostaphylos uva-ursi*), black walnut (*Juglans nigra*), red raspberry (*Rubus idaeus*), oak (*Quercus* spp.), and witch hazel (*Hamamelis virginiana*).

INTERACTIONS WITH FOODS AND OTHER COMPOUNDS

Food

Low-carbohydrate, high-protein diets, charbroiled beef, and large amounts of cruciferous vegetables (broccoli, Brussels sprouts, cabbage, and others) can reduce theophylline activity.[8] [9] High-carbohydrate, low-protein diets can increase theophylline activity and side effects.[10] Sustained-release forms of theophylline should be taken on an empty stomach and should not be crushed or chewed.[11] Liquid and non-sustained-release theophylline products are best taken on an empty stomach, but they may be taken with food if stomach upset occurs.[12] People with questions about theophylline and food should ask their prescribing doctor or pharmacist.

Caffeine

Large amounts of **caffeine** (page 33), a substance that is related to theophylline, may increase the activity and side effects of theophylline.[13] Coffee, tea, colas, chocolate, guaraná, and some supplement products contain caffeine. Limiting intake of caffeine-containing beverages and products to small amounts will avoid this interaction.

SUMMARY OF INTERACTIONS FOR THEOPHYLLINE

Depletion or interference	*Magnesium, Potassium, Vitamin B_6*
Adverse interaction	**Caffeine** *(page 33), Pepper**
Side effect reduction/prevention	*None known*
Supportive interaction	*None known*
Reduced drug absorption/bioavailability	*Tannin-containing herbs such as green tea, black tea, uva ursi, black walnut, red raspberry, oak, and witch hazel*

THIAZIDE DIURETICS

Thiazide diuretics are a family of drugs that removes water from the body. They are referred to as potassium-depleting because they cause the body to lose potassium as well as water. Potassium-depleting diuretics also cause the body to lose magnesium. Thiazide diuretics are used to lower blood pressure in people with high blood pressure. **Diuretics** (page 76) are also used to reduce water accumulation caused by other diseases.

Thiazide diuretics include chlorothiazide (Diuril and others), chlorthalidone (Hygroton and others), hydrochlorothiazide (Esidrix, HCTZ, HydroDIURIL, Oretic, and others), and metolazone (Mykrox and Zaroxolyn).

Thiazide diuretics are also combined with other drugs to treat various conditions. The combination products include the following:

- Chlorthalidone/**atenolol** (page 20) (Tenoretic and others)
- Chlorothiazide/**methyldopa** (page 141) (Aldoclor and others)
- Chlorthalidone/**clonidine** (page 53) (Combipres and others)
- Hydrochlorothiazide/**amiloride** (page 8) (Moduretic and others)
- Hydrochlorothiazide/**bisoprolol** (page 31) (Ziac)
- Hydrochlorothiazide/**captopril** (page 35) (Captozide)
- Hydrochlorothiazide/**enalapril** (page 82) (Vaseretic)
- Hydrochlorothiazide/**hydralazine** (page 109) (Apresazide and others)

- Hydrochlorothiazide/**lisinopril** (page 126) (Zestoretic and Prinizide)
- Hydrochlorothiazide/**methyldopa** (page 141) (Aldoril and others)
- Hydrochlorothiazide/**metoprolol** (page 143) (Lopressor HCT)
- Hydrochlorothiazide/**propranolol** (page 180) (Inderide and others)
- Hydrochlorothiazide/**spironolactone** (page 191) (Aldactazide and others)
- Hydrochlorothiazide/**timolol** (page 209) (Timolide)
- Hydrochlorothiazide/**triamterene** (page 214) (Dyazide, Maxzide, and others)

INTERACTIONS WITH DIETARY SUPPLEMENTS

Calcium

Thiazide diuretics decrease calcium loss in the urine due to actions on the kidneys.[1] As a result, it may be less important for some people taking thiazide diuretics to supplement calcium than for other people.

Magnesium and Potassium

Potassium-depleting diuretics, including thiazide diuretics, cause the body to lose potassium; they may also cause cellular magnesium depletion,[2] although this deficiency may not be reflected by a subnormal blood level of magnesium.[3] Magnesium loss induced by potassium-depleting diuretics can cause additional potassium loss. Evaluating whether potassium loss is increased by magnesium depletion can be difficult. Until more is known, it has been suggested that people taking potassium-depleting diuretics, including thiazide diuretics, should supplement both potassium and magnesium.[4]

People taking thiazide diuretics should be monitored by their prescribing doctor, who will prescribe potassium supplements if needed. Fruit is high in potassium, and increasing fruit intake is another way of supplementing potassium. Nutritionally oriented doctors often suggest 300 to 400 mg of magnesium per day.

Vitamin D

The reduction in urinary calcium loss resulting from treatment with thiazide diuretics is due primarily to changes in kidney function and may also be due, in part, to changes in vitamin D metabolism.[5]

Zinc

Thiazide diuretics can increase urinary zinc loss.[6]

Sodium

Diuretics, including thiazide diuretics, cause increased loss of sodium in the urine. By removing sodium from the body, diuretics also cause water to leave the body. This reduction of body water is the purpose of taking diuretics. Therefore, there is usually no reason to replace lost sodium, although strict limitation of salt intake in combination with the actions of diuretics can sometimes cause excessive sodium depletion. On the other hand, people who restrict sodium intake and in the process reduce blood pressure may need to have their dose of diuretics lowered.

INTERACTIONS WITH HERBS

Herbs that have a diuretic effect should be avoided when taking diuretic medications, as they may potentiate the effect of these drugs and lead to possible cardiovascular side effects. These herbs include dandelion, uva ursi, juniper, buchu, cleavers, horsetail, and gravel root.[7]

Digitalis (Digitalis purpurea)

Digitalis refers to a family of plants commonly called foxglove, which contains digitalis glycosides chemicals with actions and toxicities similar to the prescription drug **digoxin** (page 71). Thiazide diuretics can increase the risk of digitalis-induced heart disturbances.[8] Thiazide diuretics and digitalis-containing products should be used only under the direct supervision of a doctor trained in their use.

Ginkgo (Ginkgo biloba)

One case was reported in which ginkgo use was associated with high blood pressure in a person treated with a thiazide diuretic.[9] It was not proven that ginkgo was the cause of this reaction.

Licorice (Glycyrrhiza glabra)

Licorice may potentiate the side effects of potassium-depleting diuretics, including thiazide diuretics.[10] Thiazide diuretics and licorice should be used together only under careful medical supervision. Deglycyrrhizinated licorice (DGL) may be used safely with all diuretics.

INTERACTIONS WITH FOODS AND OTHER COMPOUNDS

Food

Thiazide diuretics may be taken with food to avoid stomach upset.[11]

SUMMARY OF INTERACTIONS FOR THIAZIDE DIURETICS

Depletion or interference	*Magnesium, Potassium, Zinc*
Adverse interaction	*Buchu, Cleavers, Dandelion, Digitalis, Ginkgo,* Gravel root, Horsetail, Juniper, Licorice, Uva ursi*
Side effect reduction/prevention	*None known*
Supportive interaction	*None known*
Reduced drug absorption/bioavailability	*None known*
Other (see text)	*Calcium, Sodium, Vitamin D*

THYROID HORMONES

Thyroid hormones are a family of drugs that include desiccated thyroid (animal thyroid, Armour Thyroid, Thyar), levothyroxine (synthetic levothyroxine, Eltroxin, Levo-T, levothroid, Levoxyl, Synthroid), liothyronine (synthetic liothyronine, Cytomel), liotrix (synthetic levothyroxine/liothyronine, Euthroid, Thyrolar), and thyroglobulin (animal levothyroxine/liothyronine, Proloid).

Thyroid medications are synthetic or animal-derived hormones used to treat people with hypothyroidism (low thyroid function), goiter, and Hashimoto's disease.

INTERACTIONS WITH DIETARY SUPPLEMENTS

Calcium

Thyroid hormones have been reported to increase urinary loss of calcium,[1] although recent research suggests that under most circumstances there may not be reduced bone density associated with taking thyroid hormones.[2] [3] Nonetheless, some doctors of natural medicine suggest that people who supplement thyroid medication for more than a few months consider having 24-hour urinary calcium levels measured. There is not yet proof that calcium supplementation for people taking long-term thyroid medication is either helpful or necessary.

Iron

The body's ability to make its own thyroid hormones is reduced during low-calorie dieting. Iron supplementation (27 mg per day) was reported to help maintain normal thyroid hormone levels in obese people despite a very low-calorie diet.[4] Moreover, iron deficiency has been associated with reduced thyroid function.[5] In this trial, iron supplementation given to iron-deficient women led to increased thyroid function and therefore a decrease in the need for thyroid medication.

Iron deficiency has also been reported to impair the body's ability to make its own thyroid hormones,[6] which could increase the need for thyroid medication. Diagnosing iron deficiency requires a doctor's help.

However, iron supplements may decrease absorption of thyroid hormone medications.[7] People taking thyroid hormone medications should talk with their prescribing doctor or a nutritionally oriented doctor before taking iron-containing products.

Soy

Ingestion of soy products simultaneously with thyroid hormones appears to reduce the absorption of the hormones.[8] To be safe, people taking thyroid medication should not consume soy products within 3 hours of taking their medication.

INTERACTIONS WITH HERBS

Bugleweed *(Lycopus virginicus, Lycopus europaeus)* and lemon balm may interfere with the action of thyroid hormones and should not be used during treatment with thyroid hormones.[9]

INTERACTIONS WITH FOODS AND OTHER COMPOUNDS

Food

Levothyroxine absorption is increased when taken on an empty stomach.[10] Thyroid hormones should be taken an hour before eating, at the same time very day.[11]

SUMMARY OF INTERACTIONS FOR THYROID HORMONES

Depletion or interference	*Calcium*
Adverse interaction	*Bugleweed,*[*] *Lemon balm*[*]
Side effect reduction/prevention	*None known*
Supportive interaction	*None known*
Reduced drug absorption/bioavailability	*Soy*
Other (see text)	*Iron*

TICLOPIDINE
(Ticlid)

Ticlopidine is a platelet inhibiting drug. It is used to prevent stroke and to treat intermittent claudication and other conditions.

INTERACTIONS WITH HERBS

Asian Ginseng *(Panax ginseng)*

Ginseng was associated with vaginal bleeding in two case reports[1] [2] and with a decrease in **warfarin** (page 224) activity in another case study.[3] These reports suggest that ginseng may effect parameters of bleeding and therefore people taking ticlopidine should consult with a physician knowledgeable about botanical medicines before taking Asian ginseng or eleuthero/Siberian ginseng *(Eleutherococcus senticosus)*.

Dan Shen *(Salvia miltiorrhiza)*

Dan shen, a Chinese herb, was associated with increased **warfarin** (page 224) activity in two cases.[4] [5] Although warfarin acts differently from ticlopidine, both affect parameters of bleeding. Until more is known, people taking ticlopidine should use dan shen only under close medical supervision. Sage *(Salvia officinalis)*, a plant relative of dan shen found in the West, has not been not associated with interactions involving warfarin.

Devil's Claw *(Harpagophytum procumbens)*

Devil's claw was associated with purpura (bleeding under the skin) in a person treated with **warfarin** (page 224).[6] As with dan shen, until more is known, caution should be exercised before people taking ticlopidine also take devil's claw.

Garlic *(Allium sativum)*

Garlic has been shown to help prevent atherosclerosis (hardening of the arteries), perhaps by reducing the ability of platelets to stick together.[7] Interfering with the action of platelets results in an increase in the tendency toward bleeding[8] and in theory could dangerously potentiate the effect of ticlopidine. Standardized extracts of garlic have been associated with bleeding in people only on rare occasions.[9] Until more is known, people taking ticlopidine are cautioned to avoid products containing standardized extracts of garlic and to avoid eating more than one clove of garlic daily.

Ginger (*Zingiber officinale*)

Ginger has been shown to reduce platelet stickiness in test tubes. Although there appear to be no reports of interactions with platelet-inhibiting drugs, people should talk with a health-care professional if they are taking a platelet inhibitor and wish to use ginger.[10]

Ginkgo (*Ginkgo biloba*)

Ginkgo extracts may reduce the ability of platelets to stick together, possibly increasing the tendency toward bleeding.[11] In a rat study, a high intake of ginkgo increased the action of ticlopidine in a way that could prove dangerous if the same effect occurred in people.[12] Standardized extracts of ginkgo have been associated with two cases of spontaneous bleeding, although the ginkgo extracts were not definitively shown to be the cause of the problem.[13] [14] People taking ticlopidine should not take ginkgo extracts until more is known about the strength of interaction between these two substances.

Herbs Containing Coumarin Derivatives

Although there are no specific studies demonstrating interactions with platelet inhibitors, the following herbs contain coumarin-like substances that may cause bleeding and therefore interact with ticlopidine. These herbs include dong quai, fenugreek, horse chestnut, red clover, sweet clover, and sweet woodruff.

Quinine (*Cinchona* species)

Quinine, a chemical found in cinchona bark and available as a drug product, has been reported to increase **warfarin** (page 224) activity.[15] Although warfarin and ticlopidine are both considered "blood thinners" they have significantly different actions. Therefore it remains unclear whether the reported interaction between quinine and warfarin would occur between ticlopidine and quinine.

Salicylate-Containing Herbs

Like ticolpidine, salicylates interfere with the action of platelets. Various herbs, including meadowsweet *(Filipendula ulmaria)*, poplar *(Populus tremuloides)*, willow *(Salix* spp.), and wintergreen *(Gaultheria procumbens)* contain salicylates. Though similar to **aspirin** (page 18), plant salicylates have been shown to have different actions in test tube studies.[16] Furthermore, salicylates are poorly absorbed and likely do not build up to levels sufficient to cause negative interactions that aspirin might.[17] No reports have been published of negative interactions between salicylate-containing plants and aspirin or aspirin-containing drugs.[18] Therefore concerns about combining salicylate-containing herbs and any drug remain theoretical, and the risk of causing bleeding problems may be low.

INTERACTIONS WITH FOODS AND OTHER COMPOUNDS

Food

Ticlopidine should be taken with food to minimize gastrointestinal upset.[19]

SUMMARY OF INTERACTIONS FOR TICLOPIDINE

Depletion or interference	*None known*
Adverse interaction	*Asian ginseng,* Dan shen, Devil's claw,* Dong quai,* Fenugreek,* Garlic,* Ginkgo,* Horse chestnut,* Quinine,* Red clover,* Salicylate-containing herbs* such as meadowsweet, poplar, willow, and wintergreen, Sweet clover,* Sweet woodruff**
Side effect reduction/prevention	*None known*
Supportive interaction	*None known*
Reduced drug absorption/bioavailability	*None known*
Other (see text)	*Ginger, Eleuthero (Siberian ginseng)*

TIMOLOL
(Blocadren, Timoptic, and Others)

TIMOLOL/HYDROCHLOROTHIAZIDE
(Timolide)

Timolol is a beta-blocker drug used to lower blood pressure in people with hypertension, treat people after heart attacks, and prevent migraine headaches. Timolol is available alone (Blocadren and others) and in the combination timolol/**hydrochlorothiazide** (page 202) (Timolide) used to lower blood pressure. Timolol is also available in eye drop and eye gel preparations (Timoptic and others) used to lower high internal eye pressure due to glaucoma and other conditions.

INTERACTIONS WITH DIETARY SUPPLEMENTS

Coenzyme Q₁₀

In a group of sixteen people with glaucoma treated with a timolol eye preparation, 6 weeks of oral coenzyme Q_{10} (90 mg per day) was reported to reduce timolol-induced cardiovascular side effects without affecting intraocular pressure treatment.[1]

INTERACTIONS WITH FOODS AND OTHER COMPOUNDS

Food

Timolol may be taken with or without food.[2]

Alcohol

Timolol may cause drowsiness, dizziness, lightheadedness, or blurred vision.[3] Alcohol may intensify these effects and increase the risk of accidental injury. To prevent problems, people taking timolol should avoid alcohol.

SUMMARY OF INTERACTIONS FOR TIMOLOL

Depletion or interference	*None known*
Adverse interaction	*None known*
Side effect reduction/prevention	*Coenzyme Q₁₀*
Supportive interaction	*None known*
Reduced drug absorption/bioavailability	*None known*

TOBRAMYCIN
(AKTob, Nebicin, Tobrex, TOBI, and Others)

TOBRAMYCIN/DEXAMETHASONE
(Tobradex)

Tobramycin is an "aminoglycoside" **antibiotic** (page 14) used to treat infections caused by many different bacteria. Tobramycin is usually administered by intravenous (IV) infusion, intramuscular (IM) injection, or inhalation. Tobramycin is available in special preparations to treat eye infections, alone (AKTob, Tobrex) and in the combination tobramycin/**dexamthasone** (page 59) (Tobradex).

INTERACTIONS WITH DIETARY SUPPLEMENTS

Minerals

Calcium, magnesium, and potassium depletion requiring prolonged replacement were reported in a child with tetany who had just completed a 3-week course of IV tobramycin.[1] The authors suggest this may have been due to kidney damage related to the drug. Seventeen people with cancer developed calcium, magnesium, and potassium depletion after treatment with aminoglycoside antibiotics, including tobramycin.[2] The authors suggested a possible potentiating action of tobramycin-induced mineral depletion by **chemotherapy** (page 40) drugs, especially **doxorubicin** (page 78) (Adriamycin).

Until more is known, people receiving IV tobramycin should ask their prescribing doctor or a nutritionally oriented doctor about monitoring calcium, magnesium, and potassium and mineral replacement.

Vitamin K

As with many antibiotics, tobramycin can deplete vitamin K.[3][4] It makes sense for people taking tobramycin to supplement vitamin K to protect against drug-induced deficiency. Doctors of natural medicine will sometimes suggest daily intake between several hundred micrograms and one milligram.

SUMMARY OF INTERACTIONS FOR TOBRAMYCIN

Depletion or interference	*Calcium,* * *Magnesium,* * *Potassium,* * *Vitamin K*
Adverse interaction	*None known*
Side effect reduction/prevention	*None known*
Supportive interaction	*None known*
Reduced drug absorption/bioavailability	*None known*

TRAMADOL
(Ultram)

Tramadol is a drug, unrelated to **nonsteroidal anti-inflammatory drugs (NSAIDs** [page 157]**)** or opiates, used to relieve moderate to moderately severe pain.

INTERACTIONS WITH DIETARY SUPPLEMENTS

5-Hydroxytryptophan (5-HTP) and L-Tryptophan

Tramadol, which blocks serotonin reuptake in the brain, has been associated with two cases of serotonin syndrome.[1] [2] 5-HTP and L-tryptophan are converted to serotonin in the brain. While no interactions have yet been reported with tramadol and 5-HTP or L-tryptophan, taking 5-HTP or L-tryptophan with tramadol may increase the risk of tramadol-induced side effects, including serotonin syndrome.

INTERACTIONS WITH FOODS AND OTHER COMPOUNDS

Food

Tramadol may be taken with or without food.[3]

Alcohol

Tramadol may impair mental ability and physical coordination.[4] Alcohol may intensify these effects and increase the risk of accidental injury. People taking tramadol are cautioned to avoid alcohol.

SUMMARY OF INTERACTIONS FOR TRAMADOL

Depletion or interference	*None known*
Adverse interaction	*5-Hydroxytryptophan (5-HTP),*[*] *L-tryptophan*[*]
Side effect reduction/prevention	*None known*
Supportive interaction	*None known*
Reduced drug absorption/bioavailability	*None known*

TRAZODONE
(Desyrel)

Trazodone is a weak serotonin reuptake inhibitor drug with other effects on brain neurotransmittors. It is used to treat people with depression. It is also used to treat people during cocaine withdrawal.

INTERACTIONS WITH HERBS

Digitalis (Digitalis lanata, Digitalis purpurea)

Digitalis refers to a family of plants commonly called foxglove that contain digitalis glycosides, chemicals with actions and toxicities similar to the prescription drug **digoxin** (page 71).

Trazodone was associated with increased serum digoxin levels in one case report.[1] No interactions between trazodone and digitalis have been reported. Until more is known, trazodone and digitalis-containing products should be used only under the direct supervision of a doctor trained in their use.

St. John's Wort (Hypericum perforatum)

Although there have been no interactions reported in the medical literature, it is best to avoid using trazodone with St. John's wort unless you are under the supervision of a qualified health-care professional.

INTERACTIONS WITH FOODS AND OTHER COMPOUNDS

Food

Trazodone should be taken with food.[2]

Alcohol

Trazodone may cause drowsiness or dizziness.[3] Alcohol may compound these effects and increase the risk of accidental injury. To prevent problems, people taking trazodone should avoid alcohol.

SUMMARY OF INTERACTIONS FOR TRAZODONE

Depletion or interference	*None known*
Adverse interaction	*St. John's wort*[*]
Side effect reduction/prevention	*None known*
Supportive interaction	*None known*
Reduced drug absorption/bioavailability	*None known*
Other (see text)	*Digitalis*

TRETINOIN
(Retin-A, Vitinoin, Vesanoid)

Tretinoin is a slightly altered version of vitamin A. Topical tretinoin is available in cream, gel, and liquid forms (Retin-A and others) to treat acne, other skin conditions, and some forms of skin cancer. Tretinoin is also available in oral capsules (Vesanoid) to induce remission in people with acute promyelocytic leukemia.

INTERACTIONS WITH DIETARY SUPPLEMENTS

Vitamin A

Large doses of vitamin A can cause side effects, and oral tretinoin can cause similar side effects. Combining vitamin A with oral tretinoin is likely to increase the risk of side effects. People taking oral tretinoin should avoid vitamin A–containing supplements.

INTERACTIONS WITH FOODS AND OTHER COMPOUNDS

Food

Food enhances absorption of retinoid drugs.[1] Tretinoin capsules (Vesanoid) should be taken with food.

SUMMARY OF INTERACTIONS FOR TRETINOIN

Depletion or interference	*None known*
Adverse interaction	*Vitamin A*
Side effect reduction/prevention	*None known*
Supportive interaction	*None known*
Reduced drug absorption/bioavailability	*None known*

TRIAMTERENE
(Dyrenium)

TRIAMTERENE/HYDROCHLOROTHIAZIDE
(Maxzide, Dyazide)

Triamterene is a potassium-sparing (prevents excess loss of potassium) **diuretic** (page 76) drug. Diuretics increase urinary water loss from the body and are used to treat high blood pressure, congestive heart failure, and some kidney or liver conditions. Triamterene is available as a single agent and in the combination of triamterene/**hydrochlorothiazide** (page 202) (Maxzide and Dyazide).

INTERACTIONS WITH DIETARY SUPPLEMENTS

Calcium

A review of the research literature indicates that triamterene may increase calcium loss.[1] The importance of this information is unclear.

Folic Acid

Triamterene is a weak folic acid antagonist that has been associated with folic acid-deficiency anemia in people already at risk for folic acid deficiency.[2] People treated long term with triamterene, without additional risk for folic acid deficiency, however, were found to have normal folic acid levels and no signs of folic acid deficiency.[3] It remains unclear whether the relationship between triamterene and folic acid is clinically important or requires supplementation.

Potassium

As a potassium-sparing drug, triamterene reduces urinary loss of potassium, which can lead to elevated potassium levels. People taking triamterene should avoid potassium supplements, potassium-containing salt substitutes (Morton Salt Substitute, No Salt, Lite Salt, and others) and even high-potassium foods (primarily fruit). Doctors should monitor potassium blood levels in patients taking triamterene to prevent problems associated with elevated potassium levels.

Sodium

Diuretics (page 76), including triamterene, cause increased loss of sodium in the urine. By removing sodium from the body, diuretics also cause water to leave the body. This reduction of body water is the purpose of taking diuretics. Therefore, there is usually no reason to replace lost sodium, although strict limitation of salt intake in combination with the actions of diuretics can sometimes cause excessive sodium depletion. On the other hand, people who restrict sodium intake and in the process reduce blood pressure may need to have their dose of diuretics lowered. People taking triamterene should talk with their prescribing doctor before severely restricting salt.

INTERACTIONS WITH HERBS

Herbs that have a diuretic effect should be avoided when taking diuretic medications, as they may potentiate the effect of these drugs and lead to possible cardiovascular side effects. These herbs include dandelion, uva ursi, juniper, buchu, cleavers, horsetail, and gravel root.[4]

INTERACTIONS WITH FOODS AND OTHER COMPOUNDS

Food

Triamterene is best taken after meals to avoid stomach upset.[5]

SUMMARY OF INTERACTIONS FOR TRIAMTERENE

Depletion or interference	*Calcium,* Folic acid**
Adverse interaction	*Buchu, Cleavers, Dandelion, Gravel root, Horsetail, Juniper, Potassium, Uva ursi*
Side effect reduction/prevention	*None known*
Supportive interaction	*None known*
Reduced drug absorption/bioavailability	*None known*
Other (see text)	*Sodium*

TRICYCLIC ANTIDEPRESSANTS

Tricyclic antidepressants are used to treat people with depression and less commonly to treat other illnesses.

The tricyclic antidepressant family of drugs includes amitriptyline (Elavil), desipramine (Norpramin), doxepin (Sinequan), imipramine (Tofranil), and others.

INTERACTIONS WITH DIETARY SUPPLEMENTS

B Vitamins

Giving 10 mg per day each of vitamins B_1, B_2, and B_6 to elderly, depressed persons already on tricyclic antidepressants improved their depression and ability to think more than placebo did.[1] The subjects in this study were institutionalized, so it is unclear if these results apply to persons living at home.

L-Tryptophan and Vitamin B_3

Combination of 6 grams per day L-tryptophan and 1,500 mg per day niacinamide (a form of vitamin B_3) with imipramine has shown to be more effective than imipramine alone for people with bipolar disorder.[2] These levels did not improve the effects of imipramine in people with depression. Lower amounts, 4 grams per day L-tryptophan and 1,000 mg per day niacinamide, did show some tendency to potentiate imipramine. The importance of the dose of L-tryptophan was confirmed in other studies, suggesting that if too much L-tryptophan (6 grams per day) is used, it is not beneficial, while levels around 4 grams per day may make tricyclic antidepressants work better.[3] [4]

Coenzyme Q$_{10}$

A number of tricyclic antidepressants have been shown to inhibit enzymes that require coenzyme Q$_{10}$ (CoQ$_{10}$), a nutrient that is needed for normal heart function.[5] It is therefore possible that CoQ$_{10}$ deficiency may be a contributing factor to the cardiac side effects that sometimes occur with tricyclic antidepressants. Until further information is available, some nutritionally oriented practitioners advise people taking tricyclic antidepressants to supplement with 30 to 100 mg of CoQ$_{10}$ per day.

INTERACTIONS WITH HERBS

St. John's Wort

Although there have been no interactions reported in the medical literature, it is best to avoid using tricyclic antidepressants with St. John's wort unless you are under the supervision of a qualified health-care professional.

Tea (*Camellia sinensis*)

Brewed black tea has been reported to cause precipitation of amitriptyline and imipramine in a test tube.[6] If this reaction occurred in the body, it could decrease absorption of these drugs. Until more is known, it makes sense to separate ingestion of tea and tricyclic antidepressants by at least 2 hours.

INTERACTIONS WITH FOODS AND OTHER COMPOUNDS

Alcohol

Tricyclic antidepressants can cause drowsiness and dizziness.[7] Alcohol may intensify these actions, increasing the risk for accidental injury. People taking tricyclic antidepressants should avoid alcohol.

SUMMARY OF INTERACTIONS FOR TRICYCLIC ANTIDEPRESSANTS

Depletion or interference	*CoQ$_{10}$**
Adverse interaction	*St. John's wort**
Side effect reduction/prevention	*None known*
Supportive interaction	*Niacinamide, Vitamin B$_1$, Vitamin B$_2$, Vitamin B$_3$, Vitamin B$_5$, Vitamin B$_6$, Vitamin B$_{12}$, Vitamin B-Complex, L-tryptophan**
Reduced drug absorption/bioavailability	*Tea**

TRIMETHOPRIM
(Proloprim, Trimpex)

TRIMETHOPRIM/SULFAMETHOXAZOLE
(Bactrim, Cotrim, Septra, Uroplus, and Others)

Trimethoprim is an antibacterial drug used to treat people with urinary tract infections. The combination drug product **trimethoprim/sulfamethoxazole (TMP/SMX)** (page 219) is used to treat a wide variety of bacterial infections and some infections due to parasites.

INTERACTIONS WITH DIETARY SUPPLEMENTS

Calcium, Magnesium, Vitamin B$_{12}$

Sulfonamides, including **sulfamethoxazole** (page 194), can decrease absorption of calcium, magnesium, and vitamin B$_{12}$.[1] This is generally not a problem when taking sulfamethoxazole for 2 weeks or less. People taking sulfamethoxazole for longer than 2 weeks should ask their prescribing doctor or a nutritionally oriented doctor about nutrient monitoring and supplementation.

Folic Acid, Vitamin B$_6$, Vitamin K

Sulfonamides, including **sulfamethoxazole** (page 194), can interfere with the activity of folic acid, vitamin B$_6$, and vitamin K.[2] This is generally not a problem when taking sulfamethoxazole for 2 weeks or less. People taking sulfamethoxazole for longer than 2 weeks should ask their prescribing doctor or a nutritionally oriented doctor about nutrient monitoring and supplementation.

   TMP/SMX (page 219) has been rarely associated with folic acid–deficiency anemia.[3] This action may be due to trimethoprim-induced folic acid depletion.[4] Trimethoprim and TMP/SMX should be used with caution in people with folic acid deficiency, for which blood tests are available. Folic acid replacement does not interfere with the antibacterial activity of trimethoprim[5] or TMP/SMX.[6]

Potassium

TMP/SMX (page 219) has been reported to elevate blood potassium and other constituents of blood (creatine and BUN).[7] In particular, people with impaired kidney function should be closely monitored by their prescribing doctor for these changes. People taking trimethoprim or TMP/SMX should talk with the prescribing doctor before taking any potassium supplements or potassium-containing products, such as No Salt, Morton Salt Substitute, Lite Salt, and even high-potassium foods (primarily fruit).

SUMMARY OF INTERACTIONS FOR TRIMETHOPRIM

Depletion or interference	*Calcium,[*] Folic acid,[*] Magnesium,[*] Vitamin B6,[*] Vitamin B12,[*] Vitamin K[*]*
Adverse interaction	*Potassium*
Side effect reduction/prevention	*None known*
Supportive interaction	*None known*
Reduced drug absorption/bioavailability	*None known*

TRIMETHOPRIM/SULFAMETHOXAZOLE, TMP/SMX

(Bactrim, Cotrim, Septra, Uroplus)

The antibiotic combination of **trimethoprim** (page 218) and **sulfamethoxazole** (page 194) (TMP/SMX) is used to treat a wide variety of bacterial infections and some infections due to parasites. Bactrim, Cotrim, and Septra are brand names for products containing identical amounts of TMP/SMX. Bactrim DS and Septra DS contain twice as much TMP and SMX as Bactrim and Septra.

INTERACTIONS WITH DIETARY SUPPLEMENTS

Folic Acid

TMP/SMX has been rarely associated with folic acid–deficiency megaloblastic anemia.[1] This action may be due to trimethoprim.[2] TMP/SMX should be used with caution in people with folic acid deficiency, for which a blood test is available. Folic acid replacement does not interfere with the antibacterial activity of TMP/SMX.[3] People with AIDS-induced pneumonia given TMP/SMX had a worse survival rate when folinic acid, an activated form of folic acid, was added.[4]

PABA (Para-Aminobenzoic Acid)

PABA may interfere with the action of sulfamethoxazole. It should not be taken together with **trimethoprim/sulfamethoxazole** (page 194) until more is known.

Potassium

TMP/SMX has been reported to increase blood potassium above normal levels.[5] Potassium supplements, potassium-containing salt substitutes (No Salt, Morton Salt Substitute, and others), and even high-potassium foods (primarily fruit) can be problematic.

SUMMARY OF INTERACTIONS FOR TRIMETHOPRIM AND SULFAMETHOXAZOLE

Depletion or interference	*Folic acid*[*]
Adverse interaction	*PABA,*[*] *Potassium*
Side effect reduction/prevention	*None known*
Supportive interaction	*None known*
Reduced drug absorption/bioavailability	*None known*

VALPROIC ACID
(Depakene)

DIVALPROEX SODIUM
(Depakote)

SODIUM VALPROATE
(Depakene Syrup)

Valproic acid, divalproex sodium, and sodium valproate are closely related drugs used to control (prevent) seizures in people with epilepsy.

INTERACTIONS WITH DIETARY SUPPLEMENTS

Antioxidants

On the basis of the biochemical actions of valproic acid, it has been suggested that people taking valproic acid should make sure they have adequate intakes of vitamin E and selenium.[1] The importance of supplementation with either nutrient has not yet been tested, however.

Carnitine

Valproic acid has been reported to cause carnitine deficiency in children,[2] which may be corrected with carnitine supplementation.[3]

Carnitine (50 mg per 2.2 pounds of body weight) supplementation has protected children from valproic acid–induced increases in blood ammonia levels.[4] A double-blind, crossover study found that carnitine (100 mg per 2.2 pounds of body weight) supplementation was no more effective than placebo in improving the sense of well-being in children treated with valproic acid.[5] The benefit of carnitine supplementation for people taking valproic acid remains unresolved.[6]

Copper and Zinc

In various studies of children treated with valproic acid for epilepsy compared with control groups, serum zinc levels remained normal[7] [8] or decreased,[9] serum copper levels remained normal[10] [11] or decreased,[12] and red blood cell zinc levels were decreased.[13] The importance of these changes and how frequently they occur remain unclear.

INTERACTIONS WITH FOODS AND OTHER COMPOUNDS

Food

Valproic acid, valproate, and divalproex may be taken with food to avoid/reduce stomach upset.[14] Capsules, tablets, and sprinkles containing these drugs should not be chewed, to avoid mouth and throat irritation.[15]

Alcohol

Valproic acid, valproate, and divalproex may all cause drowsiness and dizziness.[16] Alcohol may intensify these actions and increase the risk of accidental injury. People taking valproic acid, valproate, or divalproex should avoid alcohol.

SUMMARY OF INTERACTIONS FOR VALPROIC ACID

Depletion or interference	*Carnitine, Copper**
Adverse interaction	*None known*
Side effect reduction/prevention	*Carnitine**
Supportive interaction	*None known*
Reduced drug absorption/bioavailability	*None known*
Other (see text)	*Antioxidants (Selenium, Vitamin E), Zinc*

VENLAFAXINE

(Effexor)

Venlafaxine is a drug used to treat depression. It is unrelated to other drugs used to treat depression.

INTERACTIONS WITH DIETARY SUPPLEMENTS

5-Hydroxytryptophan (5-HTP) and L-Tryptophan

Venlafaxine, a potent serotonin reuptake inhibitor, has been associated with several cases of serotonin syndrome.[1][2][3][4] 5-HTP and L-tryptophan are converted to serotonin in the brain, and taking it with venlafaxine may increase venlafaxine-induced side effects. While no interactions with venlafaxine and 5-HTP or L-tryptophan have been reported, until more is known, people taking venlafaxine are cautioned to avoid 5-HTP or L-tryptophan.

Sodium

One case was reported of a 79-year-old woman with depression treated with venlafaxine who experienced hyponatremia (abnormally low blood levels of sodium).[5] It remains unclear whether this interaction has any but rare ramifications.

INTERACTIONS WITH HERBS

St. John's Wort (Hypericum perforatum)

Although there have been no interactions reported in the medical literature, it is best to avoid using venlafaxine with St. John's wort unless you are under the supervision of a qualified health-care professional.

INTERACTIONS WITH FOODS AND OTHER COMPOUNDS

Food

Venlafaxine is recommended to be taken with food.[6]

Alcohol

Venlafaxine may cause dizziness or drowsiness.[7] Alcohol may intensify these effects and increase the risk of accidental injury.[8] To prevent problems, people taking venlafaxine should avoid alcohol.

SUMMARY OF INTERACTIONS FOR VENLAFAXINE

Depletion or interference	*None known*
Adverse interaction	*5-Hydroxytryptophan (5-HTP),* * *L-tryptophan,* * *St. John's wort* *

Side effect reduction/prevention	*None known*
Supportive interaction	*None known*
Reduced drug absorption/bioavailability	*None known*
Other (see text)	*Sodium*

VERAPAMIL
(Calan, Isoptin, Verelan)

Verapamil is one of the calcium channel blocker drugs used to treat angina pectoris, heart arrhythmias, and high blood pressure (hypertension).

INTERACTIONS WITH DIETARY SUPPLEMENTS

Calcium

Calcium supplementation has been reported to reverse the blood pressure-lowering actions of this drug when used to treat arrhythmias.[1] [2] It remains unclear whether people taking verapamil for the purpose of lowering blood pressure should avoid calcium supplementation. These people should discuss the matter with the prescribing doctor.

On the other hand, people who take verapamil to treat other conditions, such as angina or heart arrhythmias, should discuss with their physicians the possibility of using low-level (as little as 27 mg per day) calcium supplementation, to reduce excessive blood pressure–lowering actions caused by verapamil in those who do not have high blood pressure.[3]

Vitamin D

Vitamin D may interfere with the effectiveness of verapamil.[4] People taking verapamil should ask their prescribing doctor or a nutritionally oriented doctor before using vitamin D–containing supplements.

Fluid and Fiber

Constipation is a common side effect of verapamil treatment.[5] Increasing fluid and fiber intake can ease constipation.

INTERACTIONS WITH FOODS AND OTHER COMPOUNDS

Grapefruit Juice

Grapefruit juice may increase verapamil blood levels.[6] The importance of this interaction regarding verapamil effectiveness and side effects is unknown. Until more is known, it makes sense for people taking this drug to either avoid drinking grapefruit juice entirely or drink grapefruit juice only under the careful monitoring and supervision of the prescribing doctor. In theory, this last possibility might allow for a decrease in drug dose, but it could be dangerous in the absence of diligent monitoring. The same effects might be seen from eating grapefruit as from drinking its juice.

SUMMARY OF INTERACTIONS FOR VERAPAMIL

Depletion or interference	*None known*
Adverse interaction	*Calcium (for people with high blood pressure), Vitamin D**
Side effect reduction/prevention	*Calcium (for people with high blood pressure), Fiber, Fluid*
Supportive interaction	*None known*
Reduced drug absorption/bioavailability	*None known*
Other (see text)	*Grapefruit juice*

WARFARIN
(Coumadin)

Warfarin is an anticoagulant (slows blood clotting) used to prevent and treat people with venous thrombosis (blood clots in the veins) and pulmonary embolism (blood clots in the lungs). Warfarin is also used to treat or prevent dangerous blood clotting in people with atrial fibrillation (an irregularity in heartbeat) and in some cases to prevent stroke.

INTERACTIONS WITH DIETARY SUPPLEMENTS

Bromelain

In theory, bromelain might potentiate the action of anticoagulants. This theoretical concern has not yet been substantiated by human research, however.[1]

Coenzyme Q_{10}

Coenzyme Q_{10} (CoQ_{10}) is structurally similar to vitamin K and has been reported to interfere with warfarin activity.[2] It remains unknown how common or rare this interaction is. Those taking warfarin should only take CoQ_{10} with the guidance of their doctor.

Minerals

Iron, magnesium, and zinc may bind with warfarin, potentially decreasing their absorption and activity.[3] People on warfarin therapy should take warfarin and iron/magnesium/zinc-containing products at least 2 hours apart.

Vitamin C

Although case reports have suggested that vitamin C might increase the activity of anticoagulants in a potentially dangerous way, this interaction has not been confirmed in research studies.[4]

Vitamin D

In 1975, a single letter to the *Journal of the American Medical Association* suggested that vitamin D increases the activity of anticoagulants and that this interaction could prove dangerous.[5] Perhaps because vitamin D is in multivitamins taken by tens of millions of people and other reports of problems have not surfaced, most doctors typically do not tell people taking anticoagulant medications to avoid vitamin D.

Vitamin E

An isolated case was reported in 1974 of vitamin E (up to 1,200 IU per day) associated with increased anticoagulation in a person treated with warfarin.[6] More recently, a double-blind, randomized trial found warfarin activity was unchanged in people treated with warfarin when given vitamin E (up to 1,200 per day) or placebo.[7] It now appears safe for people taking warfarin to supplement vitamin E despite the information often provided by doctors about this purported interaction to the contrary, based on the isolated case report from 1974.

Vitamin K

Warfarin slows blood clotting by interfering with vitamin K activity. People taking warfarin should avoid vitamin K–containing supplements unless specifically directed otherwise by their prescribing doctor. Some vegetables (broccoli, Brussels sprouts, kale, parsley, spinach, and others) are high in vitamin K. Eating large quantities[8] or making sudden changes in the amounts eaten of these vegetables can interfere with the effectiveness and safety of warfarin therapy.

Vitamin K supplementation can be used, however, to counteract the actions of excessive doses of anticoagulants such as warfarin.[9] Such administration requires the supervision of a doctor.

INTERACTIONS WITH HERBS

Asian Ginseng (*Panax ginseng*)

Ginseng was associated with vaginal bleeding in two case reports[10] [11] and with a decrease in warfarin activity in another case report.[12] Persons taking warfarin should consult with a physician knowledgeable about botanical medicines if they are considering taking Asian ginseng or eleuthero/Siberian ginseng (*Eleutherococcus senticosus*).

Dan Shen (*Salvia miltiorrhiza*)

Dan shen, a Chinese herb, was associated with increased warfarin activity in two cases.[13] [14] Dan shen should only be used under close medical supervision by people taking warfarin. Sage (*Salvia officinalis*), a plant relative of dan shen found in the West, is not associated with interactions involving warfarin.

Devil's Claw (*Harpagophytum procumbens*)

Devil's claw was associated with purpura (bleeding under the skin) in a person treated with warfarin.[15]

Garlic (*Allium sativum*)

Garlic has been shown to help prevent atherosclerosis (hardening of the arteries), perhaps by reducing the ability of platelets to stick together.[16] This can result in an increase in the tendency toward bleeding.[17] Standardized extracts have been associated with bleeding in people on rare occasions.[18] Garlic extracts have also been associated with two human cases of increased warfarin activity.[19] The extracts were not definitively shown to be the cause of the problem. Until more is known, people taking warfarin are cautioned to avoid products containing standardized extracts of garlic and to avoid eating more than one clove of garlic daily.

Ginger (*Zingiber officinale*)

Ginger has been shown to reduce platelet stickiness in test tubes. Although there are no reports of interactions with anticoagulant drugs, people should discuss it with a health-care professional if they are taking an anticoagulant and wish to use ginger.[20]

Ginkgo (*Ginkgo biloba*)

Ginkgo extracts may reduce the ability of platelets to stick together, possibly increasing the tendency toward bleeding.[21] Standardized extracts of ginkgo have been associated with two cases of spontaneous bleeding, although the ginkgo extracts were not definitively shown to be the cause of the problem.[22] [23] There is one case report of a person taking warfarin in whom bleeding occurred after the addition of ginkgo.[24] People taking warfarin should consult with a physician knowledgeable about botanical medicines if they are considering taking ginkgo.

Herbs Containing Coumarin Derivatives

Although there are no specific studies demonstrating interactions with anticoagulants, the following herbs contain coumarin-like substances that may interact with warfarin and may cause bleeding.[25] These herbs include dong quai, fenugreek, horse chestnut, red clover, sweet clover, and sweet woodruff. People should consult their health-care professional if they're taking an anticoagulant and wish to use one of these herbs.

Quinine (*Cinchona* species)

Quinine, a chemical found in cinchona bark and available as a drug product, has been reported to increase warfarin activity.[26] People should read labels for quinine/cinchona content. People taking warfarin should avoid quinine-containing products.

INTERACTIONS WITH FOODS AND OTHER COMPOUNDS

Food

Some vegetables (broccoli, Brussels sprouts, kale, parsley, spinach, and others) are high in vitamin K. Eating large quantities,[27] or making sudden changes in the amounts eaten of these vegetables, interferes with the effectiveness and safety of warfarin therapy. Eating char-broiled food may decrease warfarin activity[28] while eating soy meal foods and cooked onions may increase warfarin activity.[29] The significance of these last two interactions remains unclear.

Papaya (*Carica papaya*)

Papain, an enzyme extract of papaya, was associated with increased warfarin activity in one person.[30] Persons taking warfarin should consult with a physician knowledgeable about botanical medicines if they are considering taking papain-containing products.

Alcohol

Alcohol use, especially long-term heavy drinking, can decrease the effectiveness of warfarin.[31] People taking warfarin are cautioned to avoid alcohol.

SUMMARY OF INTERACTIONS FOR WARFARIN

Depletion or interference	*None known*
Adverse interaction	*Asian ginseng,* Dan shen, Devil's claw,* Dong quai,* Fenugreek,* Garlic,* Ginger,* Ginkgo,* Horse chestnut,* Papaya (papain),* Quinine,* Red clover,* Sweet clover,* Sweet woodruff,* Vitamin D,* Vitamin K*
Side effect reduction/prevention	*None known*
Supportive interaction	*None known*

Reduced drug absorption/bioavailability	*Coenzyme Q_{10}, Iron,* Magnesium,* Zinc**
Other (see text)	*Bromelain, Eleuthero (Siberian ginseng), Vitamin C, Vitamin E*

ZOLPIDEM
(Ambien)

Zolpidem is a hypnotic drug used for short-term treatment of people with insomnia.

INTERACTIONS WITH DIETARY SUPPLEMENTS

5-Hydroxytryptophan (5-HTP) and L-Tryptophan

Nine cases of zolpidem-induced hallucinations associated with serotonin reuptake inhibiting antidepressants have been reported, some lasting for several hours.[1] 5-HTP and L-tryptophan are converted to serotonin in the brain, and taking it with zolpidem may increase zolpidem-induced hallucinations, though no interactions have yet been reported with zolpidem and 5-HTP or L-tryptophan.

INTERACTIONS WITH FOODS AND OTHER COMPOUNDS

Food

Food may interfere with zolpidem absorption and slow the onset of sleep.[2] Zolpidem should be taken 1 hour before or 2 hours after food to avoid this interaction.

Alcohol

Zolpidem causes drowsiness. Alcohol may compound this effect and increase the risk of accidental injury.[3] To prevent problems, people taking zolpidem should avoid alcohol.

SUMMARY OF INTERACTIONS FOR ZOLPIDEM

Depletion or interference	*None known*
Adverse interaction	*5-Hydroxytryptophan (5-HTP),* L-tryptophan**
Side effect reduction/prevention	*None known*
Supportive interaction	*None known*
Reduced drug absorption/bioavailability	*None known*

Appendix I

COMBINATION DRUGS

ALDACTAZIDE

This drug is a combination of two or more active ingredients. Please refer to each of the ingredients for information about nutrient interactions: **Hydrochlorothiazide** (page 202); **Spironolactone** (page 191).

ALDOCLOR

This drug is a combination of two or more active ingredients. Please refer to each of the ingredients for information about nutrient interactions: **Chlorothiazide** (page 202); **Methyldopa** (page 141).

ALDORIL

This drug is a combination of two or more active ingredients. Please refer to each of the ingredients for information about nutrient interactions: **Hydrochlorothiazide** (page 202); **Methyldopa** (page 141).

ALKA-SELTZER

This drug is a combination of two or more active ingredients. Please refer to each of the ingredients for information about nutrient interactions: **Aspirin** (page 18); Citric acid; **Sodium bicarbonate** (page 190).

ALKA-SELTZER PLUS

This drug is a combination of two or more active ingredients. Please refer to each of the ingredients for information about nutrient interactions: **Acetaminophen** (page 2); **Pseudoephedrine** (page 83); **Chlorpheniramine** (page 45).

ANACIN

This drug is a combination of two or more active ingredients. Please refer to each of the ingredients for information about nutrient interactions: **Aspirin** (page 18); **Caffeine** (page 33).

APPEDRINE

This drug is a combination of two or more active ingredients. Please refer to each of the ingredients for information about nutrient interactions: Multiple vitamins and minerals; **Phenylpropanolamine** (page 172).

APRESAZIDE

This drug is a combination of two or more active ingredients. Please refer to each of the ingredients for information about nutrient interactions: **Hydralazine** (page 109); **Hydrochlorothiazide** (page 202).

CALCIUM RICH ROLAIDS

This drug is a combination of two or more active ingredients. Please refer to each of the ingredients for information about nutrient interactions: Calcium carbonate; **Magnesium hydroxide** (page 135).

CAPTOZIDE

This drug is a combination of two or more active ingredients. Please refer to each of the ingredients for information about nutrient interactions: **Captopril** (page 35); **Hydrochlorothiazide** (page 202).

CHLOR-TRIMETON 12 HOUR

This drug is a combination of two or more active ingredients. Please refer to each of the ingredients for information about nutrient interactions: **Chlorpheniramine** (page 45); **Pseudoephedrine** (page 83).

CLARITIN-D

This drug is a combination of two or more active ingredients. Please refer to each of the ingredients for information about nutrient interactions: **Loratadine** (page 131); **Pseudoephedrine** (page 83).

COMBIPRES

This drug is a combination of two or more active ingredients. Please refer to each of the ingredients for information about nutrient interactions: **Chlorthalidone** (page 202); **Clonidine** (page 53).

COMBIVENT

This drug is a combination of two or more active ingredients. Please refer to each of the ingredients for information about nutrient interactions: **Albuterol** (page 4); **Ipratropium Bromide** (page 118).

CONTAC 12 HOUR

This drug is a combination of two or more active ingredients. Please refer to each of the ingredients for information about nutrient interactions: **Chlorpheniramine** (page 45); **Phenylpropanolamine** (page 172).

COSOPT

This drug is a combination of two or more active ingredients. Please refer to each of the ingredients for information about nutrient interactions: **Dorzolamide** (page 78); **Timolol** (page 209).

DARVOCET

This drug is a combination of two or more active ingredients. Please refer to each of the ingredients for information about nutrient interactions: **Acetaminophen** (page 2); **Propoxyphene** (page 179).

DARVOCET N

This drug is a combination of two or more active ingredients. Please refer to each of the ingredients for information about nutrient interactions: **Acetaminophen** (page 2); **Propoxyphene-N** (page 179).

DARVON COMPOUND

This drug is a combination of two or more active ingredients. Please refer to each of the ingredients for information about nutrient interactions: **Aspirin** (page 18); **Caffeine** (page 33); **Propoxyphene** (page 179).

Combination Drugs

DAYQUIL ALLERGY RELIEF

This drug is a combination of two or more active ingredients. Please refer to each of the ingredients for information about nutrient interactions: **Brompheniramine** (page 31); **Phenylpropanolamine** (page 172).

DEX-A-DIET PLUS VITAMIN C

This drug is a combination of two or more active ingredients. Please refer to each of the ingredients for information about nutrient interactions: **Phenylpropanolamine** (page 172); Vitamin C.

DEXATRIM PLUS VITAMIN C

This drug is a combination of two or more active ingredients. Please refer to each of the ingredients for information about nutrient interactions: **Phenylpropanolamine** (page 172); Vitamin C.

DI-GEL TABLETS, ADVANCED FORMULA

This drug is a combination of two or more active ingredients. Please refer to each of the ingredients for information about nutrient interactions: Calcium carbonate; **Magnesium hydroxide** (page 135); **Simethicone** (page 189).

DIADEX GRAPEFRUIT DIET PLAN

This drug is a combination of two or more active ingredients. Please refer to each of the ingredients for information about nutrient interactions: Grapefruit extract; **Phenylpropanolamine** (page 172).

DIMETAPP

This drug is a combination of two or more active ingredients. Please refer to each of the ingredients for information about nutrient interactions: **Brompheniramine** (page 31); **Phenylpropanolamine** (page 172).

DYAZIDE

This drug is a combination of two or more active ingredients. Please refer to each of the ingredients for information about nutrient interactions: **Hydrochlorothiazide** (page 202); **Triamterene** (page 214).

EMPIRIN WITH CODEINE

This drug is a combination of two or more active ingredients. Please refer to each of the ingredients for information about nutrient interactions: **Aspirin** (page 18); **Codeine** (page 54).

ENTEX LA

This drug is a combination of two or more active ingredients. Please refer to each of the ingredients for information about nutrient interactions: **Guaifenesin** (page 105); **Phenylpropanolamine** (page 172).

EXCEDRIN PM

This drug is a combination of two or more active ingredients. Please refer to each of the ingredients for information about nutrient interactions: **Acetaminophen** (page 2); **Diphenhydramine** (page 75).

HELIDAC

This drug is a combination of two or more active ingredients. Please refer to each of the ingredients for information about nutrient interactions: **Bismuth subsalicylate** (page 30); **Metronidazole** (page 144); **Tetracycline** (page 199).

INDERIDE

This drug is a combination of two or more active ingredients. Please refer to each of the ingredients for information about nutrient interactions: **Hydrochlorothiazide** (page 202); **Propranolol** (page 180).

LOPRESSOR HCT

This drug is a combination of two or more active ingredients. Please refer to each of the ingredients for information about nutrient interactions: **Hydrochlorothiazide** (page 202); **Metoprolol** (page 143).

LORTAB

This drug is a combination of two or more active ingredients. Please refer to each of the ingredients for information about nutrient interactions: **Acetaminophen** (page 2); **Hydrocodone** (page 110).

Combination Drugs

MAALOX

This drug is a combination of two or more active ingredients. Please refer to each of the ingredients for information about nutrient interactions: **Aluminum hydroxide** (page 6); **Magnesium hydroxide** (page 135).

MAXZIDE

This drug is a combination of two or more active ingredients. Please refer to each of the ingredients for information about nutrient interactions: **Hydrochlorothiazide** (page 202); **Triamterene** (page 214).

MODURETIC

This drug is a combination of two or more active ingredients. Please refer to each of the ingredients for information about nutrient interactions: **Amiloride** (page 8); **Hydrochlorothiazide** (page 202).

MYLANTA

This drug is a combination of two or more active ingredients. Please refer to each of the ingredients for information about nutrient interactions: **Aluminum hydroxide** (page 6); **Magnesium hydroxide** (page 135).

NYQUIL

This drug is a combination of two or more active ingredients. Please refer to each of the ingredients for information about nutrient interactions: **Acetaminophen** (page 2); **Pseudoephedrine** (page 83); **Doxylamine** (page 81); **Dextromethorphan** (page 70); Alcohol

NYQUIL HOT THERAPY POWDER

This drug is a combination of two or more active ingredients. Please refer to each of the ingredients for information about nutrient interactions: **Acetaminophen** (page 2); **Pseudoephedrine** (page 83); **Doxylamine** (page 81); **Dextromethorphan** (page 70).

PERCOCET

This drug is a combination of two or more active ingredients. Please refer to each of the ingredients for information about nutrient interactions: **Acetaminophen** (page 2); **Oxycodone** (page 163).

PERCODAN

This drug is a combination of two or more active ingredients. Please refer to each of the ingredients for information about nutrient interactions: **Aspirin** (page 18); **Oxycodone** (page 163).

PHENERGAN WITH CODEINE

This drug is a combination of two or more active ingredients. Please refer to each of the ingredients for information about nutrient interactions: **Codeine** (page 54); **Promethazine** (page 178).

PHENERGAN VC WITH CODEINE

This drug is a combination of two or more active ingredients. Please refer to each of the ingredients for information about nutrient interactions: **Codeine** (page 54); Phenylephrine; **Promethazine** (page 178).

PREMPRO

This drug is a combination of two or more active ingredients. Please refer to each of the ingredients for information about nutrient interactions: **Conjugated estrogens** (page 57); **Medroxyprogesterone** (page 137).

PRIMATENE DUAL ACTION

This drug is a combination of two or more active ingredients. Please refer to each of the ingredients for information about nutrient interactions: **Ephedrine** (page 83); **Guaifenesin** (page 105); **Theophylline** (page 200).

PRINIZIDE

This drug is a combination of two or more active ingredients. Please refer to each of the ingredients for information about nutrient interactions: **Hydrochlorothiazide** (page 202); **Lisinopril** (page 126).

ROBITUSSIN AC

This drug is a combination of two or more active ingredients. Please refer to each of the ingredients for information about nutrient interactions: **Codeine** (page 54); **Guaifenesin** (page 105).

Combination Drugs

ROBITUSSIN CF

This drug is a combination of two or more active ingredients. Please refer to each of the ingredients for information about nutrient interactions: **Dextromethorphan** (page 70); **Guaifenesin** (page 105); **Phenylpropanolamine** (page 172).

ROBITUSSIN DM

This drug is a combination of two or more active ingredients. Please refer to each of the ingredients for information about nutrient interactions: **Dextromethorphan** (page 70); **Guaifenesin** (page 105).

ROXICET

This drug is a combination of two or more active ingredients. Please refer to each of the ingredients for information about nutrient interactions: **Acetaminophen** (page 2); **Oxycodone** (page 163).

ROXIPRIN

This drug is a combination of two or more active ingredients. Please refer to each of the ingredients for information about nutrient interactions: **Aspirin** (page 18); **Oxycodone** (page 163).

SOMA COMPOUND

This drug is a combination of two or more active ingredients. Please refer to each of the ingredients for information about nutrient interactions: **Aspirin** (page 18); **Carisoprodol** (page 38).

SOMA WITH CODEINE

This drug is a combination of two or more active ingredients. Please refer to each of the ingredients for information about nutrient interactions: **Aspirin** (page 18); **Carisoprodol** (page 38); **Codeine** (page 54).

TAVIST-D

This drug is a combination of two or more active ingredients. Please refer to each of the ingredients for information about nutrient interactions: **Clemastine** (page 52); **Phenylpropanolamine** (page 172).

Combination Drugs

TEMPO TABLETS

This drug is a combination of two or more active ingredients. Please refer to each of the ingredients for information about nutrient interactions: **Aluminum hydroxide** (page 6); Calcium carbonate; **Magnesium hydroxide** (page 135); **Simethicone** (page 189).

TENORETIC

This drug is a combination of two or more active ingredients. Please refer to each of the ingredients for information about nutrient interactions: **Atenolol** (page 20); **Chlorthalidone** (page 202).

THERAFLU

This drug is a combination of two or more active ingredients. Please refer to each of the ingredients for information about nutrient interactions: **Acetaminophen** (page 2); **Pseudoephedrine** (page 83); **Chlorpheniramine** (page 45).

TIMOLIDE

This drug is a combination of two or more active ingredients. Please refer to each of the ingredients for information about nutrient interactions: **Hydrochlorothiazide** (page 202); **Timolol** (page 209).

TOBRADEX

This drug is a combination of two or more active ingredients. Please refer to each of the ingredients for information about nutrient interactions: **Dexamethasone** (page 60); **Tobramycin** (page 210).

TRIAMINIC-12

This drug is a combination of two or more active ingredients. Please refer to each of the ingredients for information about nutrient interactions: **Chlorpheniramine** (page 45); **Phenylpropanolamine** (page 172).

TYLENOL ALLERGY SINUS

This drug is a combination of two or more active ingredients. Please refer to each of the ingredients for information about nutrient interactions: **Acetaminophen** (page 2); **Pseudoephedrine** (page 83); **Diphenhydramine** (page 75).

Combination Drugs

TYLENOL WITH CODEINE

This drug is a combination of two or more active ingredients. Please refer to each of the ingredients for information about nutrient interactions: **Acetaminophen** (page 2); **Codeine** (page 54).

TYLENOL COLD

This drug is a combination of two or more active ingredients. Please refer to each of the ingredients for information about nutrient interactions: **Acetaminophen** (page 2); **Chlorpheniramine** (page 45); **Dextromethorphan** (page 70); **Pseudoephedrine** (page 83).

TYLENOL FLU NIGHTTIME MAXIMUM STRENGTH POWDER

This drug is a combination of two or more active ingredients. Please refer to each of the ingredients for information about nutrient interactions: **Acetaminophen** (page 2); **Diphenhydramine** (page 70); **Pseudoephedrine** (page 83).

TYLENOL MULTI-SYMPTOM HOT MEDICATION

This drug is a combination of two or more active ingredients. Please refer to each of the ingredients for information about nutrient interactions: **Acetaminophen** (page 2); **Chlorpheniramine** (page 45); **Dextromethorphan** (page 70); **Pseudoephedrine** (page 83).

TYLENOL PM

This drug is a combination of two or more active ingredients. Please refer to each of the ingredients for information about nutrient interactions: **Acetaminophen** (page 2); **Diphenhydramine** (page 75).

TYLENOL SINUS

This drug is a combination of two or more active ingredients. Please refer to each of the ingredients for information about nutrient interactions: **Acetaminophen** (page 2); **Pseudoephedrine** (page 83).

VASERETIC

This drug is a combination of two or more active ingredients. Please refer to each of the ingredients for information about nutrient interactions: **Enalapril** (page 82); **Hydrochlorothiazide** (page 202).

VICODIN

This drug is a combination of two or more active ingredients. Please refer to each of the ingredients for information about nutrient interactions: **Acetaminophen** (page 2); **Hydrocodone** (page 110).

WYGESIC

This drug is a combination of two or more active ingredients. Please refer to each of the ingredients for information about nutrient interactions: **Acetaminophen** (page 2); **Propoxyphene** (page 179).

ZESTORETIC

This drug is a combination of two or more active ingredients. Please refer to each of the ingredients for information about nutrient interactions: **Hydrochlorothiazide** (page 202); **Lisinopril** (page 126).

ZIAC

This drug is a combination of two or more active ingredients. Please refer to each of the ingredients for information about nutrient interactions: **Bisoprolol** (page 31); **Hydrochlorothiazide** (page 202).

Combination Drugs

Appendix 2

DRUG INTERACTIONS BY HERB OR SUPPLEMENT

Interaction notes: The following table lists herb/supplements in the left column. The corresponding columns indicate which drugs the herb/supplement interacts with (either positively and/or negatively). Where (none) is listed, there are no listed interactions for the herb/supplement. Where multiple items are listed for the same herb and the same drug, it is to note the different generic or trade names the generic drug is known by. Where a trade name is followed by a generic name in parentheses, it means the drug is a combination of 2 or more ingredients and the interaction applies to the one listed in parentheses.

DRUG-HERB INTERACTIONS

Herb	Drug with Interaction	Generic or Trade Name(s)
Alfalfa (Medicago sativa)	*(none)*	*(none)*
Aloe (Aloe vera, Aloe barbadensis)	*Corticosteroids*	*AeroBid*
	Corticosteroids	*Aristocort*
	Corticosteroids	*Azmacort*
	Corticosteroids	*Beclomethasone*
	Corticosteroids	*Beclovent*
	Corticosteroids	*Beconase*
	Corticosteroids	*Budesonide*
	Corticosteroids	*Cortef*
	Corticosteroids	*Corticosteroids*
	Corticosteroids	*Cortisone-like drugs*
	Corticosteroids	*Cutivate*
	Corticosteroids	*Decadron*
	Corticosteroids	*Decadron Phosphate Turbinaire*
	Corticosteroids	*Delta-Cortef*
	Corticosteroids	*Deltasone*
	Corticosteroids	*Dexamethasone*

Herb	Drug with Interaction	Generic or Trade Name(s)
Aloe (continued)	Glyburide	Diabeta
	Corticosteroids	Elocon
	Corticosteroids	Flonase
	Corticosteroids	Flunisolide
	Corticosteroids	Fluticasone
	Glyburide	Glibenclamide
	Glyburide	Glyburide
	Corticosteroids	Hydrocortisone
	Corticosteroids	Hytone
	Corticosteroids	Medrol
	Corticosteroids	Methylprednisolone
	Glyburide	Micronase
	Corticosteroids	Mometasone
	Corticosteroids	Nasacort
	Corticosteroids	Nasalide
	Corticosteroids	Orasone
	Corticosteroids	Pediapred
	Corticosteroids	Prednisolone
	Corticosteroids	Prednisone
	Glyburide	Pres Tab
	Corticosteroids	Pulmicort
	Corticosteroids	Rhinocort
	Corticosteroids	Steroids (Prednisone)
	Corticosteroids	Tobradex (Dexamthasone)
	Corticosteroids	Triamcinolone
	Corticosteroids	Vancenase
	Corticosteroids	Vanceril
American Ginseng (Panax quinquefolius)	(none)	(none)
Ashwagandha (Withania somniferum)	(none)	(none)
Asian Ginseng (Panax ginseng)	Warfarin	Anticoagulant (Warfarin)
	Warfarin	Coumadin
	Influenza Vaccine	Flu vaccine
	Influenza Vaccine	FluShield
	Influenza Vaccine	Fluvirin
	Influenza Vaccine	Fluzone
	Influenza Vaccine	Influenza Virus Vaccine
	Ticlopidine	Ticlid
	Ticlopidine	Ticlopidine
	Warfarin	Warfarin
Astragalus (Astragalus membranaceus)	(none)	(none)
Barberry (Berberis vulgaris)	Tetracycline	Achromycin
	Doxycycline	Doxycycline
	Tetracycline	Helidac (Tetracycline)
	Tetracycline	Sumycin

Herb	Drug with Interaction	Generic or Trade Name(s)
Barberry (continued)	*Tetracycline*	*Tetracycline*
	Doxycycline	*Vibramycin*
Bilberry (Vaccinium myrtillus)	*(none)*	*(none)*
Bitter Melon (Momordica charantia)	*(none)*	*(none)*
Blackberry (Rubus fructicosus)	*(none)*	*(none)*
Black Cohosh (Cimicifuga racemosa)	*(none)*	*(none)*
Blessed Thistle (Cnicus benedictus)	*(none)*	*(none)*
Bloodroot (Sanguinaria canadensis)	*(none)*	*(none)*
Blueberry (Vaccinium spp.)	*(none)*	*(none)*
Blue Cohosh (Caulophyllum thalictroides)	*(none)*	*(none)*
Boneset (Eupatorium perfoliatum)	*(none)*	*(none)*
Boswellia (Boswellia serrata)	*(none)*	*(none)*
Bugleweed (Lycopus virginicus)	*Thyroid Hormones*	*Animal Levothyroxine/Liothyronine*
	Thyroid Hormones	*Animal Thyroid*
	Thyroid Hormones	*Armour Thyroid*
	Thyroid Hormones	*Cytomel*
	Thyroid Hormones	*Desiccated Thyroid*
	Thyroid Hormones	*Eltroxin*
	Thyroid Hormones	*Euthroid*
	Thyroid Hormones	*Levo-T*
	Thyroid Hormones	*Levothroid*
	Thyroid Hormones	*Levothyroxine*
	Thyroid Hormones	*Levoxyl*
	Thyroid Hormones	*Liothyronine*
	Thyroid Hormones	*Liotrix*
	Thyroid Hormones	*Proloid*
	Thyroid Hormones	*Synthetic Liothyronine*
	Thyroid Hormones	*Synthroid*
	Thyroid Hormones	*Thyar*
	Thyroid Hormones	*Thyroglobulin*
	Thyroid Hormones	*Thyroid Hormones*
	Thyroid Hormones	*Thyrolar*
Burdock (Arctium lappa)	*(none)*	*(none)*
Butcher's Broom (Ruscus aculeatus)	*(none)*	*(none)*
Calendula (Calendula officinalis)	*(none)*	*(none)*
Carob (Ceratonia siliqua)	*(none)*	*(none)*
Cascara (Rhamnus purshiani cortex)	*(none)*	*(none)*
Catnip (Nepeta cataria)	*(none)*	*(none)*
Cat's Claw (Uncaria tomentosa)	*(none)*	*(none)*
Cayenne (Capsicum annuum, Capsicum frutescens)	*Aspirin*	*Acetylsalicylic Acid*
	Aspirin	*Alka-Seltzer (Aspirin)*
	Aspirin	*Anacin (Aspirin)*
	Aspirin	*ASA*
	Aspirin	*Aspirin*
	Aspirin	*Darvon Compound (Aspirin)*

Drug Interactions

Herb	Drug with Interaction	Generic or Trade Name(s)
Cayenne (continued)	*Aspirin*	*Empirin with Codeine (Aspirin)*
	Aspirin	*Percodan (Aspirin)*
	Aspirin	*Roxiprin (Aspirin)*
	Aspirin	*Soma Compound (Aspirin)*
	Aspirin	*Soma Compound with Codeine (Aspirin)*
Chamomile (Matricaria recutita)	*(none)*	*(none)*
Chickweed (Stellaria media)	*(none)*	*(none)*
Cinnamon (Cinnamomum zeylanicum)	*(none)*	*(none)*
Cranberry (Vaccinium macrocarpon)	*Lansoprazole*	*Lansoprazole*
	Omeprazole	*Losec*
	Omeprazole	*Omeprazole*
	Lansoprazole	*Prevacid*
	Omeprazole	*Prilosec*
Cranesbill (Geranium maculatum)	*(none)*	*(none)*
Damiana (Turnera diffusa)	*(none)*	*(none)*
Dandelion (Taraxacum officinale)	*Thiazide Diuretics*	*Aldactazide (Hydrochlorothiazide)*
	Spironolactone	*Aldactazide (Spironolactone)*
	Spironolactone	*Aldactone*
	Thiazide Diuretics	*Aldoclor (Chlorothiazide)*
	Thiazide Diuretics	*Aldoril (Hydrochlorothiazide)*
	Thiazide Diuretics	*Apresazide (Hydrochlorothiazide)*
	Loop Diuretics	*Bumex*
	Thiazide Diuretics	*Captozide (Hydrochlorothiazide)*
	Thiazide Diuretics	*Chlorothiazide*
	Thiazide Diuretics	*Chlorothiazide/Methyldopa*
	Thiazide Diuretics	*Chlorthalidone*
	Thiazide Diuretics	*Combipres (Chlorthalidone)*
	Loop Diuretics	*Demadex*
	Thiazide Diuretics	*Diuril*
	Thiazide Diuretics	*Dyazide (Hydrochlorothiazide)*
	Triamterene	*Dyazide (Triamterene)*
	Triamterene	*Dyrenium*
	Loop Diuretics	*Edecrin*
	Thiazide Diuretics	*Esidrix*
	Loop Diuretics	*Ethacrynic Acid*
	Loop Diuretics	*Furosemide*
	Thiazide Diuretics	*HCTZ*
	Thiazide Diuretics	*Hydrochlorothiazide*
	Thiazide Diuretics	*HydroDIURIL*
	Thiazide Diuretics	*Hygroton*
	Thiazide Diuretics	*Inderide (Hydrochlorothiazide)*
	Loop Diuretics	*Lasix*

Drug Interactions (vertical side tab)

Herb	Drug with Interaction	Generic or Trade Name(s)
Dandelion (continued)	*Loop Diuretics*	*Loop Diuretics*
	Thiazide Diuretics	*Lopressor HCT (Hydrochlorot-hiazide)*
	Thiazide Diuretics	*Maxzide (Hydrochlorothiazide)*
	Triamterene	*Maxzide (Triamterene)*
	Thiazide Diuretics	*Metolazone*
	Thiazide Diuretics	*Moduretic (Hydrochloroth-iazide)*
	Thiazide Diuretics	*Mykros*
	Thiazide Diuretics	*Oretic*
	Thiazide Diuretics	*Prinizide (Hydrochlorothiazide)*
	Spironolactone	*Spironolactone*
	Thiazide Diuretics	*Tenoretic (Chlorthalidone)*
	Thiazide Diuretics	*Thiazide Diuretics*
	Thiazide Diuretics	*Timolide (Hydrochlorothiazide)*
	Loop Diuretics	*Torsemide*
	Triamterene	*Triamterene*
	Thiazide Diuretics	*Vaseretic (Hydrochlorothiazide)*
	Thiazide Diuretics	*Zaroxolyn*
	Thiazide Diuretics	*Zestoretic (Hydrochloroth-iazide)*
	Thiazide Diuretics	*Ziac (Hydrochlorothiazide)*
Devil's Claw (Harpogophytum procumbens)	*Warfarin*	*Anticoagulant (Warfarin)*
	Warfarin	*Coumadin*
	Ticlopidine	*Ticlid*
	Ticlopidine	*Ticlopidine*
	Warfarin	*Warfarin*
Dong quai (Angelica sinensis)	*Heparin*	*Anticoagulant (Heparin)*
	Warfarin	*Anticoagulant (Warfarin)*
	Warfarin	*Coumadin*
	Heparin	*Heparin*
	Ticlopidine	*Ticlid*
	Ticlopidine	*Ticlopidine*
	Warfarin	*Warfarin*
Echinacea (Echinacea purpurea, Echinacea angustifolia, Echinacea pallida)	*Chemotherapy*	*Cancer Chemotherapy*
	Chemotherapy	*Chemotherapy*
	Econazole	*Econazole*
	Econazole	*Spectazole*
Elderberry (Sambucus nigra)	*(none)*	*(none)*
Ephedra (Ephedra sinica, Ephedra intermedia, Ephedra equisetina)	*Phenylpropanolamine*	*Acutrim*
	Ephedrine	*Adrenaline*
	Corticosteroids	*AeroBid*
	Ephedrine	*Afrin*

Drug Interactions

Drug Interactions

Herb	Drug with Interaction	Generic or Trade Name(s)
Ephedra (continued)	*Ephedrine*	*Alka-Seltzer Plus (Pseudoephedrine)*
	Caffeine	*Anacin (Caffeine)*
	Phenylpropanolamine	*Appedrine (Phenylpropanolamine)*
	Corticosteroids	*Aristocort*
	Corticosteroids	*Azmacort*
	Corticosteroids	*Beclomethasone*
	Corticosteroids	*Beclovent*
	Corticosteroids	*Beconase*
	Epinephrine	*Bronkaid Mist*
	Epinephrine	*Brontin Mist*
	Corticosteroids	*Budesonide*
	Caffeine	*Caffedrine*
	Caffeine	*Caffeine*
	Ephedrine	*Chlor-Trimeton 12 Hour (Pseudoephedrine)*
	Ephedrine	*Claritin-D (Pseudoephedrine)*
	Phenylpropanolamine	*Contac 12 Hour (Phenylpropanolamine)*
	Corticosteroids	*Cortef*
	Corticosteroids	*Corticosteroids*
	Corticosteroids	*Cortisone-like drugs*
	Corticosteroids	*Cutivate*
	Caffeine	*Darvon Compound (Caffeine)*
	Phenylpropanolamine	*DayQuil Allergy Relief (Phenylpropanolamine)*
	Corticosteroids	*Decadron*
	Corticosteroids	*Decadron Phosphate Turbinaire*
	Corticosteroids	*Delta-Cortef*
	Corticosteroids	*Deltasone*
	Phenylpropanolamine	*Dex-A-Diet*
	Phenylpropanolamine	*Dex-A-Diet Plus Vitamin C (Phenylpropanolamine)*
	Corticosteroids	*Dexamethasone*
	Phenylpropanolamine	*Dexatrim*
	Phenylpropanolamine	*Dexatrim Plus Vitamin C (Phenylpropanolamine)*
	Phenylpropanolamine	*Diadex Grapefruit Diet Plan (Phenylpropanolamine)*
	Phenylpropanolamine	*Dimetapp (Phenylpropanolamine)*
	Corticosteroids	*Elocon*
	Phenylpropanolamine	*Entex LA (Phenylpropanolamine)*
	Ephedrine	*Ephedrine*
	Epinephrine	*Epinephrine*

Herb	**Drug with Interaction**	**Generic or Trade Name(s)**
Ephedra (continued)	*Corticosteroids*	*Flonase*
	Corticosteroids	*Flunisolide*
	Corticosteroids	*Fluticasone*
	Corticosteroids	*Hydrocortisone*
	Corticosteroids	*Hytone*
	Corticosteroids	*Medrol*
	Corticosteroids	*Methylprednisolone*
	Corticosteroids	*Mometasone*
	Phenelzine	*Nardil*
	Corticosteroids	*Nasacort*
	Corticosteroids	*Nasalide*
	Caffeine	*NoDoz*
	Ephedrine	*Nyquil (Pseudoephedrine)*
	Ephedrine	*Nyquil Hot Therapy Powder (Pseudoephedrine)*
	Corticosteroids	*Orasone*
	Corticosteroids	*Pediapred*
	Phenelzine	*Phenelzine*
	Phenylpropanolamine	*Phenylpropanolamine*
	Phenylpropanolamine	*PPA*
	Corticosteroids	*Prednisolone*
	Corticosteroids	*Prednisone*
	Ephedrine	*Pretz-D*
	Ephedrine	*Primatene Dual Action (Ephedrine)*
	Epinephrine	*Primatene Mist*
	Phenylpropanolamine	*Propagest*
	Ephedrine	*Pseudoephedrine*
	Corticosteroids	*Pulmicort*
	Caffeine	*Quick Pep*
	Phenylpropanolamine	*Rhindecon*
	Corticosteroids	*Rhinocort*
	Phenylpropanolamine	*Robitussin CF (Phenyl-propanolamine)*
	Corticosteroids	*Steroids (Prednisone)*
	Ephedrine	*Sudafed*
	Phenylpropanolamine	*Tavist-D (Phenylpropanolamine)*
	Ephedrine	*Theraflu (Pseudoephedrine)*
	Ephedrine	*Theraflu Flu and Cold (Pseu-doephedrine)*
	Corticosteroids	*Tobradex (Dexamethasone)*
	Corticosteroids	*Triamcinolone*
	Phenylpropanolamine	*Triaminic-12 (Phenyl-propanolamine)*
	Ephedrine	*Tylenol Allergy Sinus (Pseu-doephedrine)*
	Ephedrine	*Tylenol Cold (Pseudoephedrine)*

Drug Interactions

Herb	Drug with Interaction	Generic or Trade Name(s)
Ephedra (continued)	Ephedrine	Tylenol Flu NightTime Maximum Strength Powder (Pseudoephedrine)
	Ephedrine	Tylenol Multi-Symptom Hot Medication (Pseudoephedrine)
	Ephedrine	Tylenol Sinus (Pseudoephedrine)
	Phenylpropanolamine	Unitrol
	Corticosteroids	Vancenase
	Corticosteroids	Vanceril
	Ephedrine	Vick Vatronol
	Caffeine	Vivarin
Eyebright (Euphrasia officinalis)	(none)	(none)
False Unicorn (Chamaelirium luteum)	(none)	(none)
Fennel (Foeniculum vulgare)	(none)	(none)
Fenugreek (Trigonella foenum-graecum)	Insulin	Animal-Source Insulin
	Heparin	Anticoagulant (Heparin)
	Warfarin	Anticoagulant (Warfarin)
	Warfarin	Coumadin
	Glipizide	Glipizide
	Glipizide	Glucotrol
	Heparin	Heparin
	Insulin	Human Analog Insulin
	Insulin	Human Insulin
	Insulin	Humanlog
	Insulin	Humulin
	Insulin	Iletin
	Insulin	Insulin
	Insulin	Novolin
	Ticlopidine	Ticlid
	Ticlopidine	Ticlopidine
	Warfarin	Warfarin
Feverfew (Tanacetum parthenium)	(none)	(none)
Fo-Ti (Polygonum multiflorum)	(none)	(none)
Garlic (Allium sativum)	Warfarin	Anticoagulant (Warfarin)
	Warfarin	Coumadin
	Ticlopidine	Ticlid
	Ticlopidine	Ticlopidine
	Warfarin	Warfarin
Gentian (Gentiana lutea)	(none)	(none)
Ginger (Zingiber officinale)	Anesthetic Major	Anesthetics, Major
	Heparin	Anticoagulant (Heparin)
	Warfarin	Anticoagulant (Warfarin)
	Chemotherapy	Cancer Chemotherapy
	Chemotherapy	Chemotherapy
	Warfarin	Coumadin
	Heparin	Heparin

Drug Interactions

Herb	Drug with Interaction	Generic or Trade Name(s)
Ginger (continued)	*Ticlopidine*	*Ticlid*
	Ticlopidine	*Ticlopidine*
	Warfarin	*Warfarin*
Ginkgo biloba	*Thiazide Diuretics*	*Aldactazide (Hydrochloroth-iazide)*
	Thiazide Diuretics	*Aldoclor (Chlorothiazide)*
	Thiazide Diuretics	*Aldoril (Hydrochlorothiazide)*
	Heparin	*Anticoagulant (Heparin)*
	Warfarin	*Anticoagulant (Warfarin)*
	Thiazide Diuretics	*Apresazide (Hydrochloroth-iazide)*
	Thiazide Diuretics	*Captozide (Hydrochloroth-iazide)*
	Thiazide Diuretics	*Chlorothiazide*
	Thiazide Diuretics	*Chlorothiazide/Methyldopa*
	Thiazide Diuretics	*Chlorthalidone*
	Thiazide Diuretics	*Combipres (Chlorthalidone)*
	Warfarin	*Coumadin*
	Cyclosporine	*Cyclosporine*
	Thiazide Diuretics	*Diuril*
	Thiazide Diuretics	*Dyazide (Hydrochlorothiazide)*
	Thiazide Diuretics	*Esidrix*
	Fluvoxamine	*Faurin*
	Fluoxetine	*Fluoxetine*
	Fluvoxamine	*Fluvoxamine*
	Thiazide Diuretics	*HCTZ*
	Heparin	*Heparin*
	Thiazide Diuretics	*Hydrochlorothiazide*
	Thiazide Diuretics	*HydroDIURIL*
	Thiazide Diuretics	*Hygroton*
	Thiazide Diuretics	*Inderide (Hydrochlorothiazide)*
	Thiazide Diuretics	*Lopressor HCT (Hydrochloroth-iazide)*
	Fluvoxamine	*Luvox*
	Thiazide Diuretics	*Maxzide (Hydrochlorothiazide)*
	Thiazide Diuretics	*Metolazone*
	Thiazide Diuretics	*Moduretic (Hydrochloroth-iazide)*
	Thiazide Diuretics	*Mykros*
	Cyclosporine	*Neoral*
	Thiazide Diuretics	*Oretic*
	Paroxetine	*Paroxetine*
	Paroxetine	*Paxil*
	Thiazide Diuretics	*Prinizide (Hydrochlorothiazide)*
	Fluoxetine	*Prozac*
	Cyclosporine	*Sandimmune*
	Sertraline	*Sertraline*

Herb	Drug with Interaction	Generic or Trade Name(s)
Ginkgo biloba (continued)	*Thiazide Diuretics*	*Tenoretic (Chlorthalidone)*
	Thiazide Diuretics	*Thiazide Diuretics*
	Ticlopidine	*Ticlid*
	Ticlopidine	*Ticlopidine*
	Thiazide Diuretics	*Timolide (Hydrochlorothiazide)*
	Thiazide Diuretics	*Vaseretic (Hydrochlorothiazide)*
	Warfarin	*Warfarin*
	Thiazide Diuretics	*Zaroxolyn*
	Thiazide Diuretics	*Zestoretic (Hydrochlorothiazide)*
	Thiazide Diuretics	*Ziac (Hydrochlorothiazide)*
	Sertraline	*Zoloft*
Goldenseal (Hydrastis canadensis)	*Tetracycline*	*Achromycin*
	Doxycycline	*Doxycycline*
	Tetracycline	*Helidac (Tetracycline)*
	Tetracycline	*Sumycin*
	Tetracycline	*Tetracycline*
	Doxycycline	*Vibramycin*
Gotu Kola (Centella asiatica)	*(none)*	*(none)*
Green Tea (Camellia sinensis)	*Ephedrine*	*Adrenaline*
	Ephedrine	*Afrin*
	Ephedrine	*Alka-Seltzer Plus (Pseudoephedrine)*
	Theophylline	*Aminophylline*
	Atropine	*Atropine*
	Ephedrine	*Chlor-Trimeton 12 Hour (Pseudoephedrine)*
	Ephedrine	*Claritin-D (Pseudoephedrine)*
	Codeine	*Codeine*
	Codeine	*Empirin with Codeine (Codeine)*
	Ephedrine	*Ephedrine*
	Atropine	*Isopto Atropine*
	Ephedrine	*Nyquil (Pseudoephedrine)*
	Ephedrine	*Nyquil Hot Therapy Powder (Pseudoephedrine)*
	Codeine	*Phenergan VC with Codeine (Codeine)*
	Codeine	*Phenergan with Codeine (Codeine)*
	Theophylline	*Phyllocontin*
	Ephedrine	*Pretz-D*
	Ephedrine	*Primatene Dual Action (Ephedrine)*
	Theophylline	*Primatene Dual Action (Theophylline)*
	Ephedrine	*Pseudoephedrine*

Herb	Drug with Interaction	Generic or Trade Name(s)
Green Tea (continued)	Codeine	Robitussin AC (Codeine)
	Theophylline	Slo-Bid
	Theophylline	Slo-Phyllin
	Codeine	Soma Compound with Codeine (Codeine)
	Ephedrine	Sudafed
	Theophylline	Theo-Dur
	Theophylline	Theolair
	Theophylline	Theophylline
	Ephedrine	Theraflu (Pseudoephedrine)
	Ephedrine	Theraflu Flu and Cold (Pseudoephedrine)
	Theophylline	Truphylline
	Ephedrine	Tylenol Allergy Sinus (Pseudoephedrine)
	Ephedrine	Tylenol Cold (Pseudoephedrine)
	Ephedrine	Tylenol Flu NightTime Maximum Strength Powder (Pseudoephedrine)
	Ephedrine	Tylenol Multi-Symptom Hot Medication (Pseudoephedrine)
	Ephedrine	Tylenol Sinus (Pseudoephedrine)
	Codeine	Tylenol with Codeine (Codeine)
	Theophylline	Uniphyl
	Ephedrine	Vick Vatronol
Guaraná (Paullinia cupana)	Phenylpropanolamine	Acutrim
	Ephedrine	Adrenaline
	Ephedrine	Afrin
	Ephedrine	Alka-Seltzer Plus (Pseudoephedrine)
	Theophylline	Aminophylline
	Caffeine	Anacin (Caffeine)
	Phenylpropanolamine	Appedrine (Phenylpropanolamine)
	Epinephrine	Bronkaid Mist
	Epinephrine	Brontin Mist
	Caffeine	Caffedrine
	Caffeine	Caffeine
	Ephedrine	Chlor-Trimeton 12 Hour (Pseudoephedrine)
	Cimetidine	Cimetidine
	Ciprofloxacin	Cipro
	Ciprofloxacin	Ciprofloxacin
	Ephedrine	Claritin-D (Pseudoephedrine)

Drug Interactions

Herb	Drug with Interaction	Generic or Trade Name(s)
Guaraná (continued)	*Phenylpropanolamine*	*Contac 12 Hour (Phenyl-propanolamine)*
	Caffeine	*Darvon Compound (Caffeine)*
	Phenylpropanolamine	*DayQuil Allergy Relief (Phenyl-propanolamine)*
	Phenylpropanolamine	*Dex-A-Diet*
	Phenylpropanolamine	*Dex-A-Diet Plus Vitamin C (Phenylpropanolamine)*
	Phenylpropanolamine	*Dexatrim*
	Phenylpropanolamine	*Dexatrim Plus Vitamin C (Phenylpropanolamine)*
	Phenylpropanolamine	*Diadex Grapefruit Diet Plan (Phenylpropanolamine)*
	Phenylpropanolamine	*Dimetapp (Phenyl-propanolamine)*
	Phenylpropanolamine	*Entex LA (Phenyl-propanolamine)*
	Ephedrine	*Ephedrine*
	Epinephrine	*Epinephrine*
	Caffeine	*NoDoz*
	Ephedrine	*Nyquil (Pseudoephedrine)*
	Ephedrine	*Nyquil Hot Therapy Powder (Pseudoephedrine)*
	Phenylpropanolamine	*Phenylpropanolamine*
	Theophylline	*Phyllocontin*
	Phenylpropanolamine	*PPA*
	Ephedrine	*Pretz-D*
	Ephedrine	*Primatene Dual Action (Ephedrine)*
	Theophylline	*Primatene Dual Action (Theo-phylline)*
	Epinephrine	*Primatene Mist*
	Phenylpropanolamine	*Propagest*
	Ephedrine	*Pseudoephedrine*
	Caffeine	*Quick Pep*
	Phenylpropanolamine	*Rhindecon*
	Phenylpropanolamine	*Robitussin CF (Phenyl-propanolamine)*
	Theophylline	*Slo-Bid*
	Theophylline	*Slo-Phyllin*
	Ephedrine	*Sudafed*
	Cimetidine	*Tagamet*
	Cimetidine	*Tagamet HB*
	Phenylpropanolamine	*Tavist-D (Phenylpropanolamine)*
	Theophylline	*Theo-Dur*
	Theophylline	*Theolair*
	Theophylline	*Theophylline*

Drug Interactions

Herb	Drug with Interaction	Generic or Trade Name(s)
Guaraná (continued)	*Ephedrine*	*Theraflu (Pseudoephedrine)*
	Ephedrine	*Theraflu Flu and Cold (Pseudoephedrine)*
	Phenylpropanolamine	*Triaminic-12 (Phenylpropanolamine)*
	Theophylline	*Truphylline*
	Ephedrine	*Tylenol Allergy Sinus (Pseudoephedrine)*
	Ephedrine	*Tylenol Cold (Pseudoephedrine)*
	Ephedrine	*Tylenol Flu NightTime Maximum Strength Powder (Pseudoephedrine)*
	Ephedrine	*Tylenol Multi-Symptom Hot - Medication (Pseudoephedrine)*
	Ephedrine	*Tylenol Sinus (Pseudoephedrine)*
	Theophylline	*Uniphyl*
	Phenylpropanolamine	*Unitrol*
	Ephedrine	*Vick Vatronol*
	Caffeine	*Vivarin*
Guggul (Commiphora mukul)	*(none)*	*(none)*
Gymnema (Gymnema sylvestre)	*Insulin*	*Animal-Source Insulin*
	Glyburide	*Diabeta*
	Glyburide	*Glibenclamide*
	Glipizide	*Glipizide*
	Glipizide	*Glucotrol*
	Glyburide	*Glyburide*
	Insulin	*Human Analog Insulin*
	Insulin	*Human Insulin*
	Insulin	*Humanlog*
	Insulin	*Humulin*
	Insulin	*Iletin*
	Insulin	*Insulin*
	Glyburide	*Micronase*
	Insulin	*Novolin*
	Glyburide	*Pres Tab*
Hawthorn (Crataegus laevigata, Crataegus oxyacantha, Crataegus monogyna)	*Digoxin*	*Digoxin*
	Digoxin	*Lanoxin*
Hops (Humulus lupulus)	*(none)*	*(none)*
Horseradish (Cochlearia armoracia)	*(none)*	*(none)*
Horsetail (Equisetum arvense)	*Thiazide Diuretics*	*Aldactazide (Hydrochlorothiazide)*
	Spironolactone	*Aldactazide (Spironolactone)*
	Spironolactone	*Aldactone*

Drug Interactions

Herb	Drug with Interaction	Generic or Trade Name(s)
Horsetail (continued)	*Thiazide Diuretics*	Aldoclor (Chlorothiazide)
	Thiazide Diuretics	Aldoril (Hydrochlorothiazide)
	Thiazide Diuretics	Apresazide (Hydrochlorothiazide)
	Loop Diuretics	Bumex
	Thiazide Diuretics	Captozide (Hydrochlorothiazide)
	Thiazide Diuretics	Chlorothiazide
	Thiazide Diuretics	Chlorothiazide/Methyldopa
	Thiazide Diuretics	Chlorthalidone
	Thiazide Diuretics	Combipres (Chlorthalidone)
	Loop Diuretics	Demadex
	Thiazide Diuretics	Diuril
	Thiazide Diuretics	Dyazide (Hydrochlorothiazide)
	Triamterene	Dyazide (Triamterene)
	Triamterene	Dyrenium
	Loop Diuretics	Edecrin
	Thiazide Diuretics	Esidrix
	Loop Diuretics	Ethacrynic Acid
	Loop Diuretics	Furosemide
	Thiazide Diuretics	HCTZ
	Thiazide Diuretics	Hydrochlorothiazide
	Thiazide Diuretics	HydroDIURIL
	Thiazide Diuretics	Hygroton
	Thiazide Diuretics	Inderide (Hydrochlorothiazide)
	Loop Diuretics	Lasix
	Loop Diuretics	Loop Diuretics
	Thiazide Diuretics	Lopressor HCT (Hydrochlorothiazide)
	Thiazide Diuretics	Maxzide (Hydrochlorothiazide)
	Triamterene	Maxzide (Triamterene)
	Thiazide Diuretics	Metolazone
	Thiazide Diuretics	Moduretic (Hydrochlorothiazide)
	Thiazide Diuretics	Mykros
	Thiazide Diuretics	Oretic
	Thiazide Diuretics	Prinizide (Hydrochlorothiazide)
	Spironolactone	Spironolactone
	Thiazide Diuretics	Tenoretic (Chlorthalidone)
	Thiazide Diuretics	Thiazide Diuretics
	Thiazide Diuretics	Timolide (Hydrochlorothiazide)
	Loop Diuretics	Torsemide
	Triamterene	Triamterene
	Thiazide Diuretics	Vaseretic (Hydrochlorothiazide)
	Thiazide Diuretics	Zaroxolyn
	Thiazide Diuretics	Zestoretic (Hydrochlorothiazide)
	Thiazide Diuretics	Ziac (Hydrochlorothiazide)

Herb	Drug with Interaction	Generic or Trade Name(s)
Horse Chestnut (Aesculus hippocastanum)	*Heparin*	*Anticoagulant (Heparin)*
	Warfarin	*Anticoagulant (Warfarin)*
	Warfarin	*Coumadin*
	Heparin	*Heparin*
	Ticlopidine	*Ticlid*
	Ticlopidine	*Ticlopidine*
	Warfarin	*Warfarin*
Juniper (Juniperus communis)	*Thiazide Diuretics*	*Aldactazide (Hydrochlorothiazide)*
	Spironolactone	*Aldactazide (Spironolactone)*
	Spironolactone	*Aldactone*
	Thiazide Diuretics	*Aldoclor (Chlorothiazide)*
	Thiazide Diuretics	*Aldoril (Hydrochlorothiazide)*
	Thiazide Diuretics	*Apresazide (Hydrochlorothiazide)*
	Loop Diuretics	*Bumex*
	Thiazide Diuretics	*Captozide (Hydrochlorothiazide)*
	Thiazide Diuretics	*Chlorothiazide*
	Thiazide Diuretics	*Chlorothiazide/Methyldopa*
	Thiazide Diuretics	*Chlorthalidone*
	Thiazide Diuretics	*Combipres (Chlorthalidone)*
	Loop Diuretics	*Demadex*
	Thiazide Diuretics	*Diuril*
	Thiazide Diuretics	*Dyazide (Hydrochlorothiazide)*
	Triamterene	*Dyazide (Triamterene)*
	Triamterene	*Dyrenium*
	Loop Diuretics	*Edecrin*
	Thiazide Diuretics	*Esidrix*
	Loop Diuretics	*Ethacrynic Acid*
	Loop Diuretics	*Furosemide*
	Thiazide Diuretics	*HCTZ*
	Thiazide Diuretics	*Hydrochlorothiazide*
	Thiazide Diuretics	*HydroDIURIL*
	Thiazide Diuretics	*Hygroton*
	Thiazide Diuretics	*Inderide (Hydrochlorothiazide)*
	Loop Diuretics	*Lasix*
	Loop Diuretics	*Loop Diuretics*
	Thiazide Diuretics	*Lopressor HCT (Hydrochlorothiazide)*
	Thiazide Diuretics	*Maxzide (Hydrochlorothiazide)*
	Triamterene	*Maxzide (Triamterene)*
	Thiazide Diuretics	*Metolazone*
	Thiazide Diuretics	*Moduretic (Hydrochlorothiazide)*
	Thiazide Diuretics	*Mykros*

Drug Interactions

Herb	Drug with Interaction	Generic or Trade Name(s)
Juniper (continued)	*Thiazide Diuretics*	*Oretic*
	Thiazide Diuretics	*Prinizide (Hydrochlorothiazide)*
	Spironolactone	*Spironolactone*
	Thiazide Diuretics	*Tenoretic (Chlorthalidone)*
	Thiazide Diuretics	*Thiazide Diuretics*
	Thiazide Diuretics	*Timolide (Hydrochlorothiazide)*
	Loop Diuretics	*Torsemide*
	Triamterene	*Triamterene*
	Thiazide Diuretics	*Vaseretic (Hydrochlorothiazide)*
	Thiazide Diuretics	*Zaroxolyn*
	Thiazide Diuretics	*Zestoretic (Hydrochlorothiazide)*
	Thiazide Diuretics	*Ziac (Hydrochlorothiazide)*
Kava (Piper methysticum)	*Benzodiazepines*	*Alprazolam*
	Benzodiazepines	*Ativan*
	Benzodiazepines	*Benzodiazepines*
	Buspirone	*Buspar Buspirone*
	Benzodiazepines	*Chlordiazepoxide*
	Benzodiazepines	*Clonazepam*
	Benzodiazepines	*Dalmane*
	Benzodiazepines	*Diazepam*
	Benzodiazepines	*Flurazepam*
	Benzodiazepines	*Halcion*
	Benzodiazepines	*Klonopin*
	Benzodiazepines	*Librium*
	Benzodiazepines	*Lorazepam*
	Benzodiazepines	*Restoril*
	Benzodiazepines	*Temazepam*
	Benzodiazepines	*Triazolam*
	Benzodiazepines	*Valium*
	Benzodiazepines	*Xanax*
Kudzu (Pueraria lobata)	*(none)*	*(none)*
Lavender (Lavandula officinalis)	*(none)*	*(none)*
Lemon Balm (Melissa officinalis)	*Thyroid Hormones*	*Animal Levothyroxine/Liothyronine*
	Thyroid Hormones	*Animal Thyroid*
	Thyroid Hormones	*Armour Thyroid*
	Thyroid Hormones	*Cytomel*
	Thyroid Hormones	*Desiccated Thyroid*
	Thyroid Hormones	*Eltroxin*
	Thyroid Hormones	*Euthroid*
	Thyroid Hormones	*Levo-T*
	Thyroid Hormones	*Levothroid*
	Thyroid Hormones	*Levothyroxine*
	Thyroid Hormones	*Levoxyl*
	Thyroid Hormones	*Liothyronine*
	Thyroid Hormones	*Liotrix*

Drug Interactions

Herb	**Drug with Interaction**	**Generic or Trade Name(s)**
Lemon Balm (continued)	*Thyroid Hormones*	*Proloid*
	Thyroid Hormones	*Synthetic Liothyronine*
	Thyroid Hormones	*Synthroid*
	Thyroid Hormones	*Thyar*
	Thyroid Hormones	*Thyroglobulin*
	Thyroid Hormones	*Thyroid Hormones*
	Thyroid Hormones	*Thyrolar*
Licorice (Glycyrrhiza glabra, Glycyrrhiza uralensis)	*Aspirin*	*Acetylsalicylic Acid*
	Interferon	*Actimmune*
	Ibuprofen	*Advil*
	Corticosteroids	*AeroBid*
	Thiazide Diuretics	*Aldactazide (Hydrochloroth-iazide)*
	Thiazide Diuretics	*Aldoclor (Chlorothiazide)*
	Thiazide Diuretics	*Aldoril (Hydrochlorothiazide)*
	Naproxen	*Aleve*
	Interferon	*Alferon N*
	Aspirin	*Alka-Seltzer (Aspirin)*
	Aspirin	*Anacin (Aspirin)*
	Naproxen	*Anaprox*
	Thiazide Diuretics	*Apresazide (Hydrochloroth-iazide)*
	Corticosteroids	*Aristocort*
	Aspirin	*ASA*
	Aspirin	*Aspirin*
	Interferon	*Avonex*
	Corticosteroids	*Azmacort*
	Corticosteroids	*Beclomethasone*
	Corticosteroids	*Beclovent*
	Corticosteroids	*Beconase*
	Interferon	*Betaseron*
	Ibuprofen	*Brufin*
	Corticosteroids	*Budesonide*
	Loop Diuretics	*Bumex*
	Thiazide Diuretics	*Captozide (Hydrochloroth-iazide)*
	Thiazide Diuretics	*Chlorothiazide*
	Thiazide Diuretics	*Chlorothiazide/Methyldopa*
	Thiazide Diuretics	*Chlorthalidone*
	Thiazide Diuretics	*Combipres (Chlorthalidone)*
	Corticosteroids	*Cortef*
	Corticosteroids	*Corticosteroids*
	Corticosteroids	*Cortisone-like drugs*
	Corticosteroids	*Cutivate*
	Aspirin	*Darvon Compound (Aspirin)*
	Oxaprozin	*Daypro*

Herb	Drug with Interaction	Generic or Trade Name(s)
Licorice (continued)	Corticosteroids	Decadron
	Corticosteroids	Decadron Phosphate Turbinaire
	Corticosteroids	Delta-Cortef
	Corticosteroids	Deltasone
	Loop Diuretics	Demadex
	Corticosteroids	Dexamethasone
	Digoxin	Digoxin
	Thiazide Diuretics	Diuril
	Thiazide Diuretics	Dyazide (Hydrochlorothiazide)
	Loop Diuretics	Edecrin
	Corticosteroids	Elocon
	Aspirin	Empirin with Codeine (Aspirin)
	Thiazide Diuretics	Esidrix
	Loop Diuretics	Ethacrynic Acid
	Etodolac	Etodolac
	Ibuprofen	Feldene
	Corticosteroids	Flonase
	Ibuprofen	Froben
	Corticosteroids	Flunisolide
	Corticosteroids	Fluticasone
	Loop Diuretics	Furosemide
	Thiazide Diuretics	HCTZ
	Thiazide Diuretics	Hydrochlorothiazide
	Corticosteroids	Hydrocortisone
	Thiazide Diuretics	HydroDIURIL
	Thiazide Diuretics	Hygroton
	Corticosteroids	Hytone
	Ibuprofen	Ibuprofen
	Thiazide Diuretics	Inderide (Hydrochlorothiazide)
	Isoniazid	INH
	Interferon	Interferon
	Interferon	Intron
	Isoniazid	Isoniazid
	Isoniazid	Laniazid
	Digoxin	Lanoxin
	Loop Diuretics	Lasix
	Etodolac	Lodine
	Loop Diuretics	Loop Diuretics
	Thiazide Diuretics	Lopressor HCT (Hydrochlorothiazide)
	Thiazide Diuretics	Maxzide (Hydrochlorothiazide)
	Corticosteroids	Medrol
	Corticosteroids	Methylprednisolone
	Thiazide Diuretics	Metolazone
	Thiazide Diuretics	Moduretic (Hydrochlorothiazide)
	Corticosteroids	Mometasone

Herb	Drug with Interaction	Generic or Trade Name(s)
Licorice (continued)	*Ibuprofen*	*Motrin*
	Ibuprofen	*Motrin IB*
	Thiazide Diuretics	*Mykros*
	Nabumetone	*Nabumetone*
	Naproxen	*Napralen Naprosyn Naproxen*
	Naproxen	*Naproxen Sodium*
	Corticosteroids	*Nasacort*
	Corticosteroids	*Nasalide*
	Ibuprofen	*Nuprin*
	Corticosteroids	*Orasone*
	Thiazide Diuretics	*Oretic*
	Oxaprozin	*Oxaprozin*
	Corticosteroids	*Pediapred*
	Aspirin	*Percodan (Aspirin)*
	Corticosteroids	*Prednisolone*
	Corticosteroids	*Prednisone*
	Thiazide Diuretics	*Prinizide (Hydrochlorothiazide)*
	Corticosteroids	*Pulmicort*
	Interferon	*Rebif*
	Nabumetone	*Relafen*
	Corticosteroids	*Rhinocort*
	Isoniazid	*Rifamate*
	Isoniazid	*Rimactane*
	Interferon	*Roferon-A*
	Aspirin	*Roxiprin (Aspirin)*
	Aspirin	*Soma Compound (Aspirin)*
	Aspirin	*Soma Compound with Codeine (Aspirin)*
	Corticosteroids	*Steroids (Prednisone)*
	Thiazide Diuretics	*Tenoretic (Chlorthalidone)*
	Thiazide Diuretics	*Thiazide Diuretics*
	Thiazide Diuretics	*Timolide (Hydrochlorothiazide)*
	Corticosteroids	*Tobradex (Dexamthasone)*
	Loop Diuretics	*Torsemide*
	Corticosteroids	*Triamcinolone*
	Corticosteroids	*Vancenase*
	Corticosteroids	*Vanceril*
	Thiazide Diuretics	*Vaseretic (Hydrochlorothiazide)*
	Ibuprofen	*Voltarol*
	Interferon	*Weferon*
	Thiazide Diuretics	*Zaroxolyn*
	Thiazide Diuretics	*Zestoretic (Hydrochlorothiazide)*
	Thiazide Diuretics	*Ziac (Hydrochlorothiazide)*
Ligustrum (Ligustrum lucidum)	*(none)*	*(none)*
Lomatium (Lomatium dissectum)	*(none)*	*(none)*
Maitake (Grifola frondosa)	*(none)*	*(none)*

Drug Interactions

Herb	Drug with Interaction	Generic or Trade Name(s)
Marshmallow (Althea officinalis)	*(none)*	*(none)*
Milk Thistle (Silybum marianum)	*Acetaminophen*	*Acetaminophen*
	Acetaminophen	*Alka-Seltzer Plus (Acetaminophen)*
	Anesthetic Major	*Anesthetics, Major*
	Acetaminophen	*APAP*
	Clofibrate	*Atromid-S*
	Chemotherapy	*Cancer Chemotherapy*
	Chemotherapy	*Chemotherapy*
	Clofibrate	*Clofibrate*
	Acetaminophen	*Darvocet (Acetaminophen)*
	Acetaminophen	*Darvocet N (Acetaminophen)*
	Acetaminophen	*Excedrin PM (Acetaminophen)*
	Metronidazole	*Flagyl*
	Haloperidol	*Haldol*
	Haloperidol	*Haloperidol*
	Metronidazole	*Helidac (Metronidazole)*
	Acetaminophen	*Lortab (Acetaminophen)*
	Lovastatin	*Lovastatin*
	Metronidazole	*Metronidazole*
	Lovastatin	*Mevacor*
	Acetaminophen	*Nyquil (Acetaminophen)*
	Acetaminophen	*Nyquil Hot Therapy Powder (Acetaminophen)*
	Acetaminophen	*Paracetemol*
	Acetaminophen	*Percocet (Acetaminophen)*
	Pravastatin	*Pravachol*
	Pravastatin	*Pravastatin*
	Metronidazole	*Protostat*
	Acetaminophen	*Roxicet (Acetaminophen)*
	Acetaminophen	*Theraflu (Acetaminophen)*
	Acetaminophen	*Theraflu Flu and Cold (Acetaminophen)*
	Acetaminophen	*Tylenol*
	Acetaminophen	*Tylenol Allergy Sinus (Acetaminophen)*
	Acetaminophen	*Tylenol Cold (Acetaminophen)*
	Acetaminophen	*Tylenol Flu NightTime Maximum Strength Powder (Acetaminophen)*
	Acetaminophen	*Tylenol Multi-Symptom Hot Medication (Acetaminophen)*
	Acetaminophen	*Tylenol PM (Acetaminophen)*
	Acetaminophen	*Tylenol PM Extra Strength (Acetaminophen)*
	Acetaminophen	*Tylenol Sinus (Acetaminophen)*
	Acetaminophen	*Tylenol with Codeine (Acetaminophen)*

Drug Interactions

Herb	Drug with Interaction	Generic or Trade Name(s)
Milk Thistle (continued)	*Acetaminophen*	*Tylenol Allergy Sinus*
	Acetaminophen	*Vicodin (Acetaminophen)*
	Acetaminophen	*Wygesic (Acetaminophen)*
Mullein (Verbascum thapsus)	*(none)*	*(none)*
Myrrh (Commiphora molmol)	*(none)*	*(none)*
Nettle (Urtica dioica)	*(none)*	*(none)*
Oak (Quercus spp.)	*Ephedrine*	*Adrenaline*
	Ephedrine	*Afrin*
	Ephedrine	*Alka-Seltzer Plus (Pseudoephedrine)*
	Theophylline	*Aminophylline*
	Atropine	*Atropine*
	Ephedrine	*Chlor-Trimeton 12 Hour (Pseudoephedrine)*
	Ephedrine	*Claritin-D (Pseudoephedrine)*
	Codeine	*Codeine*
	Codeine	*Empirin with Codeine (Codeine)*
	Ephedrine	*Ephedrine*
	Atropine	*Isopto Atropine*
	Ephedrine	*Nyquil (Pseudoephedrine)*
	Ephedrine	*Nyquil Hot Therapy Powder (Pseudoephedrine)*
	Codeine	*Phenergan VC with Codeine (Codeine)*
	Codeine	*Phenergan with Codeine (Codeine)*
	Theophylline	*Phyllocontin*
	Ephedrine	*Pretz-D*
	Ephedrine	*Primatene Dual Action (Ephedrine)*
	Theophylline	*Primatene Dual Action (Theophylline)*
	Ephedrine	*Pseudoephedrine*
	Codeine	*Robitussin AC (Codeine)*
	Theophylline	*Slo-Bid*
	Theophylline	*Slo-Phyllin*
	Codeine	*Soma Compound with Codeine (Codeine)*
	Ephedrine	*Sudafed*
	Theophylline	*Theo-Dur*
	Theophylline	*Theolair*
	Theophylline	*Theophylline*
	Ephedrine	*Theraflu (Pseudoephedrine)*
	Ephedrine	*Theraflu Flu and Cold (Pseudoephedrine)*
	Theophylline	*Truphylline*

Drug Interactions

Drug Interactions

Herb	Drug with Interaction	Generic or Trade Name(s)
Oak (continued)	*Ephedrine*	*Tylenol Allergy Sinus (Pseudoephedrine)*
	Ephedrine	*Tylenol Cold (Pseudoephedrine)*
	Ephedrine	*Tylenol Flu NightTime Maximum Strength Powder (Pseudoephedrine)*
	Ephedrine	*Tylenol Multi-Symptom Hot Medication (Pseudoephedrine)*
	Ephedrine	*Tylenol Sinus (Pseudoephedrine)*
	Codeine	*Tylenol with Codeine (Codeine)*
	Theophylline	*Uniphyl*
	Ephedrine	*Vick Vatronol*
Oats (Avena sativa)	*(none)*	*(none)*
Oregon Grape (Berberis aquifolium)	*Tetracycline*	*Achromycin*
	Doxycycline	*Doxycycline*
	Tetracycline	*Helidac (Tetracycline)*
	Tetracycline	*Sumycin*
	Tetracycline	*Tetracycline*
	Doxycycline	*Vibramycin*
Passion Flower (Passiflora incarnata)	*(none)*	*(none)*
Pau D'arco (Tabebuia avellanedae)	*(none)*	*(none)*
Peppermint (Mentha piperita)	*Cisapride*	*Cisapride*
	Menthol	*Menthol*
	Cisapride	*Propulsid*
Phyllanthus (Phyllanthus niruri)	*(none)*	*(none)*
Psyllium (Plantago ovata or Plantago ispaghula)	*Psyllium*	*Effer-syllium*
	Lithium	*Eskalith*
	Psyllium	*Fiberal*
	Psyllium	*Konsyl*
	Lithium	*Lithium*
	Lithium	*Lithobid*
	Lithium	*Lithonate*
	Lithium	*Lithotabs*
	Psyllium	*Metamucil*
	Psyllium	*Modane Bulk*
	Psyllium	*Perdiem Fiber*
	Psyllium	*Psyllium*
	Psyllium	*Reguloid*
	Psyllium	*Serutan*
	Psyllium	*Siblin*
	Psyllium	*Syllact*
	Psyllium	*V-Lax*
Pygeum (Prunus africanum)	*(none)*	*(none)*
Red Clover (Trifolium pratense)	*Heparin*	*Anticoagulant (Heparin)*
	Warfarin	*Anticoagulant (Warfarin)*
	Conjugated Estrogens	*Conjugated Estrogens*

Herb	Drug with Interaction	Generic or Trade Name(s)
Red Clover (continued)	*Warfarin*	*Coumadin*
	Heparin	*Heparin*
	Conjugated Estrogens	*Premarin*
	Conjugated Estrogens	*Prempro (Conjugated estrogens)*
	Ticlopidine	*Ticlid*
	Ticlopidine	*Ticlopidine*
	Warfarin	*Warfarin*
Red Raspberry (Rubus idaeus)	*Ephedrine*	*Adrenaline*
	Ephedrine	*Afrin*
	Ephedrine	*Alka-Seltzer Plus (Pseudoephedrine)*
	Theophylline	*Aminophylline*
	Atropine	*Atropine*
	Ephedrine	*Chlor-Trimeton 12 Hour (Pseudoephedrine)*
	Ephedrine	*Claritin-D (Pseudoephedrine)*
	Codeine	*Codeine*
	Codeine	*Empirin with Codeine (Codeine)*
	Ephedrine	*Ephedrine*
	Atropine	*Isopto Atropine*
	Ephedrine	*Nyquil (Pseudoephedrine)*
	Ephedrine	*Nyquil Hot Therapy Powder (Pseudoephedrine)*
	Codeine	*Phenergan VC with Codeine (Codeine)*
	Codeine	*Phenergan with Codeine (Codeine)*
	Theophylline	*Phyllocontin*
	Ephedrine	*Pretz-D*
	Ephedrine	*Primatene Dual Action (Ephedrine)*
	Theophylline	*Primatene Dual Action (Theophylline)*
	Ephedrine	*Pseudoephedrine*
	Codeine	*Robitussin AC (Codeine)*
	Theophylline	*Slo-Bid*
	Theophylline	*Slo-Phyllin*
	Codeine	*Soma Compound with Codeine (Codeine)*
	Ephedrine	*Sudafed*
	Theophylline	*Theo-Dur*
	Theophylline	*Theolair*
	Theophylline	*Theophylline*
	Ephedrine	*Theraflu (Pseudoephedrine)*
	Ephedrine	*Theraflu Flu and Cold (Pseudoephedrine)*

Herb	Drug with Interaction	Generic or Trade Name(s)
Red Raspberry (continued)	Theophylline	Truphylline
	Ephedrine	Tylenol Allergy Sinus (Pseudoephedrine)
	Ephedrine	Tylenol Cold (Pseudoephedrine)
	Ephedrine	Tylenol Flu NightTime Maximum Strength Powder (Pseudoephedrine)
	Ephedrine	Tylenol Multi-Symptom Hot Medication (Pseudoephedrine)
	Ephedrine	Tylenol Sinus (Pseudoephedrine)
	Codeine	Tylenol with Codeine (Codeine)
	Theophylline	Uniphyl
	Ephedrine	Vick Vatronol
Reishi (Ganoderma lucidum)	(none)	(none)
Rosemary (Rosmarinus officinalis)	(none)	(none)
Sage (Salvia officinalis)	Warfarin	Anticoagulant (Warfarin)
	Warfarin	Coumadin
	Ticlopidine	Ticlid
	Ticlopidine	Ticlopidine
	Warfarin	Warfarin
Sandalwood (Santalum album)	(none)	(none)
Sarsaparilla (Smilax spp.)	(none)	(none)
Saw Palmetto (Serenoa repens, Sabal serrulata)	(none)	(none)
Schisandra (Schisandra chinensis)	Acetaminophen	Acetaminophen
	Acetaminophen	Alka-Seltzer Plus (Aceta-minophen)
	Acetaminophen	APAP
	Acetaminophen	Darvocet (Acetaminophen)
	Acetaminophen	Darvocet N (Acetaminophen)
	Acetaminophen	Excedrin PM (Acetaminophen)
	Acetaminophen	Lortab (Acetaminophen)
	Acetaminophen	Nyquil (Acetaminophen)
	Acetaminophen	Nyquil Hot Therapy Powder (Acetaminophen)
	Acetaminophen	Paracetemol
	Acetaminophen	Percocet (Acetaminophen)
	Acetaminophen	Roxicet (Acetaminophen)
	Acetaminophen	Theraflu (Acetaminophen)
	Acetaminophen	Theraflu Flu and Cold (Acetaminophen)
	Acetaminophen	Tylenol
	Acetaminophen	Tylenol Allergy Sinus (Acetaminophen)
	Acetaminophen	Tylenol Cold (Acetaminophen)
	Acetaminophen	Tylenol Flu NightTime Maximum Strength Powder (Acetaminophen)

Herb	Drug with Interaction	Generic or Trade Name(s)
Schisandra (continued)	*Acetaminophen*	*Tylenol Multi-Symptom Hot Medication (Acetaminophen)*
	Acetaminophen	*Tylenol PM (Acetaminophen)*
	Acetaminophen	*Tylenol PM Extra Strength (Acetaminophen)*
	Acetaminophen	*Tylenol Sinus (Acetaminophen)*
	Acetaminophen	*Tylenol with Codeine (Acetaminophen)*
	Acetaminophen	*Tylenol Allergy Sinus*
	Acetaminophen	*Vicodin (Acetaminophen)*
	Acetaminophen	*Wygesic (Acetaminophen)*
Scullcap (Scutellaria lateriflora, Scutellaria baicalensis)	*(none)*	*(none)*
Senna (Cassia senna, Cassia angustifolia)	*Senna*	*Black-Draught*
	Digoxin	*Digoxin*
	Senna	*Fletcher's Castoria*
	Senna	*Gentlax*
	Digoxin	*Lanoxin*
	Senna	*Senexon*
	Senna	*Senna*
	Senna	*Senna-Gen*
	Senna	*Senokot*
	Senna	*Senolax*
Shiitake (Lentinan edodes)	*Didanosine*	*DDI*
	Didanosine	*Didanosine*
	Didanosine	*Dideoxyinosine*
	Didanosine	*Videx*
Siberian Ginseng—Eleuthero (Eleutherococcus senticosus, Acanthopanax senticosus)	*Warfarin*	*Anticoagulant (Warfarin)*
	Chemotherapy	*Cancer Chemotherapy*
	Chemotherapy	*Chemotherapy*
	Warfarin	*Coumadin*
	Digoxin	*Digoxin*
	Influenza Vaccine	*Flu vaccine*
	Influenza Vaccine	*FluShield*
	Influenza Vaccine	*Fluvirin*
	Influenza Vaccine	*Fluzone*
	Influenza Vaccine	*Influenza Virus Vaccine*
	Digoxin	*Lanoxin*
	Ticlopidine	*Ticlid*
	Ticlopidine	*Ticlopidine*
	Warfarin	*Warfarin*
Slippery Elm (Ulmus rubra)	*(none)*	*(none)*
Stevia (Stevia rebaudiana)	*(none)*	*(none)*
St. John's Wort (Hypericum) perforatum)	*Tricyclic Antidepressants*	*Amitriptyline*
	Tricyclic Antidepressants	*Desipramine*
	Trazodone	*Desyrel*
	Tricyclic Antidepressants	*Doxepin*

Drug Interactions

Herb	Drug with Interaction	Generic or Trade Name(s)
St. John's Wort (continued)	Venlafaxine	Effexor
	Tricyclic Antidepressants	Elavil
	Fluvoxamine	Faurin
	Fluoxetine	Fluoxetine
	Fluvoxamine	Fluvoxamine
	Tricyclic Antidepressants	Imipramine
	Fluvoxamine	Luvox
	Phenelzine	Nardil
	Nefazodone	Nefazodone
	Tricyclic Antidepressants	Norpramin
	Paroxetine	Paroxetine
	Paroxetine	Paxil
	Phenelzine	Phenelzine
	Fluoxetine	Prozac
	Sertraline	Sertraline
	Nefazodone	Serzone
	Tricyclic Antidepressants	Sinequan
	Tricyclic Antidepressants	Tofranil
	Trazodone	Trazodone
	Tricyclic Antidepressants	Tricyclic Antidepressants
	Venlafaxine	Venlafaxine
	Sertraline	Zoloft
Tea Tree (Melaleuca alternifolia)	(none)	(none)
Turmeric (Curcuma longa)	(none)	(none)
Usnea (Usnea barbata)	(none)	(none)
Uva ursi (Arctostaphylos uva-ursi)	Ephedrine	Adrenaline
	Ephedrine	Afrin
	Thiazide Diuretics	Aldactazide (Hydrochlorothiazide)
	Spironolactone	Aldactazide (Spironolactone)
	Spironolactone	Aldactone
	Thiazide Diuretics	Aldoclor (Chlorothiazide)
	Thiazide Diuretics	Aldoril (Hydrochlorothiazide)
	Ephedrine	Alka-Seltzer Plus (Pseudoephedrine)
	Theophylline	Aminophylline
	Thiazide Diuretics	Apresazide (Hydrochlorothiazide)
	Atropine	Atropine
	Loop Diuretics	Bumex
	Thiazide Diuretics	Captozide (Hydrochlorothiazide)
	Thiazide Diuretics	Chlorothiazide
	Thiazide Diuretics	Chlorothiazide/Methyldopa
	Thiazide Diuretics	Chlorthalidone
	Ephedrine	Chlor-Trimeton 12 Hour (Pseudoephedrine)

Herb	Drug with Interaction	Generic or Trade Name(s)
Uva ursi (continued)	*Ephedrine*	*Claritin-D (Pseudoephedrine)*
	Codeine	*Codeine*
	Thiazide Diuretics	*Combipres (Chlorthalidone)*
	Loop Diuretics	*Demadex*
	Thiazide Diuretics	*Diuril*
	Thiazide Diuretics	*Dyazide (Hydrochlorothiazide)*
	Triamterene	*Dyazide (Triamterene)*
	Triamterene	*Dyrenium*
	Loop Diuretics	*Edecrin*
	Codeine	*Empirin with Codeine (Codeine)*
	Ephedrine	*Ephedrine*
	Thiazide Diuretics	*Esidrix*
	Loop Diuretics	*Ethacrynic Acid*
	Loop Diuretics	*Furosemide*
	Thiazide Diuretics	*HCTZ*
	Thiazide Diuretics	*Hydrochlorothiazide*
	Thiazide Diuretics	*HydroDIURIL*
	Thiazide Diuretics	*Hygroton*
	Thiazide Diuretics	*Inderide (Hydrochlorothiazide)*
	Atropine	*Isopto Atropine*
	Loop Diuretics	*Lasix*
	Loop Diuretics	*Loop Diuretics*
	Thiazide Diuretics	*Lopressor HCT (Hydrochlorothiazide)*
	Thiazide Diuretics	*Maxzide (Hydrochlorothiazide)*
	Triamterene	*Maxzide (Triamterene)*
	Thiazide Diuretics	*Metolazone*
	Thiazide Diuretics	*Moduretic (Hydrochlorothiazide)*
	Thiazide Diuretics	*Mykros*
	Ephedrine	*Nyquil (Pseudoephedrine)*
	Ephedrine	*Nyquil Hot Therapy Powder (Pseudoephedrine)*
	Thiazide Diuretics	*Oretic*
	Codeine	*Phenergan VC with Codeine (Codeine)*
	Codeine	*Phenergan with Codeine (Codeine)*
	Theophylline	*Phyllocontin*
	Ephedrine	*Pretz-D*
	Ephedrine	*Primatene Dual Action (Ephedrine)*
	Theophylline	*Primatene Dual Action (Theophylline)*
	Thiazide Diuretics	*Prinizide (Hydrochlorothiazide)*
	Ephedrine	*Pseudoephedrine*

Drug Interactions

Herb	Drug with Interaction	Generic or Trade Name(s)
Uva ursi (continued)	*Codeine*	*Robitussin AC (Codeine)*
	Theophylline	*Slo-Bid*
	Theophylline	*Slo-Phyllin*
	Codeine	*Soma Compound with Codeine (Codeine)*
	Spironolactone	*Spironolactone*
	Ephedrine	*Sudafed*
	Thiazide Diuretics	*Tenoretic (Chlorthalidone)*
	Theophylline	*Theo-Dur*
	Theophylline	*Theolair*
	Theophylline	*Theophylline*
	Ephedrine	*Theraflu (Pseudoephedrine)*
	Ephedrine	*Theraflu Flu and Cold (Pseudoephedrine)*
	Thiazide Diuretics	*Thiazide Diuretics*
	Thiazide Diuretics	*Timolide (Hydrochlorothiazide)*
	Loop Diuretics	*Torsemide*
	Triamterene	*Triamterene*
	Theophylline	*Truphylline*
	Ephedrine	*Tylenol Allergy Sinus (Pseudoephedrine)*
	Ephedrine	*Tylenol Cold (Pseudoephedrine)*
	Ephedrine	*Tylenol Flu NightTime Maximum Strength Powder (Pseudoephedrine)*
	Ephedrine	*Tylenol Multi-Symptom Hot Medication (Pseudoephedrine)*
	Ephedrine	*Tylenol Sinus (Pseu-doephedrine)*
	Codeine	*Tylenol with Codeine (Codeine)*
	Theophylline	*Uniphyl*
	Thiazide Diuretics	*Vaseretic (Hydrochlorothiazide)*
	Ephedrine	*Vick Vatronol*
	Thiazide Diuretics	*Zaroxolyn*
	Thiazide Diuretics	*Zestoretic (Hydrochlorothiazide)*
	Thiazide Diuretics	*Ziac (Hydrochlorothiazide)*
Valerian (Valeriana officinalis)	*(none)*	*(none)*
Vitex (Vitex agnus-castus)	*(none)*	*(none)*
White Willow (Salix alba)	*Bismuth Subsalicylate*	*Bismatrol*
	Bismuth Subsalicylate	*Bismuth Subsalicylate*
	Bismuth Subsalicylate	*BSS*
	Bismuth Subsalicylate	*Helidac (Bismuth subsalicylate)*
	Bismuth Subsalicylate	*Pepto-Bismol*
	Ticlopidine	*Ticlid*
	Ticlopidine	*Ticlopidine*
Wild Cherry (Prunus serotina)	*(none)*	*(none)*
Wild Indigo (Baptisia tinctoria)	*(none)*	*(none)*

Herb	Drug with Interaction	Generic or Trade Name(s)
Wild Yam (Dioscorea villosa)	*(none)*	*(none)*
Witch Hazel (Hamamelis virginiana)	*Ephedrine*	*Adrenaline*
	Ephedrine	*Afrin*
	Ephedrine	*Alka-Seltzer Plus (Pseudoephedrine)*
	Theophylline	*Aminophylline*
	Atropine	*Atropine*
	Ephedrine	*Chlor-Trimeton 12 Hour (Pseudoephedrine)*
	Ephedrine	*Claritin-D (Pseudoephedrine)*
	Codeine	*Codeine*
	Codeine	*Empirin with Codeine (Codeine)*
	Ephedrine	*Ephedrine*
	Atropine	*Isopto Atropine*
	Ephedrine	*Nyquil (Pseudoephedrine)*
	Ephedrine	*Nyquil Hot Therapy Powder - (Pseudoephedrine)*
	Codeine	*Phenergan VC with Codeine (Codeine)*
	Codeine	*Phenergan with Codeine (Codeine)*
	Theophylline	*Phyllocontin*
	Ephedrine	*Pretz-D*
	Ephedrine	*Primatene Dual Action (Ephedrine)*
	Theophylline	*Primatene Dual Action (Theophylline)*
	Ephedrine	*Pseudoephedrine*
	Codeine	*Robitussin AC (Codeine)*
	Theophylline	*Slo-Bid*
	Theophylline	*Slo-Phyllin*
	Codeine	*Soma Compound with Codeine (Codeine)*
	Ephedrine	*Sudafed*
	Theophylline	*Theo-Dur*
	Theophylline	*Theolair*
	Theophylline	*Theophylline*
	Ephedrine	*Theraflu (Pseudoephedrine)*
	Ephedrine	*Theraflu Flu and Cold (Pseudoephedrine)*
	Theophylline	*Truphylline*
	Ephedrine	*Tylenol Allergy Sinus (Pseudoephedrine)*
	Ephedrine	*Tylenol Cold (Pseudoephedrine)*
	Ephedrine	*Tylenol Flu NightTime Maximum Strength Powder (Pseudoephedrine)*

Herb	Drug with Interaction	Generic or Trade Name(s)
Witch Hazel (continued)	*Ephedrine*	*Tylenol Multi-Symptom Hot Medication (Pseudoephedrine)*
	Ephedrine	*Tylenol Sinus (Pseu-doephedrine)*
	Codeine	*Tylenol with Codeine (Codeine)*
	Theophylline	*Uniphyl*
	Ephedrine	*Vick Vatronol*
Wormwood (Artemisia absinthium)	*(none)*	*(none)*
Yarrow (Achillea millefolium)	*(none)*	*(none)*
Yellow Dock (Rumex crispus)	*(none)*	*(none)*
Yohimbe (Pausinystalia yohimbe)	*Fluvoxamine*	*Faurin*
	Fluvoxamine	*Fluvoxamine*
	Fluvoxamine	*Luvox*
Yucca (Yucca schidigera and other species)	*(none)*	*(none)*

DRUG-SUPPLEMENT INTERACTIONS

Supplement	Drug with Interaction	Generic or Trade Name(s)
5-Hydroxytryptophan (5-HTP)	*Carbidopa*	*Aldamet*
	Zolpidem	*Ambien*
	Tricyclic Antidepressants	*Amitriptyline*
	Carbidopa	*Carbidopa*
	Carbidopa Levodopa	*Carbidopa/Levodopa*
	Tricyclic Antidepressants	*Desipramine*
	Tricyclic Antidepressants	*Doxepin*
	Venlafaxine	*Effexor*
	Tricyclic Antidepressants	*Elavil*
	Lithium	*Eskalith*
	Fluvoxamine	*Faurin*
	Fluoxetine	*Fluoxetine*
	Fluvoxamine	*Fluvoxamine*
	Tricyclic Antidepressants	*Imipramine*
	Sumatriptan	*Imitrex*
	Lithium	*Lithium*
	Lithium	*Lithobid*
	Lithium	*Lithonate*
	Lithium	*Lithotabs*
	Carbidopa	*Lodosyn*
	Fluvoxamine	*Luvox*

Supplement	Drug with Interaction	Generic or Trade Name(s)
5-HTP (continued)	*Tricyclic Antidepressants*	*Norpramin*
	Paroxetine	*Paroxetine*
	Paroxetine	*Paxil*
	Fluoxetine	*Prozac*
	Sertraline	*Sertraline*
	Carbidopa Levodopa	*Sinemet*
	Tricyclic Antidepressants	*Sinequan*
	Sumatriptan	*Sumatriptan*
	Tricyclic Antidepressants	*Tofranil*
	Tramadol	*Tramadol*
	Tricyclic Antidepressants	*Tricyclic Antidepressants*
	Tramadol	*Ultram*
	Venlafaxine	*Venlafaxine*
	Sertraline	*Zoloft*
	Zolpidem	*Zolpidem*
Acetyl-L-Carnitine	*(none)*	*(none)*
Acidophilus (Probiotics) and Fructo-oligosaccharides (FOS)	*Tetracycline*	*Achromycin*
	Amoxicillin	*Amoxicillin*
	Amoxicillin	*Amoxil*
	Antibiotics	*Antibiotics*
	Amoxicillin	*Augmentin*
	Erythromycin	*EES*
	Erythromycin	*E-Mycin*
	Erythromycin	*Eryc Ery-Tab Erythromycin*
	Tetracycline	*Helidac (Tetracycline)*
	Erythromycin	*Ilosone*
	Amoxicillin	*Polymox*
	Tetracycline	*Sumycin*
	Tetracycline	*Tetracycline*
Adenosine Monophosphate (AMP)	*(none)*	*(none)*
Alanine	*(none)*	*(none)*
Alpha Lipoic Acid	*(none)*	*(none)*
Amino Acids (Overview)	*(none)*	*(none)*
Arginine	*(none)*	*(none)*
Beta-Sitosterol	*(none)*	*(none)*
Betaine Hydrochloride (Hydrochloric Acid)	*(none)*	*(none)*
Bioflavonoids	*(none)*	*(none)*
Biotin	*Insulin*	*Animal-Source Insulin*
	Anticonvulsants	*Anticonvulsants*
	Anticonvulsants	*Carbamazepine*
	Glyburide	*Diabeta*
	Anticonvulsants	*Dilantin*
	Glyburide	*Glibenclamide*
	Glyburide	*Glyburide*

Supplement	Drug with Interaction	Generic or Trade Name(s)
Biotin (continued)	*Insulin*	*Human Analog Insulin*
	Insulin	*Human Insulin*
	Insulin	*Humanlog*
	Insulin	*Humulin*
	Insulin	*Iletin*
	Insulin	*Insulin*
	Glyburide	*Micronase*
	Anticonvulsants	*Mysoline*
	Insulin	*Novolin*
	Anticonvulsants	*Phenobarbital*
	Anticonvulsants	*Phenytoin*
	Glyburide	*Pres Tab*
	Anticonvulsants	*Primidone*
	Anticonvulsants	*Tegretol*
Boric Acid	*(none)*	*(none)*
Boron	*(none)*	*(none)*
Branched-Chain Amino Acids (BCAAs)	*(none)*	*(none)*
Brewer's Yeast	*Antibiotics*	*Antibiotics*
Bromelain	*Amoxicillin*	*Amoxicillin*
	Amoxicillin	*Amoxil*
	Warfarin	*Anticoagulant (Warfarin)*
	Amoxicillin	*Augmentin*
	Warfarin	*Coumadin*
	Erythromycin	*EES*
	Erythromycin	*E-Mycin*
	Erythromycin	*Eryc Ery-Tab Erythromycin*
	Erythromycin	*Ilosone*
	Penicillin V	*Penicillin V*
	Penicillin V	*Pen-Vee K*
	Amoxicillin	*Polymox*
	Penicillin V	*Veetids*
	Warfarin	*Warfarin*
Calcium	*Tetracycline*	*Achromycin*
	Corticosteroids	*AeroBid*
	Tobramycin	*AKTob*
	Albuterol	*Albuterol*
	Thiazide Diuretics	*Aldactazide (Hydrochloroth-iazide)*
	Thiazide Diuretics	*Aldoclor (Chlorothiazide)*
	Thiazide Diuretics	*Aldoril (Hydrochlorothiazide)*
	Alendronate	*Alendronate*
	Aluminum Hydroxide	*Aluminum Hydroxide*
	Caffeine	*Anacin (Caffeine)*
	Thyroid Hormones	*Animal Levothyroxine/Liothyro-nine*
	Thyroid Hormones	*Animal Thyroid*

Supplement	**Drug with Interaction**	**Generic or Trade Name(s)**
Calcium (continued)	Antacids	Antacids
	Multi Vitamin	Appedrine (Multiple vitamins and minerals)
	Thiazide Diuretics	Apresazide (Hydrochlorothiazide)
	Corticosteroids	Aristocort
	Thyroid Hormones	Armour Thyroid
	Corticosteroids	Azmacort
	Sulfamethoxazole	Azulfidine
	Corticosteroids	Beclomethasone
	Corticosteroids	Beclovent
	Corticosteroids	Beconase
	Trimethoprim	Bethaprim
	Bile Acid Sequestrants	Bile Acid Sequestrants
	Oral Contraceptives	Birth Control Pill
	Oral Contraceptives	Brevicon
	Corticosteroids	Budesonide
	Caffeine	Caffedrine
	Caffeine	Caffeine
	Verapamil	Calan
	Thiazide Diuretics	Captozide (Hydrochlorothiazide)
	Thiazide Diuretics	Chlorothiazide
	Thiazide Diuretics	Chlorothiazide/Methyldopa
	Thiazide Diuretics	Chlorthalidone
	Bile Acid Sequestrants	Cholestyramine
	Ciprofloxacin	Cipro
	Ciprofloxacin	Ciprofloxacin
	Cisplatin	Cisplatin
	Thiazide Diuretics	Combipres (Chlorthalidone)
	Albuterol	Combivent (Albuterol)
	Trimethoprim	Comoxol
	Conjugated Estrogens	Conjugated Estrogens
	Corticosteroids	Cortef
	Corticosteroids	Corticosteroids
	Corticosteroids	Cortisone-like drugs
	Losartan	Cozaar
	Corticosteroids	Cutivate
	Cycloserine	Cycloserine
	Medroxyprogesterone	Cycrin
	Thyroid Hormones	Cytomel
	Lactase	Dairy Ease
	Caffeine	Darvon Compound (Caffeine)
	Corticosteroids	Decadron
	Corticosteroids	Decadron Phosphate Turbinaire
	Corticosteroids	Delta-Cortef

Supplement	Drug with Interaction	Generic or Trade Name(s)
Calcium (continued)	Corticosteroids	Deltasone
	Oral Contraceptives	Demulen
	Medroxyprogesterone	Depo-Provera
	Thyroid Hormones	Desiccated Thyroid
	Corticosteroids	Dexamethasone
	Aluminum Hydroxide	Di-Gel
	Thiazide Diuretics	Diuril
	Doxycycline	Doxycycline
	Thiazide Diuretics	Dyazide (Hydrochlorothiazide)
	Triamterene	Dyazide (Triamterene)
	Triamterene	Dyrenium
	Erythromycin	EES
	Corticosteroids	Elocon
	Thyroid Hormones	Eltroxin
	Erythromycin	E-Mycin
	Oral Contraceptives	Enovid
	Erythromycin	Eryc Ery-Tab Erythromycin
	Thiazide Diuretics	Esidrix
	Thyroid Hormones	Euthroid
	Corticosteroids	Flonase
	Ofloxacin	Floxin
	Alendronate	Fosamax
	Corticosteroids	Flunisolide
	Corticosteroids	Fluticasone
	Sulfamethoxazole	Gantanol
	Gentamicin	Garamycin
	Oral Contraceptives	Genora
	Gentamicin	Gentamicin
	Thiazide Diuretics	HCTZ
	Tetracycline	Helidac (Tetracycline)
	Thiazide Diuretics	Hydrochlorothiazide
	Corticosteroids	Hydrocortisone
	Thiazide Diuretics	HydroDIURIL
	Thiazide Diuretics	Hygroton
	Corticosteroids	Hytone
	Erythromycin	Ilosone
	Thiazide Diuretics	Inderide (Hydrochlorothiazide)
	Indomethacin	Indocin
	Indomethacin	Indomethacin
	Isoniazid	INH
	Isoniazid	Isoniazid
	Verapamil	Isoptin
	Lactase	LactAid
	Lactase	Lactase
	Lactase	Lactrase
	Isoniazid	Laniazid

Drug Interactions

Supplement	Drug with Interaction	Generic or Trade Name(s)
Calcium (continued)	Oral Contraceptives	Levlen
	Thyroid Hormones	Levo-T
	Thyroid Hormones	Levothroid
	Thyroid Hormones	Levothyroxine
	Thyroid Hormones	Levoxyl
	Thyroid Hormones	Liothyronine
	Thyroid Hormones	Liotrix
	Oral Contraceptives	Loestrin
	Thiazide Diuretics	Lopressor HCT (Hydrochlorothiazide)
	Losartan	Losartan
	Aluminum Hydroxide	Maalox (Aluminum hydroxide)
	Thiazide Diuretics	Maxzide (Hydrochlorothiazide)
	Triamterene	Maxzide (Triamterene)
	Corticosteroids	Medrol
	Medroxyprogesterone	Medroxyprogesterone
	Corticosteroids	Methylprednisolone
	Thiazide Diuretics	Metolazone
	Oral Contraceptives	Micronor
	Mineral Oil	Mineral Oil
	Oral Contraceptives	Modicon
	Thiazide Diuretics	Moduretic (Hydrochlorothiazide)
	Corticosteroids	Mometasone
	Thiazide Diuretics	Mykros
	Aluminum Hydroxide	Mylanta (Aluminum hydroxide)
	Corticosteroids	Nasacort
	Corticosteroids	Nasalide
	Tobramycin	Nebicin
	Neomycin	Neomycin
	Caffeine	NoDoz
	Oral Contraceptives	Nordette
	Oral Contraceptives	Norinyl
	Ofloxacin	Oculflox Ofloxacin
	Oral Contraceptives	Oral Contraceptives
	Corticosteroids	Orasone
	Thiazide Diuretics	Oretic
	Oral Contraceptives	Ortho-Novum
	Oral Contraceptives	Ovcon
	Oral Contraceptives	Ovral
	Oral Contraceptives	Ovrette
	Corticosteroids	Pediapred
	Cisplatin	Platinol
	Corticosteroids	Prednisolone
	Corticosteroids	Prednisone
	Conjugated Estrogens	Premarin

Drug Interactions

Supplement	Drug with Interaction	Generic or Trade Name(s)
Calcium (continued)	*Conjugated Estrogens*	*Prempro (Conjugated estrogens)*
	Medroxyprogesterone	*Prempro (Medroxyprogesterone)*
	Thiazide Diuretics	*Prinizide (Hydrochlorothiazide)*
	Thyroid Hormones	*Proloid*
	Trimethoprim	*Proloprim*
	Albuterol	*Proventil*
	Medroxyprogesterone	*Provera*
	Corticosteroids	*Pulmicort*
	Bile Acid Sequestrants	*Questran*
	Caffeine	*Quick Pep*
	Corticosteroids	*Rhinocort*
	Isoniazid	*Rifamate*
	Isoniazid	*Rimactane*
	Aluminum Hydroxide	*Riopan*
	Aluminum Hydroxide	*Rolaids*
	Cycloserine	*Seromycin*
	Corticosteroids	*Steroids (Prednisone)*
	Sulfamethoxazole	*Sulfamethoxazole*
	Tetracycline	*Sumycin*
	Lactase	*SureLac*
	Thyroid Hormones	*Synthetic Liothyronine*
	Thyroid Hormones	*Synthroid*
	Aluminum Hydroxide	*Tempo tablets (Aluminum hydroxide)*
	Thiazide Diuretics	*Tenoretic (Chlorthalidone)*
	Tetracycline	*Tetracycline*
	Thiazide Diuretics	*Thiazide Diuretics*
	Thyroid Hormones	*Thyar*
	Thyroid Hormones	*Thyroglobulin*
	Thyroid Hormones	*Thyroid Hormones*
	Thyroid Hormones	*Thyrolar*
	Thiazide Diuretics	*Timolide (Hydrochlorothiazide)*
	Tobramycin	*TOBI*
	Corticosteroids	*Tobradex (Dexamthasone)*
	Tobramycin	*Tobradex (Tobramycin)*
	Tobramycin	*Tobramycin*
	Tobramycin	*Tobrex*
	Corticosteroids	*Triamcinolone*
	Triamterene	*Triamterene*
	Trimethoprim	*Trimethoprim*
	Trimethoprim	*Trimpex*
	Oral Contraceptives	*Triphasil*
	Corticosteroids	*Vancenase*
	Corticosteroids	*Vanceril*

Supplement	Drug with Interaction	Generic or Trade Name(s)
Calcium (continued)	Thiazide Diuretics	Vaseretic (Hydrochlorothiazide)
	Albuterol	Ventolin
	Verapamil	Verapamil
	Verapamil	Verelan
	Doxycycline	Vibramycin
	Caffeine	Vivarin
	Thiazide Diuretics	Zaroxolyn
	Thiazide Diuretics	Zestoretic (Hydrochlorothiazide)
	Thiazide Diuretics	Ziac (Hydrochlorothiazide)
L-Carnitine	Doxorubicin	Adriamycin
	Anticonvulsants	Anticonvulsants
	AZT	Azidothymidine
	AZT	AZT
	Anticonvulsants	Carbamazepine
	Valproic Acid	Depakene Syrup
	Valproic Acid	Depakene
	Valproic Acid	Depakote
	Anticonvulsants	Dilantin
	Valproic Acid	Divalproex sodium
	Doxorubicin	Doxorubicin
	Anticonvulsants	Mysoline
	Anticonvulsants	Phenobarbital
	Anticonvulsants	Phenytoin
	Anticonvulsants	Primidone
	AZT	Retrovir
	Valproic Acid	Sodium Valproate
	Anticonvulsants	Tegretol
	Valproic Acid	Valproic Acid
	AZT	Zidovudine
Cartilage (Bovine and Shark)	(none)	(none)
Chlorophyll	(none)	(none)
Chondroitin Sulfate	(none)	(none)
Chromium	Insulin	Animal-Source Insulin
	Glyburide	Diabeta
	Glyburide	Glibenclamide
	Glyburide	Glyburide
	Insulin	Human Analog Insulin
	Insulin	Human Insulin
	Insulin	Humanlog
	Insulin	Humulin
	Insulin	Iletin
	Insulin	Insulin
	Glyburide	Micronase
	Insulin	Novolin
	Glyburide	Pres Tab

Supplement	Drug with Interaction	Generic or Trade Name(s)
Conjugated Linoleic Acid (CLA)	(none)	(none)
Coenzyme Q₁₀	Doxorubicin	Adriamycin
	Tricyclic Antidepressants	Amitriptyline
	Warfarin	Anticoagulant (Warfarin)
	Gemfibrozil	Apo-Gemfibrozil
	Atorvastatin	Atorvastatin
	Timolol	Blocadren
	Timolol	Cosopt (Timolol)
	Warfarin	Coumadin
	Tricyclic Antidepressants	Desipramine
	Tricyclic Antidepressants	Doxepin
	Doxorubicin	Doxorubicin
	Tricyclic Antidepressants	Elavil
	Fluvastatin	Fluvastatin
	Gemfibrozil	Gemfibrozil
	Tricyclic Antidepressants	Imipramine
	Propranolol	Inderal
	Propranolol	Inderide (Propranolol)
	Fluvastatin	Lescol
	Atorvastatin	Lipitor
	Gemfibrozil	Lopid
	Lovastatin	Lovastatin
	Lovastatin	Mevacor
	Tricyclic Antidepressants	Norpramin
	Gemfibrozil	Novo-Gemfibrozil
	Pravastatin	Pravachol
	Pravastatin	Pravastatin
	Propranolol	Propranolol
	Simvastatin	Simvastatin
	Tricyclic Antidepressants	Sinequan
	Timolol	Timolide (Timolol)
	Timolol	Timolol
	Timolol	Timoptic
	Tricyclic Antidepressants	Tofranil
	Tricyclic Antidepressants	Tricyclic Antidepressants
	Warfarin	Warfarin
	Simvastatin	Zocor
Copper	Quinapril	Accupril
	ACE Inhibitors	ACE Inhibitors
	Ibuprofen	Advil
	Naproxen	Aleve
	Ramipril	Altace
	Naproxen	Anaprox
	ACE Inhibitors	Angiotensin Converting Enzyme Inhibitors
	Antacids	Antacids

Supplement	Drug with Interaction	Generic or Trade Name(s)
Copper (continued)	Multi Vitamin	Appedrine (Multiple vitamins and minerals)
	Nizatidine	Axid
	Nizatidine	Axid AR
	AZT	Azidothymidine
	AZT	AZT
	Benazepril	Benazepril
	Oral Contraceptives	Birth Control Pill
	Oral Contraceptives	Brevicon
	Ibuprofen	Brufin
	Captopril	Capoten
	Captopril	Captopril
	Captopril	Captozide (Captopril)
	Ciprofloxacin	Cipro
	Ciprofloxacin	Ciprofloxacin
	Penicillamine	Cuprimine
	Oxaprozin	Daypro
	Oral Contraceptives	Demulen
	Valproic Acid	Depakene Syrup
	Valproic Acid	Depakene
	Valproic Acid	Depakote
	Penicillamine	Depen
	Vitamin C	Dex-A-Diet Plus Vitamin C (Vitamin C)
	Vitamin C	Dexatrim Plus Vitamin C (Vitamin C)
	Valproic Acid	Divalproex sodium
	Oral Contraceptives	Enovid
	Etodolac	Etodolac
	Famotidine	Famotidine
	Ibuprofen	Feldene
	Ibuprofen	Froben
	Oral Contraceptives	Genora
	Ibuprofen	Ibuprofen
	Oral Contraceptives	Levlen
	Lisinopril	Lisinopril
	Etodolac	Lodine
	Oral Contraceptives	Loestrin
	Benazepril	Lotensin
	Oral Contraceptives	Micronor
	Oral Contraceptives	Modicon
	Ibuprofen	Motrin
	Ibuprofen	Motrin IB
	Nabumetone	Nabumetone
	Naproxen	Napralen Naprosyn Naproxen
	Naproxen	Naproxen Sodium

Supplement	Drug with Interaction	Generic or Trade Name(s)
Copper (continued)	Nizatidine	Nizatidine
	Oral Contraceptives	Nordette
	Oral Contraceptives	Norinyl
	Ibuprofen	Nuprin
	Oral Contraceptives	Oral Contraceptives
	Oral Contraceptives	Ortho-Novum
	Oral Contraceptives	Ovcon
	Oral Contraceptives	Ovral
	Oral Contraceptives	Ovrette
	Oxaprozin	Oxaprozin
	Penicillamine	Penicillamine
	Famotidine	Pepcid
	Famotidine	Pepcid AC
	Lisinopril	Prinivil
	Lisinopril	Prinizide (Lisinopril)
	Quinapril	Quinapril
	Ramipril	Ramipril
	Nabumetone	Relafen
	AZT	Retrovir
	Valproic Acid	Sodium Valproate
	Oral Contraceptives	Triphasil
	Valproic Acid	Valproic Acid
	Ibuprofen	Voltarol
	Lisinopril	Zestoretic (Lisinopril)
	AZT	Zidovudine
Creatine Monohydrate	(none)	(none)
Cysteine	Acetaminophen	Acetaminophen
	Interferon	Actimmune
	Doxorubicin	Adriamycin
	Corticosteroids	AeroBid
	Interferon	Alferon N
	Acetaminophen	Alka-Seltzer Plus (Acetaminophen)
	Acetaminophen	APAP
	Corticosteroids	Aristocort
	Interferon	Avonex
	Corticosteroids	Azmacort
	Corticosteroids	Beclomethasone
	Corticosteroids	Beclovent
	Corticosteroids	Beconase
	Interferon	Betaseron
	Corticosteroids	Budesonide
	Chemotherapy	Cancer Chemotherapy
	Chemotherapy	Chemotherapy
	Corticosteroids	Cortef
	Corticosteroids	Corticosteroids
	Corticosteroids	Cortisone-like drugs

Supplement	Drug with Interaction	Generic or Trade Name(s)
Cysteine (continued)	Corticosteroids	Cutivate
	Acetaminophen	Darvocet (Acetaminophen)
	Acetaminophen	Darvocet N (Acetaminophen)
	Corticosteroids	Decadron
	Corticosteroids	Decadron Phosphate Turbinaire
	Corticosteroids	Delta-Cortef
	Corticosteroids	Deltasone
	Nitroglycerin	Deponit
	Corticosteroids	Dexamethasone
	Doxorubicin	Doxorubicin
	Corticosteroids	Elocon
	Acetaminophen	Excedrin PM (Acetaminophen)
	Corticosteroids	Flonase
	Corticosteroids	Flunisolide
	Corticosteroids	Fluticasone
	Nitroglycerin	Glycerly Trinitrate
	Corticosteroids	Hydrocortisone
	Corticosteroids	Hytone
	Isosorbide Mononitrate	Imdur
	Interferon	Interferon
	Interferon	Intron
	Isosorbide Mononitrate	ISMO
	Isosorbide Mononitrate	Isosorbide Mononitrate
	Acetaminophen	Lortab (Acetaminophen)
	Corticosteroids	Medrol
	Corticosteroids	Methylprednisolone
	Nitroglycerin	Minitran
	Corticosteroids	Mometasone
	Isosorbide Mononitrate	Monoket
	Corticosteroids	Nasacort
	Corticosteroids	Nasalide
	Nitroglycerin	Nitro-Bid
	Nitroglycerin	Nitrodisc
	Nitroglycerin	Nitro-Dur
	Nitroglycerin	Nitrogard
	Nitroglycerin	Nitroglycerin
	Nitroglycerin	Nitrolingual
	Nitroglycerin	Nitrostat
	Acetaminophen	Nyquil (Acetaminophen)
	Acetaminophen	Nyquil Hot Therapy Powder (Acetaminophen)
	Corticosteroids	Orasone
	Acetaminophen	Paracetemol
	Corticosteroids	Pediapred
	Acetaminophen	Percocet (Acetaminophen)
	Corticosteroids	Prednisolone
	Corticosteroids	Prednisone

Drug Interactions

Supplement	Drug with Interaction	Generic or Trade Name(s)
Cysteine (continued)	Corticosteroids	Pulmicort
	Interferon	Rebif
	Corticosteroids	Rhinocort
	Interferon	Roferon-A
	Acetaminophen	Roxicet (Acetaminophen)
	Corticosteroids	Steroids (Prednisone)
	Acetaminophen	Theraflu (Acetaminophen)
	Acetaminophen	Theraflu Flu and Cold (Acetaminophen)
	Corticosteroids	Tobradex (Dexamthasone)
	Nitroglycerin	Transderm-Nitro
	Corticosteroids	Triamcinolone
	Acetaminophen	Tylenol
	Acetaminophen	Tylenol Allergy Sinus (Acetaminophen)
	Acetaminophen	Tylenol Cold (Acetaminophen)
	Acetaminophen	Tylenol Flu NightTime Maximum Strength Powder (Acetaminophen)
	Acetaminophen	Tylenol Multi-Symptom Hot Medication (Acetaminophen)
	Acetaminophen	Tylenol PM (Acetaminophen)
	Acetaminophen	Tylenol PM Extra Strength (Acetaminophen)
	Acetaminophen	Tylenol Sinus (Acetaminophen)
	Acetaminophen	Tylenol with Codeine (Acetaminophen)
	Acetaminophen	Tylenol Allergy Sinus
	Corticosteroids	Vancenase
	Corticosteroids	Vanceril
	Acetaminophen	Vicodin (Acetaminophen)
	Interferon	Weferon
	Acetaminophen	Wygesic (Acetaminophen)
Docosahexaenoic Acid (DHA)	Cyclosporine	Cyclosporine
	Cyclosporine	Neoral
	Cyclosporine	Sandimmune
	Corticosteroids	AeroBid
	Corticosteroids	Aristocort
	Corticosteroids	Azmacort
	Corticosteroids	Beclomethasone
	Corticosteroids	Beclovent
	Corticosteroids	Beconase
	Corticosteroids	Budesonide
	Corticosteroids	Cortef
	Corticosteroids	Corticosteroids
	Corticosteroids	Cortisone-like drugs
	Corticosteroids	Cutivate

Supplement	Drug with Interaction	Generic or Trade Name(s)
DHA (continued)	Corticosteroids	Decadron
	Corticosteroids	Decadron Phosphate Turbinaire
	Corticosteroids	Delta-Cortef
	Corticosteroids	Deltasone
	Corticosteroids	Dexamethasone
	Corticosteroids	Elocon
	Corticosteroids	Flonase
	Corticosteroids	Flunisolide
	Corticosteroids	Fluticasone
	Corticosteroids	Hydrocortisone
	Corticosteroids	Hytone
	Corticosteroids	Medrol
	Corticosteroids	Methylprednisolone
	Corticosteroids	Mometasone
	Corticosteroids	Nasacort
	Corticosteroids	Nasalide
	Corticosteroids	Orasone
	Corticosteroids	Pediapred
	Corticosteroids	Prednisolone
	Corticosteroids	Prednisone
	Corticosteroids	Pulmicort
	Corticosteroids	Rhinocort
	Corticosteroids	Steroids (Prednisone)
	Corticosteroids	Tobradex (Dexamthasone)
	Corticosteroids	Triamcinolone
	Corticosteroids	Vancenase
	Corticosteroids	Vanceril
DMAE (2-Dimethylaminoethanol)	(none)	(none)
DMSO (Dimethyl Sulfoxide)	(none)	(none)
Digestive Enzymes	Warfarin	Anticoagulant (Warfarin)
	Warfarin	Coumadin
	Warfarin	Warfarin
Evening Primrose Oil (GLA)	Ibuprofen	Advil
	Naproxen	Aleve
	Naproxen	Anaprox
	Ibuprofen	Brufin
	Oxaprozin	Daypro
	Etodolac	Etodolac
	Ibuprofen	Feldene
	Ibuprofen	Froben
	Ibuprofen	Ibuprofen
	Indomethacin	Indocin
	Indomethacin	Indomethacin
	Etodolac	Lodine
	Ibuprofen	Motrin
	Ibuprofen	Motrin IB
	Nabumetone	Nabumetone

Supplement	Drug with Interaction	Generic or Trade Name(s)
Evening Primrose Oil (continued)	Naproxen	Napralen Naprosyn Naproxen
	Naproxen	Naproxen Sodium
	Ibuprofen	Nuprin
	Oxaprozin	Oxaprozin
	Nabumetone	Relafen
	Ibuprofen	Voltarol
Fiber	Verapamil	Calan
	Propoxyphene	Darvocet (Propoxyphene)
	Propoxyphene	Darvocet N (Propoxyphene-N)
	Propoxyphene	Darvon Compound (Propoxyphene)
	Propoxyphene	Darvon-N
	Verapamil	Isoptin
	Lovastatin	Lovastatin
	Lovastatin	Mevacor
	Propoxyphene	Propoxyphene
	Verapamil	Verapamil
	Verapamil	Verelan
	Propoxyphene	Wygesic (Propoxyphene)
Fish Oil (EPA and DHA) and Cod Liver Oil	Cyclosporine	Cyclosporine
	Cyclosporine	Neoral
	Cyclosporine	Sandimmune
Flaxseed Oil	(none)	(none)
Folic Acid	Aspirin	Acetylsalicylic Acid
	Tetracycline	Achromycin
	Aspirin	Alka-Seltzer (Aspirin)
	Aspirin	Anacin (Aspirin)
	Antacids	Antacids
	Anticonvulsants	Anticonvulsants
	Aspirin	ASA
	Aspirin	Aspirin
	Nizatidine	Axid
	Nizatidine	Axid AR
	Sulfamethoxazole	Azulfidine
	Trimethoprim Sulfamethoxazole	Bactrim
	Trimethoprim	Bethaprim
	Bile Acid Sequestrants	Bile Acid Sequestrants
	Oral Contraceptives	Birth Control Pill
	Oral Contraceptives	Brevicon
	Chemotherapy	Cancer Chemotherapy
	Anticonvulsants	Carbamazepine
	Chemotherapy	Chemotherapy
	Bile Acid Sequestrants	Cholestyramine
	Colestipol	Colestid
	Colestipol	Colestipol
	Trimethoprim	Comoxol

Supplement	Drug with Interaction	Generic or Trade Name(s)
Folic Acid (continued)	Trimethoprim Sulfamethoxazole	Cotrim (Co-Trimoxazole)
	Cycloserine	Cycloserine
	Medroxyprogesterone	Cycrin
	Aspirin	Darvon Compound (Aspirin)
	Oral Contraceptives	Demulen
	Medroxyprogesterone	Depo-Provera
	Anticonvulsants	Dilantin
	Triamterene	Dyazide (Triamterene)
	Triamterene	Dyrenium
	Erythromycin	EES
	Aspirin	Empirin with Codeine (Aspirin)
	Erythromycin	E-Mycin
	Oral Contraceptives	Enovid
	Erythromycin	Eryc Ery-Tab Erythromycin
	Lithium	Eskalith
	Famotidine	Famotidine
	Fluoxetine	Fluoxetine
	Methotrexate	Folex
	Sulfamethoxazole	Gantanol
	Oral Contraceptives	Genora
	Metformin	Glucophage
	Tetracycline	Helidac (Tetracycline)
	Erythromycin	Ilosone
	Indomethacin	Indocin
	Indomethacin	Indomethacin
	Isoniazid	INH
	Isoniazid	Isoniazid
	Isoniazid	Laniazid
	Oral Contraceptives	Levlen
	Lithium	Lithium
	Lithium	Lithobid
	Lithium	Lithonate
	Lithium	Lithotabs
	Oral Contraceptives	Loestrin
	Triamterene	Maxzide (Triamterene)
	Medroxyprogesterone	Medroxyprogesterone
	Metformin	Metformin
	Methotrexate	Methotrexate
	Oral Contraceptives	Micronor
	Oral Contraceptives	Modicon
	Anticonvulsants	Mysoline
	Neomycin	Neomycin
	Nitrous Oxide	Nitrous Oxide
	Nizatidine	Nizatidine
	Oral Contraceptives	Nordette
	Oral Contraceptives	Norinyl
	Oral Contraceptives	Oral Contraceptives

Supplement	Drug with Interaction	Generic or Trade Name(s)
Folic Acid (continued)	Oral Contraceptives	Ortho-Novum
	Oral Contraceptives	Ovcon
	Oral Contraceptives	Ovral
	Oral Contraceptives	Ovrette
	Famotidine	Pepcid
	Famotidine	Pepcid AC
	Aspirin	Percodan (Aspirin)
	Anticonvulsants	Phenobarbital
	Anticonvulsants	Phenytoin
	Medroxyprogesterone	Prempro (Medroxyprogesterone)
	Anticonvulsants	Primidone
	Trimethoprim	Proloprim
	Medroxyprogesterone	Provera
	Fluoxetine	Prozac
	Bile Acid Sequestrants	Questran
	Methotrexate	Rheumatrex
	Isoniazid	Rifamate
	Isoniazid	Rimactane
	Aspirin	Roxiprin (Aspirin)
	Trimethoprim Sulfamethoxazole	Septra
	Cycloserine	Seromycin
	Aspirin	Soma Compound (Aspirin)
	Aspirin	Soma Compound with Codeine (Aspirin)
	Sulfamethoxazole	Sulfamethoxazole
	Sulfasalazine	Sulfasalazine
	Tetracycline	Sumycin
	Anticonvulsants	Tegretol
	Tetracycline	Tetracycline
	Triamterene	Triamterene
	Trimethoprim	Trimethoprim
	Trimethoprim Sulfamethoxazole	Trimethoprim/Sulfamethoxazole
	Trimethoprim	Trimpex
	Oral Contraceptives	Triphasil
	Trimethoprim Sulfamethoxazole	Uroplus
Fumaric Acid	(none)	(none)
Gamma Oryzanol	(none)	(none)
Glucosamine Sulfate	(none)	(none)
Glutamic Acid	(none)	(none)
Glutamine	Chemotherapy	Cancer Chemotherapy
	Chemotherapy	Chemotherapy
	Paclitaxel	Paclitaxel
	Paclitaxel	Taxol
Glycine	Haloperidol	Haldol
Glycine	Haloperidol	Haloperidol
Histidine	(none)	(none)

Supplement	Drug with Interaction	Generic or Trade Name(s)
HMB (Beta Hydroxy-Beta-Methylbutyrate)	(none)	(none)
Hydroxycitric acid (HCA)	(none)	(none)
Inosine	(none)	(none)
Inositol	(none)	(none)
Iodine	(none)	(none)
Iron	Aspirin	Acetylsalicylic Acid
	Tetracycline	Achromycin
	Ibuprofen	Advil
	Carbidopa	Aldamet
	Methyldopa	Aldoclor (Methyldopa)
	Methyldopa	Aldomet
	Methyldopa	Aldoril (Methyldopa)
	Naproxen	Aleve
	Aspirin	Alka-Seltzer (Aspirin)
	Sodium Bicarbonate	Alka-Seltzer (Sodium bicarbonate)
	Aspirin	Anacin (Aspirin)
	Naproxen	Anaprox
	Thyroid Hormones	Animal Levothyroxine/Liothyronine
	Thyroid Hormones	Animal Thyroid
	Warfarin	Anticoagulant (Warfarin)
	Multi Vitamin	Appedrine (Multiple vitamins and minerals)
	Thyroid Hormones	Armour Thyroid
	Aspirin	ASA
	Aspirin	Aspirin
	Nizatidine	Axid
	Nizatidine	Axid AR
	AZT	Azidothymidine
	AZT	AZT
	Oral Contraceptives	Birth Control Pill
	Oral Contraceptives	Brevicon
	Ibuprofen	Brufin
	Magnesium Hydroxide	Calcium Rich Rolaids (Magnesium hydroxide)
	Carbidopa	Carbidopa
	Carbidopa Levodopa	Carbidopa/Levodopa
	Cimetidine	Cimetidine
	Ciprofloxacin	Cipro
	Ciprofloxacin	Ciprofloxacin
	Warfarin	Coumadin
	Penicillamine	Cuprimine
	Thyroid Hormones	Cytomel
	Aspirin	Darvon Compound (Aspirin)
	Oxaprozin	Daypro

Drug Interactions

Supplement	Drug with Interaction	Generic or Trade Name(s)
Iron (continued)	Deferoxamine	Deferoxamine
	Oral Contraceptives	Demulen
	Penicillamine	Depen
	Deferoxamine	Desferal
	Thyroid Hormones	Desiccated Thyroid
	Vitamin C	Dex-A-Diet Plus Vitamin C (Vitamin C)
	Vitamin C	Dexatrim Plus Vitamin C (Vitamin C)
	Magnesium Hydroxide	Di-Gel Tablets (Magnesium hydroxide)
	Doxycycline	Doxycycline
	Thyroid Hormones	Eltroxin
	Aspirin	Empirin with Codeine (Aspirin)
	Oral Contraceptives	Enovid
	Etodolac	Etodolac
	Thyroid Hormones	Euthroid
	Famotidine	Famotidine
	Ibuprofen	Feldene
	Ofloxacin	Floxin
	Ibuprofen	Froben
	Oral Contraceptives	Genora
	Haloperidol	Haldol
	Haloperidol	Haloperidol
	Tetracycline	Helidac (Tetracycline)
	Ibuprofen	Ibuprofen
	Indomethacin	Indocin
	Indomethacin	Indomethacin
	Oral Contraceptives	Levlen
	Thyroid Hormones	Levo-T
	Thyroid Hormones	Levothroid
	Thyroid Hormones	Levothyroxine
	Thyroid Hormones	Levoxyl
	Thyroid Hormones	Liothyronine
	Thyroid Hormones	Liotrix
	Etodolac	Lodine
	Carbidopa	Lodosyn
	Oral Contraceptives	Loestrin
	Magnesium Hydroxide	Maalox (Magnesium hydroxide)
	Magnesium Hydroxide	Magnesium Hydroxide
	Methyldopa	Methyldopa
	Oral Contraceptives	Micronor
	Magnesium Hydroxide	Milk of Magnesia
	Oral Contraceptives	Modicon
	Magnesium Hydroxide	MOM
	Ibuprofen	Motrin

Supplement	Drug with Interaction	Generic or Trade Name(s)
Iron (continued)	*Ibuprofen*	*Motrin IB*
	Magnesium Hydroxide	*Mylanta (Magnesium hydroxide)*
	Nabumetone	*Nabumetone*
	Naproxen	*Napralen Naprosyn Naproxen*
	Naproxen	*Naproxen Sodium*
	Neomycin	*Neomycin*
	Nizatidine	*Nizatidine*
	Oral Contraceptives	*Nordette*
	Oral Contraceptives	*Norinyl*
	Ibuprofen	*Nuprin*
	Ofloxacin	*Oculflox Ofloxacin*
	Oral Contraceptives	*Oral Contraceptives*
	Oral Contraceptives	*Ortho-Novum*
	Oral Contraceptives	*Ovcon*
	Oral Contraceptives	*Ovral*
	Oral Contraceptives	*Ovrette*
	Oxaprozin	*Oxaprozin*
	Penicillamine	*Penicillamine*
	Famotidine	*Pepcid*
	Famotidine	*Pepcid AC*
	Aspirin	*Percodan (Aspirin)*
	Thyroid Hormones	*Proloid*
	Ranitidine	*Ranitidine*
	Nabumetone	*Relafen*
	AZT	*Retrovir*
	Aspirin	*Roxiprin (Aspirin)*
	Carbidopa Levodopa	*Sinemet*
	Sodium Bicarbonate	*Sodium Bicarbonate*
	Aspirin	*Soma Compound (Aspirin)*
	Aspirin	*Soma Compound with Codeine (Aspirin)*
	Stanozolol	*Stanozolol*
	Sulfasalazine	*Sulfasalazine*
	Tetracycline	*Sumycin*
	Thyroid Hormones	*Synthetic Liothyronine*
	Thyroid Hormones	*Synthroid*
	Cimetidine	*Tagamet*
	Cimetidine	*Tagamet HB*
	Magnesium Hydroxide	*Tempo tablets (Magnesium hydroxide)*
	Tetracycline	*Tetracycline*
	Thyroid Hormones	*Thyar*
	Thyroid Hormones	*Thyroglobulin*
	Thyroid Hormones	*Thyroid Hormones*
	Thyroid Hormones	*Thyrolar*
	Oral Contraceptives	*Triphasil*

Supplement	Drug with Interaction	Generic or Trade Name(s)
Iron (continued)	*Doxycycline*	*Vibramycin*
	Ibuprofen	*Voltarol*
	Warfarin	*Warfarin*
	Stanozolol	*Winstrol*
	Ranitidine	*Zantac*
	Ranitidine	*Zantac 75*
	AZT	*Zidovudine*
Isoleucine	*(none)*	*(none)*
Kelp	*(none)*	*(none)*
Lactase	*Lactase*	*Dairy Ease*
	Lactase	*LactAid*
	Lactase	*Lactase*
	Lactase	*Lactrase*
	Lactase	*SureLac*
Lecithin/Phosphatidylcholine/Choline	*(none)*	*(none)*
Leucine	*(none)*	*(none)*
Lipase	*(none)*	*(none)*
Lutein	*(none)*	*(none)*
Lycopene	*(none)*	*(none)*
Lysine	*(none)*	*(none)*
Magnesium	*Tetracycline*	*Achromycin*
	Corticosteroids	*AeroBid*
	Tobramycin	*AKTob*
	Albuterol	*Albuterol*
	Thiazide Diuretics	*Aldactazide (Hydrochloroth-iazide)*
	Spironolactone	*Aldactazide (Spironolactone)*
	Spironolactone	*Aldactone*
	Thiazide Diuretics	*Aldoclor (Chlorothiazide)*
	Thiazide Diuretics	*Aldoril (Hydrochlorothiazide)*
	Alendronate	*Alendronate*
	Amiloride	*Amiloride*
	Theophylline	*Aminophylline*
	Amphotericin B	*Amphotericin B*
	Warfarin	*Anticoagulant (Warfarin)*
	Multi Vitamin	*Appedrine (Multiple vitamins and minerals)*
	Thiazide Diuretics	*Apresazide (Hydrochloroth-iazide)*
	Corticosteroids	*Aristocort*
	Atorvastatin	*Atorvastatin*
	Nizatidine	*Axid*
	Nizatidine	*Axid AR*
	Azithromycin	*Azithromycin*
	Corticosteroids	*Azmacort*
	Sulfamethoxazole	*Azulfidine*
	Corticosteroids	*Beclomethasone*

Supplement	Drug with Interaction	Generic or Trade Name(s)
Magnesium (continued)	Corticosteroids	Beclovent
	Corticosteroids	Beconase
	Trimethoprim	Bethaprim
	Oral Contraceptives	Birth Control Pill
	Oral Contraceptives	Brevicon
	Epinephrine	Bronkaid Mist
	Epinephrine	Brontin Mist
	Corticosteroids	Budesonide
	Loop Diuretics	Bumex
	Thiazide Diuretics	Captozide (Hydrochloroth-iazide)
	Thiazide Diuretics	Chlorothiazide
	Thiazide Diuretics	Chlorothiazide/Methyldopa
	Thiazide Diuretics	Chlorthalidone
	Cimetidine	Cimetidine
	Ciprofloxacin	Cipro
	Ciprofloxacin	Ciprofloxacin
	Cisplatin	Cisplatin
	Thiazide Diuretics	Combipres (Chlorthalidone)
	Albuterol	Combivent (Albuterol)
	Trimethoprim	Comoxol
	Conjugated Estrogens	Conjugated Estrogens
	Corticosteroids	Cortef
	Corticosteroids	Corticosteroids
	Corticosteroids	Cortisone-like drugs
	Warfarin	Coumadin
	Losartan	Cozaar
	Corticosteroids	Cutivate
	Cycloserine	Cycloserine
	Cyclosporine	Cyclosporine
	Medroxyprogesterone	Cycrin
	Corticosteroids	Decadron
	Corticosteroids	Decadron Phosphate Turbinaire
	Corticosteroids	Delta-Cortef
	Corticosteroids	Deltasone
	Loop Diuretics	Demadex
	Oral Contraceptives	Demulen
	Medroxyprogesterone	Depo-Provera
	Corticosteroids	Dexamethasone
	Digoxin	Digoxin
	Thiazide Diuretics	Diuril
	Doxycycline	Doxycycline
	Thiazide Diuretics	Dyazide (Hydrochlorothiazide)
	Loop Diuretics	Edecrin
	Erythromycin	EES
	Corticosteroids	Elocon
	Erythromycin	E-Mycin

Drug Interactions

Supplement	Drug with Interaction	Generic or Trade Name(s)
Magnesium (continued)	Oral Contraceptives	Enovid
	Epinephrine	Epinephrine
	Erythromycin	Eryc Ery-Tab Erythromycin
	Thiazide Diuretics	Esidrix
	Loop Diuretics	Ethacrynic Acid
	Famotidine	Famotidine
	Corticosteroids	Flonase
	Ofloxacin	Floxin
	Alendronate	Fosamax
	Amphotericin B	Fungizone
	Corticosteroids	Flunisolide
	Corticosteroids	Fluticasone
	Loop Diuretics	Furosemide
	Sulfamethoxazole	Gantanol
	Gentamicin	Garamycin
	Oral Contraceptives	Genora
	Gentamicin	Gentamicin
	Glipizide	Glipizide
	Metformin	Glucophage
	Glipizide	Glucotrol
	Thiazide Diuretics	HCTZ
	Tetracycline	Helidac (Tetracycline)
	Thiazide Diuretics	Hydrochlorothiazide
	Corticosteroids	Hydrocortisone
	Thiazide Diuretics	HydroDIURIL
	Thiazide Diuretics	Hygroton
	Corticosteroids	Hytone
	Erythromycin	Ilosone
	Thiazide Diuretics	Inderide (Hydrochlorothiazide)
	Isoniazid	INH
	Isoniazid	Isoniazid
	Isoniazid	Laniazid
	Digoxin	Lanoxin
	Loop Diuretics	Lasix
	Oral Contraceptives	Levlen
	Atorvastatin	Lipitor
	Oral Contraceptives	Loestrin
	Loop Diuretics	Loop Diuretics
	Thiazide Diuretics	Lopressor HCT (Hydrochlorothiazide)
	Losartan	Losartan
	Nitrofurantoin	Macrobid
	Nitrofurantoin	Macrodantin
	Thiazide Diuretics	Maxzide (Hydrochlorothiazide)
	Corticosteroids	Medrol
	Medroxyprogesterone	Medroxyprogesterone
	Metformin	Metformin

Supplement	Drug with Interaction	Generic or Trade Name(s)
Magnesium (continued)	Corticosteroids	Methylprednisolone
	Thiazide Diuretics	Metolazone
	Oral Contraceptives	Micronor
	Amiloride	Midamor
	Oral Contraceptives	Modicon
	Amiloride	Moduretic (Amiloride)
	Thiazide Diuretics	Moduretic (Hydrochloroth- iazide)
	Corticosteroids	Mometasone
	Thiazide Diuretics	Mykros
	Corticosteroids	Nasacort
	Corticosteroids	Nasalide
	Tobramycin	Nebicin
	Neomycin	Neomycin
	Cyclosporine	Neoral
	Nitrofurantoin	Nitrofurantoin
	Nizatidine	Nizatidine
	Oral Contraceptives	Nordette
	Oral Contraceptives	Norinyl
	Ofloxacin	Oculflox Ofloxacin
	Oral Contraceptives	Oral Contraceptives
	Corticosteroids	Orasone
	Thiazide Diuretics	Oretic
	Oral Contraceptives	Ortho-Novum
	Oral Contraceptives	Ovcon
	Oral Contraceptives	Ovral
	Oral Contraceptives	Ovrette
	Corticosteroids	Pediapred
	Famotidine	Pepcid
	Famotidine	Pepcid AC
	Theophylline	Phyllocontin
	Cisplatin	Platinol
	Corticosteroids	Prednisolone
	Corticosteroids	Prednisone
	Conjugated Estrogens	Premarin
	Conjugated Estrogens	Prempro (Conjugated estro- gens)
	Medroxyprogesterone	Prempro (Medroxyproges- terone)
	Theophylline	Primatene Dual Action (Theo- phylline)
	Epinephrine	Primatene Mist
	Thiazide Diuretics	Prinizide (Hydrochlorothiazide)
	Trimethoprim	Proloprim
	Albuterol	Proventil
	Medroxyprogesterone	Provera
	Corticosteroids	Pulmicort

Supplement	Drug with Interaction	Generic or Trade Name(s)
Magnesium (continued)	*Ranitidine*	*Ranitidine*
	Corticosteroids	*Rhinocort*
	Isoniazid	*Rifamate*
	Isoniazid	*Rimactane*
	Cyclosporine	*Sandimmune*
	Cycloserine	*Seromycin*
	Theophylline	*Slo-Bid*
	Theophylline	*Slo-Phyllin*
	Spironolactone	*Spironolactone*
	Corticosteroids	*Steroids (Prednisone)*
	Sulfamethoxazole	*Sulfamethoxazole*
	Tetracycline	*Sumycin*
	Cimetidine	*Tagamet*
	Cimetidine	*Tagamet HB*
	Thiazide Diuretics	*Tenoretic (Chlorthalidone)*
	Tetracycline	*Tetracycline*
	Theophylline	*Theo-Dur*
	Theophylline	*Theolair*
	Theophylline	*Theophylline*
	Thiazide Diuretics	*Thiazide Diuretics*
	Thiazide Diuretics	*Timolide (Hydrochlorothiazide)*
	Tobramycin	*TOBI*
	Corticosteroids	*Tobradex (Dexamthasone)*
	Tobramycin	*Tobradex (Tobramycin)*
	Tobramycin	*Tobramycin*
	Tobramycin	*Tobrex*
	Loop Diuretics	*Torsemide*
	Corticosteroids	*Triamcinolone*
	Trimethoprim	*Trimethoprim*
	Trimethoprim	*Trimpex*
	Oral Contraceptives	*Triphasil*
	Theophylline	*Truphylline*
	Theophylline	*Uniphyl*
	Corticosteroids	*Vancenase*
	Corticosteroids	*Vanceril*
	Thiazide Diuretics	*Vaseretic (Hydrochlorothiazide)*
	Albuterol	*Ventolin*
	Doxycycline	*Vibramycin*
	Warfarin	*Warfarin*
	Ranitidine	*Zantac*
	Ranitidine	*Zantac 75*
	Thiazide Diuretics	*Zaroxolyn*
	Thiazide Diuretics	*Zestoretic (Hydrochlorothiazide)*
	Thiazide Diuretics	*Ziac (Hydrochlorothiazide)*
	Azithromycin	*Zithromax*
Malic Acid	*(none)*	*(none)*

Supplement	Drug with Interaction	Generic or Trade Name(s)
Manganese	*Oral Contraceptives*	*Birth Control Pill*
	Oral Contraceptives	*Brevicon*
	Ciprofloxacin	*Cipro*
	Ciprofloxacin	*Ciprofloxacin*
	Oral Contraceptives	*Demulen*
	Oral Contraceptives	*Enovid*
	Oral Contraceptives	*Genora*
	Oral Contraceptives	*Levlen*
	Oral Contraceptives	*Loestrin*
	Oral Contraceptives	*Micronor*
	Oral Contraceptives	*Modicon*
	Oral Contraceptives	*Nordette*
	Oral Contraceptives	*Norinyl*
	Oral Contraceptives	*Oral Contraceptives*
	Oral Contraceptives	*Ortho-Novum*
	Oral Contraceptives	*Ovcon*
	Oral Contraceptives	*Ovral*
	Oral Contraceptives	*Ovrette*
	Oral Contraceptives	*Triphasil*
Medium Chain Triglycerides	*(none)*	*(none)*
Melatonin	*Corticosteroids*	*AeroBid*
	Benzodiazepines	*Alprazolam*
	Anticonvulsants	*Anticonvulsants*
	Corticosteroids	*Aristocort*
	Benzodiazepines	*Ativan*
	Corticosteroids	*Azmacort*
	Corticosteroids	*Beclomethasone*
	Corticosteroids	*Beclovent*
	Corticosteroids	*Beconase*
	Benzodiazepines	*Benzodiazepines*
	Corticosteroids	*Budesonide*
	Chemotherapy	*Cancer Chemotherapy*
	Anticonvulsants	*Carbamazepine*
	Chemotherapy	*Chemotherapy*
	Benzodiazepines	*Chlordiazepoxide*
	Benzodiazepines	*Clonazepam*
	Corticosteroids	*Cortef*
	Corticosteroids	*Corticosteroids*
	Corticosteroids	*Cortisone-like drugs*
	Corticosteroids	*Cutivate*
	Benzodiazepines	*Dalmane*
	Corticosteroids	*Decadron*
	Corticosteroids	*Decadron Phosphate Turbinaire*
	Corticosteroids	*Delta-Cortef*
	Corticosteroids	*Deltasone*
	Corticosteroids	*Dexamethasone*
	Benzodiazepines	*Diazepam*

Supplement	Drug with Interaction	Generic or Trade Name(s)
Melatonin (continued)	*Anticonvulsants*	*Dilantin*
	Corticosteroids	*Elocon*
	Corticosteroids	*Flonase*
	Fluoxetine	*Fluoxetine*
	Benzodiazepines	*Flurazepam*
	Corticosteroids	*Flunisolide*
	Corticosteroids	*Fluticasone*
	Benzodiazepines	*Halcion*
	Corticosteroids	*Hydrocortisone*
	Corticosteroids	*Hytone*
	Benzodiazepines	*Klonopin*
	Benzodiazepines	*Librium*
	Benzodiazepines	*Lorazepam*
	Corticosteroids	*Medrol*
	Corticosteroids	*Methylprednisolone*
	Corticosteroids	*Mometasone*
	Anticonvulsants	*Mysoline*
	Corticosteroids	*Nasacort*
	Corticosteroids	*Nasalide*
	Tamoxifen	*Nolvadex*
	Corticosteroids	*Orasone*
	Corticosteroids	*Pediapred*
	Anticonvulsants	*Phenobarbital*
	Anticonvulsants	*Phenytoin*
	Corticosteroids	*Prednisolone*
	Corticosteroids	*Prednisone*
	Anticonvulsants	*Primidone*
	Fluoxetine	*Prozac*
	Corticosteroids	*Pulmicort*
	Benzodiazepines	*Restoril*
	Corticosteroids	*Rhinocort*
	Corticosteroids	*Steroids (Prednisone)*
	Tamoxifen	*Tamoxifen*
	Anticonvulsants	*Tegretol*
	Benzodiazepines	*Temazepam*
	Corticosteroids	*Tobradex (Dexamethasone)*
	Corticosteroids	*Triamcinolone*
	Benzodiazepines	*Triazolam*
	Benzodiazepines	*Valium*
	Corticosteroids	*Vancenase*
	Corticosteroids	*Vanceril*
	Benzodiazepines	*Xanax*
Methionine	*(none)*	*(none)*
Molybdenum	*(none)*	*(none)*
Multiple Vitamin/Mineral	*Quinapril*	*Accupril*
	Isotretinoin	*Accutane*
	ACE Inhibitors	*ACE Inhibitors*

Supplement	Drug with Interaction	Generic or Trade Name(s)
Multiple Vitamin/Mineral (continued)	Aspirin	Acetylsalicylic Acid
	Phenylpropanolamine	Acutrim
	Aspirin	Alka-Seltzer (Aspirin)
	Ramipril	Altace
	Aspirin	Anacin (Aspirin)
	ACE Inhibitors	Angiotensin Converting Enzyme Inhibitors
	Antacids	Antacids
	Antibiotics	Antibiotics
	Warfarin	Anticoagulant (Warfarin)
	Phenylpropanolamine	Appedrine (Phenyl-propanolamine)
	Aspirin	ASA
	Aspirin	Aspirin
	Nizatidine	Axid
	Nizatidine	Axid AR
	Chemotherapy	Cancer Chemotherapy
	Captopril	Capoten
	Captopril	Captopril
	Captopril	Captozide (Captopril)
	Cephalosporins	Ceclor
	Cephalosporins	Cefanex
	Cephalosporins	Cefixime
	Cephalosporins	Cefpodoxime
	Cephalosporins	Ceftin
	Cephalosporins	Ceftriaxone
	Cephalosporins	Cefuroxime
	Cephalosporins	Cephaclor
	Cephalosporins	Cephadroxil
	Cephalosporins	Cephalexin
	Cephalosporins	Cephalosporins
	Chemotherapy	Chemotherapy
	Phenylpropanolamine	Contac 12 Hour (Phenyl-propanolamine)
	Warfarin	Coumadin
	Penicillamine	Cuprimine
	Aspirin	Darvon Compound (Aspirin)
	Phenylpropanolamine	DayQuil Allergy Relief (Phenyl-propanolamine)
	Penicillamine	Depen
	Phenylpropanolamine	Dex-A-Diet
	Phenylpropanolamine	Dex-A-Diet Plus Vitamin C (Phenylpropanolamine)
	Vitamin C	Dex-A-Diet Plus Vitamin C (Vitamin C)
	Phenylpropanolamine	Dexatrim
	Phenylpropanolamine	Dexatrim Plus Vitamin C (Phenylpropanolamine)

Supplement	Drug with Interaction	Generic or Trade Name(s)
Multiple Vitamin/Mineral (continued)	Vitamin C	Dexatrim Plus Vitamin C (Vitamin C)
	Phenylpropanolamine	Diadex Grapefruit Diet Plan (Phenylpropanolamine)
	Phenylpropanolamine	Dimetapp (Phenylpropanolamine)
	Doxycycline	Doxycycline
	Cephalosporins	Duricef
	Erythromycin	EES
	Aspirin	Empirin with Codeine (Aspirin)
	Erythromycin	E-Mycin
	Phenylpropanolamine	Entex LA (Phenylpropanolamine)
	Erythromycin	Eryc Ery-Tab Erythromycin
	Famotidine	Famotidine
	Ofloxacin	Floxin
	Erythromycin	Ilosone
	Isoniazid	INH
	Isoniazid	Isoniazid
	Isotretinoin	Isotretinoin
	Cephalosporins	Keflet
	Cephalosporins	Keflex
	Cephalosporins	Keftab
	Isoniazid	Laniazid
	Lisinopril	Lisinopril
	Mineral Oil	Mineral Oil
	Neomycin	Neomycin
	Nizatidine	Nizatidine
	Ofloxacin	Oculflox Ofloxacin
	Penicillamine	Penicillamine
	Famotidine	Pepcid
	Famotidine	Pepcid AC
	Aspirin	Percodan (Aspirin)
	Phenylpropanolamine	Phenylpropanolamine
	Phenylpropanolamine	PPA
	Lisinopril	Prinivil
	Lisinopril	Prinizide (Lisinopril)
	Phenylpropanolamine	Propagest
	Quinapril	Quinapril
	Ramipril	Ramipril
	Ranitidine	Ranitidine
	Phenylpropanolamine	Rhindecon
	Isoniazid	Rifamate
	Isoniazid	Rimactane
	Phenylpropanolamine	Robitussin CF (Phenylpropanolamine)
	Cephalosporins	Rocephin

Supplement	Drug with Interaction	Generic or Trade Name(s)
Multiple Vitamin/Mineral (continued)	Aspirin	Roxiprin (Aspirin)
	Aspirin	Soma Compound (Aspirin)
	Aspirin	Soma Compound with Codeine (Aspirin)
	Sulfasalazine	Sulfasalazine
	Cephalosporins	Suprax
	Phenylpropanolamine	Tavist-D (Phenylpropanolamine)
	Phenylpropanolamine	Triaminic-12 (Phenyl-propanolamine)
	Cephalosporins	Ulracef
	Phenylpropanolamine	Unitrol
	Cephalosporins	Vantin
	Doxycycline	Vibramycin
	Warfarin	Warfarin
	Ranitidine	Zantac
	Ranitidine	Zantac 75
	Lisinopril	Zestoretic (Lisinopril)
N-Acetyl Cysteine (NAC)	Acetaminophen	Acetaminophen
	Interferon	Actimmune
	Doxorubicin	Adriamycin
	Corticosteroids	AeroBid
	Interferon	Alferon N
	Acetaminophen	Alka-Seltzer Plus (Aceta-minophen)
	Acetaminophen	APAP
	Corticosteroids	Aristocort
	Interferon	Avonex
	Corticosteroids	Azmacort
	Corticosteroids	Beclomethasone
	Corticosteroids	Beclovent
	Corticosteroids	Beconase
	Interferon	Betaseron
	Corticosteroids	Budesonide
	Chemotherapy	Cancer Chemotherapy
	Chemotherapy	Chemotherapy
	Corticosteroids	Cortef
	Corticosteroids	Corticosteroids
	Corticosteroids	Cortisone-like drugs
	Corticosteroids	Cutivate
	Acetaminophen	Darvocet (Acetaminophen)
	Acetaminophen	Darvocet N (Acetaminophen)
	Corticosteroids	Decadron
	Corticosteroids	Decadron Phosphate Turbinaire
	Corticosteroids	Delta-Cortef
	Corticosteroids	Deltasone
	Nitroglycerin	Deponit
	Corticosteroids	Dexamethasone

Supplement	Drug with Interaction	Generic or Trade Name(s)
NAC (continued)	Doxorubicin	Doxorubicin
	Corticosteroids	Elocon
	Acetaminophen	Excedrin PM (Acetaminophen)
	Corticosteroids	Flonase
	Corticosteroids	Flunisolide
	Corticosteroids	Fluticasone
	Nitroglycerin	Glycerly Trinitrate
	Corticosteroids	Hydrocortisone
	Corticosteroids	Hytone
	Isosorbide Mononitrate	Imdur
	Interferon	Interferon
	Interferon	Intron
	Isosorbide Mononitrate	ISMO
	Isosorbide Mononitrate	Isosorbide Mononitrate
	Acetaminophen	Lortab (Acetaminophen)
	Corticosteroids	Medrol
	Corticosteroids	Methylprednisolone
	Nitroglycerin	Minitran
	Corticosteroids	Mometasone
	Isosorbide Mononitrate	Monoket
	Corticosteroids	Nasacort
	Corticosteroids	Nasalide
	Nitroglycerin	Nitro-Bid
	Nitroglycerin	Nitrodisc
	Nitroglycerin	Nitro-Dur
	Nitroglycerin	Nitrogard
	Nitroglycerin	Nitroglycerin
	Nitroglycerin	Nitrolingual
	Nitroglycerin	Nitrostat
	Acetaminophen	Nyquil (Acetaminophen)
	Acetaminophen	Nyquil Hot Therapy Powder (Acetaminophen)
	Corticosteroids	Orasone
	Acetaminophen	Paracetemol
	Corticosteroids	Pediapred
	Acetaminophen	Percocet (Acetaminophen)
	Corticosteroids	Prednisolone
	Corticosteroids	Prednisone
	Corticosteroids	Pulmicort
	Interferon	Rebif
	Corticosteroids	Rhinocort
	Interferon	Roferon-A
	Acetaminophen	Roxicet (Acetaminophen)
	Corticosteroids	Steroids (Prednisone)
	Acetaminophen	Theraflu (Acetaminophen)
	Acetaminophen	Theraflu Flu and Cold (Acetaminophen)

Supplement	Drug with Interaction	Generic or Trade Name(s)
NAC (continued)	Corticosteroids	Tobradex (Dexamthasone)
	Nitroglycerin	Transderm-Nitro
	Corticosteroids	Triamcinolone
	Acetaminophen	Tylenol
	Acetaminophen	Tylenol Allergy Sinus (Acetaminophen)
	Acetaminophen	Tylenol Cold (Acetaminophen)
	Acetaminophen	Tylenol Flu NightTime Maximum Strength Powder (Acetaminophen)
	Acetaminophen	Tylenol Multi-Symptom Hot Medication (Acetaminophen)
	Acetaminophen	Tylenol PM (Acetaminophen)
	Acetaminophen	Tylenol PM Extra Strength (Acetaminophen)
	Acetaminophen	Tylenol Sinus (Acetaminophen)
	Acetaminophen	Tylenol with Codeine (Acetaminophen)
	Acetaminophen	Tylenol Allergy Sinus
	Corticosteroids	Vancenase
	Corticosteroids	Vanceril
	Acetaminophen	Vicodin (Acetaminophen)
	Interferon	Weferon
	Acetaminophen	Wygesic (Acetaminophen)
NADH (Nicotinamide Adenine Dinucleotide)	(none)	(none)
Octacosanol	(none)	(none)
Ornithine alpha-ketoglutarate (OKG)	(none)	(none)
Ornithine	(none)	(none)
PABA (Paraaminobenzoic Acid)	Sulfamethoxazole	Azulfidine
	Trimethoprim Sulfamethoxazole	Bactrim
	Trimethoprim Sulfamethoxazole	Cotrim (Co-Trimoxazole)
	Dapsone	Dapsone
	Methotrexate	Folex
	Sulfamethoxazole	Gantanol
	Methotrexate	Methotrexate
	Methotrexate	Rheumatrex
	Trimethoprim Sulfamethoxazole	Septra
	Sulfamethoxazole	Sulfamethoxazole
	Sulfasalazine	Sulfasalazine
	Trimethoprim Sulfamethoxazole	Trimethoprim/Sulfamethoxazole
	Trimethoprim Sulfamethoxazole	Uroplus
L-Phenylalanine and D,L-Phenylalanine (DLPA)	(none)	(none)
Phosphatidylserine	(none)	(none)
Pollen	(none)	(none)

Supplement	Drug with Interaction	Generic or Trade Name(s)
Potassium	Quinapril	Accupril
	ACE Inhibitors	ACE Inhibitors
	Tetracycline	Achromycin
	Ibuprofen	Advil
	Corticosteroids	AeroBid
	Tobramycin	AKTob
	Albuterol	Albuterol
	Thiazide Diuretics	Aldactazide (Hydrochloroth-iazide)
	Spironolactone	Aldactazide (Spironolactone)
	Spironolactone	Aldactone
	Thiazide Diuretics	Aldoclor (Chlorothiazide)
	Thiazide Diuretics	Aldoril (Hydrochlorothiazide)
	Naproxen	Aleve
	Ramipril	Altace
	Amiloride	Amiloride
	Theophylline	Aminophylline
	Naproxen	Anaprox
	ACE Inhibitors	Angiotensin Converting Enzyme Inhibitors
	Heparin	Anticoagulant (Heparin)
	Thiazide Diuretics	Apresazide (Hydrochloroth-iazide)
	Corticosteroids	Aristocort
	Corticosteroids	Azmacort
	Sulfamethoxazole	Azulfidine
	Trimethoprim Sulfamethoxazole	Bactrim
	Corticosteroids	Beclomethasone
	Corticosteroids	Beclovent
	Corticosteroids	Beconase
	Benazepril	Benazepril
	Trimethoprim	Bethaprim
	Bisacodyl	Bisacodyl
	Senna	Black-Draught
	Epinephrine	Bronkaid Mist
	Epinephrine	Brontin Mist
	Ibuprofen	Brufin
	Corticosteroids	Budesonide
	Loop Diuretics	Bumex
	Magnesium Hydroxide	Calcium Rich Rolaids (Magne-sium hydroxide)
	Captopril	Capoten
	Captopril	Captopril
	Captopril	Captozide (Captopril)
	Thiazide Diuretics	Captozide (Hydrochloroth-iazide)
	Thiazide Diuretics	Chlorothiazide

Supplement	**Drug with Interaction**	**Generic or Trade Name(s)**
Potassium (continued)	*Thiazide Diuretics*	*Chlorothiazide/Methyldopa*
	Thiazide Diuretics	*Chlorthalidone*
	Cisplatin	*Cisplatin*
	Colchicine	*Colchicine*
	Thiazide Diuretics	*Combipres (Chlorthalidone)*
	Albuterol	*Combivent (Albuterol)*
	Trimethoprim	*Comoxol*
	Corticosteroids	*Cortef*
	Corticosteroids	*Corticosteroids*
	Corticosteroids	*Cortisone-like drugs*
	Trimethoprim Sulfamethoxazole	*Cotrim (Co-Trimoxazole)*
	Losartan	*Cozaar*
	Corticosteroids	*Cutivate*
	Oxaprozin	*Daypro*
	Corticosteroids	*Decadron*
	Corticosteroids	*Decadron Phosphate Turbinaire*
	Corticosteroids	*Delta-Cortef*
	Corticosteroids	*Deltasone*
	Loop Diuretics	*Demadex*
	Corticosteroids	*Dexamethasone*
	Magnesium Hydroxide	*Di-Gel Tablets (Magnesium hydroxide)*
	Digoxin	*Digoxin*
	Thiazide Diuretics	*Diuril*
	Bisacodyl	*Dulcolax*
	Thiazide Diuretics	*Dyazide (Hydrochlorothiazide)*
	Triamterene	*Dyazide (Triamterene)*
	Triamterene	*Dyrenium*
	Loop Diuretics	*Edecrin*
	Corticosteroids	*Elocon*
	Enalapril	*Enalapril*
	Epinephrine	*Epinephrine*
	Thiazide Diuretics	*Esidrix*
	Loop Diuretics	*Ethacrynic Acid*
	Etodolac	*Etodolac*
	Ibuprofen	*Feldene*
	Senna	*Fletcher's Castoria*
	Corticosteroids	*Flonase*
	Ibuprofen	*Froben*
	Corticosteroids	*Flunisolide*
	Corticosteroids	*Fluticasone*
	Loop Diuretics	*Furosemide*
	Sulfamethoxazole	*Gantanol*
	Gentamicin	*Garamycin*
	Gentamicin	*Gentamicin*
	Senna	*Gentlax*
	Haloperidol	*Haldol*

Supplement	Drug with Interaction	Generic or Trade Name(s)
Potassium (continued)	*Haloperidol*	*Haloperidol*
	Thiazide Diuretics	*HCTZ*
	Tetracycline	*Helidac (Tetracycline)*
	Heparin	*Heparin*
	Thiazide Diuretics	*Hydrochlorothiazide*
	Corticosteroids	*Hydrocortisone*
	Thiazide Diuretics	*HydroDIURIL*
	Thiazide Diuretics	*Hygroton*
	Corticosteroids	*Hytone*
	Ibuprofen	*Ibuprofen*
	Thiazide Diuretics	*Inderide (Hydrochlorothiazide)*
	Indomethacin	*Indocin*
	Indomethacin	*Indomethacin*
	Digoxin	*Lanoxin*
	Loop Diuretics	*Lasix*
	Lisinopril	*Lisinopril*
	Etodolac	*Lodine*
	Loop Diuretics	*Loop Diuretics*
	Thiazide Diuretics	*Lopressor HCT (Hydrochlorothiazide)*
	Losartan	*Losartan*
	Benazepril	*Lotensin*
	Magnesium Hydroxide	*Maalox (Magnesium hydroxide)*
	Magnesium Hydroxide	*Magnesium Hydroxide*
	Thiazide Diuretics	*Maxzide (Hydrochlorothiazide)*
	Triamterene	*Maxzide (Triamterene)*
	Corticosteroids	*Medrol*
	Corticosteroids	*Methylprednisolone*
	Thiazide Diuretics	*Metolazone*
	Amiloride	*Midamor*
	Magnesium Hydroxide	*Milk of Magnesia*
	Mineral Oil	*Mineral Oil*
	Amiloride	*Moduretic (Amiloride)*
	Thiazide Diuretics	*Moduretic (Hydrochlorothiazide)*
	Magnesium Hydroxide	*MOM*
	Corticosteroids	*Mometasone*
	Ibuprofen	*Motrin*
	Ibuprofen	*Motrin IB*
	Thiazide Diuretics	*Mykros*
	Magnesium Hydroxide	*Mylanta (Magnesium hydroxide)*
	Nabumetone	*Nabumetone*
	Naproxen	*Napralen Naprosyn Naproxen*
	Naproxen	*Naproxen Sodium*
	Corticosteroids	*Nasacort*

Supplement	Drug with Interaction	Generic or Trade Name(s)
Potassium (continued)	Corticosteroids	Nasalide
	Tobramycin	Nebicin
	Neomycin	Neomycin
	Ibuprofen	Nuprin
	Corticosteroids	Orasone
	Thiazide Diuretics	Oretic
	Oxaprozin	Oxaprozin
	Corticosteroids	Pediapred
	Theophylline	Phyllocontin
	Cisplatin	Platinol
	Corticosteroids	Prednisolone
	Corticosteroids	Prednisone
	Theophylline	Primatene Dual Action (Theophylline)
	Epinephrine	Primatene Mist
	Lisinopril	Prinivil
	Thiazide Diuretics	Prinizide (Hydrochlorothiazide)
	Lisinopril	Prinizide (Lisinopril)
	Trimethoprim	Proloprim
	Albuterol	Proventil
	Corticosteroids	Pulmicort
	Quinapril	Quinapril
	Ramipril	Ramipril
	Nabumetone	Relafen
	Corticosteroids	Rhinocort
	Senna	Senexon
	Senna	Senna
	Senna	Senna-Gen
	Senna	Senokot
	Senna	Senolax
	Trimethoprim Sulfamethoxazole	Septra
	Theophylline	Slo-Bid
	Theophylline	Slo-Phyllin
	Spironolactone	Spironolactone
	Corticosteroids	Steroids (Prednisone)
	Sulfamethoxazole	Sulfamethoxazole
	Tetracycline	Sumycin
	Magnesium Hydroxide	Tempo tablets (Magnesium hydroxide)
	Thiazide Diuretics	Tenoretic (Chlorthalidone)
	Tetracycline	Tetracycline
	Theophylline	Theo-Dur
	Theophylline	Theolair
	Theophylline	Theophylline
	Thiazide Diuretics	Thiazide Diuretics
	Thiazide Diuretics	Timolide (Hydrochlorothiazide)
	Tobramycin	TOBI

Supplement	Drug with Interaction	Generic or Trade Name(s)
Potassium (continued)	*Corticosteroids*	*Tobradex (Dexamethasone)*
	Tobramycin	*Tobradex (Tobramycin)*
	Tobramycin	*Tobramycin*
	Tobramycin	*Tobrex*
	Loop Diuretics	*Torsemide*
	Corticosteroids	*Triamcinolone*
	Triamterene	*Triamterene*
	Trimethoprim	*Trimethoprim*
	Trimethoprim Sulfamethoxazole	*Trimethoprim/Sulfamethoxazole*
	Trimethoprim	*Trimpex*
	Theophylline	*Truphylline*
	Theophylline	*Uniphyl*
	Trimethoprim Sulfamethoxazole	*Uroplus*
	Corticosteroids	*Vancenase*
	Corticosteroids	*Vanceril*
	Enalapril	*Vaseretic (Enalapril)*
	Thiazide Diuretics	*Vaseretic (Hydrochlorothiazide)*
	Enalapril	*Vasotec*
	Albuterol	*Ventolin*
	Ibuprofen	*Voltarol*
	Thiazide Diuretics	*Zaroxolyn*
	Thiazide Diuretics	*Zestoretic (Hydrochlorothiazide)*
	Lisinopril	*Zestoretic (Lisinopril)*
	Thiazide Diuretics	*Ziac (Hydrochlorothiazide)*
Pregnenolone	*(none)*	*(none)*
Proanthocyanidins	*(none)*	*(none)*
Progesterone	*Conjugated Estrogens*	*Conjugated Estrogens*
	Medroxyprogesterone	*Cycrin*
	Medroxyprogesterone	*Depo-Provera*
	Medroxyprogesterone	*Medroxyprogesterone*
	Conjugated Estrogens	*Premarin*
	Conjugated Estrogens	*Prempro (Conjugated estrogens)*
	Medroxyprogesterone	*Prempro (Medroxyprogesterone)*
	Medroxyprogesterone	*Provera*
Pyruvate	*(none)*	*(none)*
Quercetin	*Estradiol*	*Alora*
	Estradiol	*Climara*
	Estradiol	*Esclim*
	Estradiol	*Estrace Estraderm Estradiol*
	Estradiol	*FemPatch*
	Estradiol	*Vivelle*
Resveratrol	*(none)*	*(none)*
Royal Jelly	*(none)*	*(none)*
SAM (S-adenosyl-L-methionine)	*(none)*	*(none)*

Supplement	Drug with Interaction	Generic or Trade Name(s)
Selenium	Cisplatin	Cisplatin
	Valproic Acid	Depakene Syrup
	Valproic Acid	Depakene
	Valproic Acid	Depakote
	Valproic Acid	Divalproex sodium
	Cisplatin	Platinol
	Valproic Acid	Sodium Valproate
	Valproic Acid	Valproic Acid
Silicon	(none)	(none)
Soy	Thyroid Hormones	Animal Levothyroxine/Liothyronine
	Thyroid Hormones	Animal Thyroid
	Warfarin	Anticoagulant (Warfarin)
	Thyroid Hormones	Armour Thyroid
	Ipratropium Bromide	Atrovent
	Ipratropium Bromide	Combivent (Ipratropium Bromide)
	Conjugated Estrogens	Conjugated Estrogens
	Warfarin	Coumadin
	Thyroid Hormones	Cytomel
	Thyroid Hormones	Desiccated Thyroid
	Thyroid Hormones	Eltroxin
	Thyroid Hormones	Euthroid
	Ipratropium Bromide	Ipratropium Bromide
	Thyroid Hormones	Levo-T
	Thyroid Hormones	Levothroid
	Thyroid Hormones	Levothyroxine
	Thyroid Hormones	Levoxyl
	Thyroid Hormones	Liothyronine
	Thyroid Hormones	Liotrix
	Conjugated Estrogens	Premarin
	Conjugated Estrogens	Prempro (Conjugated estrogens)
	Thyroid Hormones	Proloid
	Thyroid Hormones	Synthetic Liothyronine
	Thyroid Hormones	Synthroid
	Thyroid Hormones	Thyar
	Thyroid Hormones	Thyroglobulin
	Thyroid Hormones	Thyroid Hormones
	Thyroid Hormones	Thyrolar
	Warfarin	Warfarin
Spirulina	(none)	(none)
Strontium	(none)	(none)
Sulfur (Methylsulfonylmethane, MSM)	(none)	(none)
Taurine	Chemotherapy	Cancer Chemotherapy
	Chemotherapy	Chemotherapy
Tyrosine	(none)	(none)

Supplement	Drug with Interaction	Generic or Trade Name(s)
Valine	*(none)*	*(none)*
Vanadium	*(none)*	*(none)*
Vitamin A and Beta-Carotene	*Isotretinoin*	*Accutane*
	Corticosteroids	*AeroBid*
	Multi Vitamin	*Appedrine (Multiple vitamins and minerals)*
	Corticosteroids	*Aristocort*
	Atorvastatin	*Atorvastatin*
	Corticosteroids	*Azmacort*
	Corticosteroids	*Beclomethasone*
	Corticosteroids	*Beclovent*
	Corticosteroids	*Beconase*
	Bile Acid Sequestrants	*Bile Acid Sequestrants*
	Oral Contraceptives	*Birth Control Pill*
	Oral Contraceptives	*Brevicon*
	Corticosteroids	*Budesonide*
	Chemotherapy	*Cancer Chemotherapy*
	Chemotherapy	*Chemotherapy*
	Bile Acid Sequestrants	*Cholestyramine*
	Colchicine	*Colchicine*
	Colestipol	*Colestid*
	Colestipol	*Colestipol*
	Corticosteroids	*Cortef*
	Corticosteroids	*Corticosteroids*
	Corticosteroids	*Cortisone-like drugs*
	Corticosteroids	*Cutivate*
	Cyclophosphamide	*Cyclophosphamide*
	Medroxyprogesterone	*Cycrin*
	Cyclophosphamide	*Cytoxan*
	Corticosteroids	*Decadron*
	Corticosteroids	*Decadron Phosphate Turbinaire*
	Corticosteroids	*Delta-Cortef*
	Corticosteroids	*Deltasone*
	Oral Contraceptives	*Demulen*
	Medroxyprogesterone	*Depo-Provera*
	Corticosteroids	*Dexamethasone*
	Corticosteroids	*Elocon*
	Oral Contraceptives	*Enovid*
	Corticosteroids	*Flonase*
	Fluvastatin	*Fluvastatin*
	Corticosteroids	*Flunisolide*
	Corticosteroids	*Fluticasone*
	Oral Contraceptives	*Genora*
	Corticosteroids	*Hydrocortisone*
	Corticosteroids	*Hytone*
	Isotretinoin	*Isotretinoin*
	Lansoprazole	*Lansoprazole*

Supplement	Drug with Interaction	Generic or Trade Name(s)
Vitamin A (continued)	*Fluvastatin*	*Lescol*
	Oral Contraceptives	*Levlen*
	Atorvastatin	*Lipitor*
	Oral Contraceptives	*Loestrin*
	Lovastatin	*Lovastatin*
	Corticosteroids	*Medrol*
	Medroxyprogesterone	*Medroxyprogesterone*
	Corticosteroids	*Methylprednisolone*
	Lovastatin	*Mevacor*
	Oral Contraceptives	*Micronor*
	Mineral Oil	*Mineral Oil*
	Oral Contraceptives	*Modicon*
	Corticosteroids	*Mometasone*
	Corticosteroids	*Nasacort*
	Corticosteroids	*Nasalide*
	Neomycin	*Neomycin*
	Cyclophosphamide	*Neosar*
	Oral Contraceptives	*Nordette*
	Oral Contraceptives	*Norinyl*
	Oral Contraceptives	*Oral Contraceptives*
	Corticosteroids	*Orasone*
	Oral Contraceptives	*Ortho-Novum*
	Oral Contraceptives	*Ovcon*
	Oral Contraceptives	*Ovral*
	Oral Contraceptives	*Ovrette*
	Corticosteroids	*Pediapred*
	Pravastatin	*Pravachol*
	Pravastatin	*Pravastatin*
	Corticosteroids	*Prednisolone*
	Corticosteroids	*Prednisone*
	Medroxyprogesterone	*Prempro (Medroxyprogesterone)*
	Lansoprazole	*Prevacid*
	Medroxyprogesterone	*Provera*
	Corticosteroids	*Pulmicort*
	Bile Acid Sequestrants	*Questran*
	Tretinoin	*Retin-A*
	Corticosteroids	*Rhinocort*
	Simvastatin	*Simvastatin*
	Corticosteroids	*Steroids (Prednisone)*
	Corticosteroids	*Tobradex (Dexamthasone)*
	Tretinoin	*Tretinoin*
	Corticosteroids	*Triamcinolone*
	Oral Contraceptives	*Triphasil*
	Corticosteroids	*Vancenase*
	Corticosteroids	*Vanceril*
	Tretinoin	*Vesanoid*

Drug Interactions

Supplement	Drug with Interaction	Generic or Trade Name(s)
Vitamin A (continued)	Tretinoin	Vitinoin
	Simvastatin	Zocor
Vitamin B Complex	Tricyclic Antidepressants	Amitriptyline
	Multi Vitamin	Appedrine (Multiple vitamins and minerals)
	Tricyclic Antidepressants	Desipramine
	Tricyclic Antidepressants	Doxepin
	Tricyclic Antidepressants	Elavil
	Tricyclic Antidepressants	Imipramine
	Tricyclic Antidepressants	Norpramin
	Tricyclic Antidepressants	Sinequan
	Sulfasalazine	Sulfasalazine
	Tricyclic Antidepressants	Tofranil
	Tricyclic Antidepressants	Tricyclic Antidepressants
Vitamin B₁ (Thiamin)	Tricyclic Antidepressants	Amitriptyline
	Oral Contraceptives	Birth Control Pill
	Oral Contraceptives	Brevicon
	Loop Diuretics	Bumex
	Loop Diuretics	Demadex
	Oral Contraceptives	Demulen
	Tricyclic Antidepressants	Desipramine
	Tricyclic Antidepressants	Doxepin
	Loop Diuretics	Edecrin
	Tricyclic Antidepressants	Elavil
	Oral Contraceptives	Enovid
	Loop Diuretics	Ethacrynic Acid
	Loop Diuretics	Furosemide
	Oral Contraceptives	Genora
	Tricyclic Antidepressants	Imipramine
	Loop Diuretics	Lasix
	Oral Contraceptives	Levlen
	Oral Contraceptives	Loestrin
	Loop Diuretics	Loop Diuretics
	Oral Contraceptives	Micronor
	Oral Contraceptives	Modicon
	Oral Contraceptives	Nordette
	Oral Contraceptives	Norinyl
	Tricyclic Antidepressants	Norpramin
	Oral Contraceptives	Oral Contraceptives
	Oral Contraceptives	Ortho-Novum
	Oral Contraceptives	Ovcon
	Oral Contraceptives	Ovral
	Oral Contraceptives	Ovrette
	Tricyclic Antidepressants	Sinequan
	Tricyclic Antidepressants	Tofranil
	Loop Diuretics	Torsemide

Supplement	Drug with Interaction	Generic or Trade Name(s)
Vitamin B₁ (continued)	*Tricyclic Antidepressants*	*Tricyclic Antidepressants*
	Oral Contraceptives	*Triphasil*
Vitamin B₁₂ (Cobalamin)	*Tetracycline*	*Achromycin*
	Methyldopa	*Aldoclor (Methyldopa)*
	Methyldopa	*Aldomet*
	Methyldopa	*Aldoril (Methyldopa)*
	Tricyclic Antidepressants	*Amitriptyline*
	Clofibrate	*Atromid-S*
	Nizatidine	*Axid*
	Nizatidine	*Axid AR*
	AZT	*Azidothymidine*
	AZT	*AZT*
	Sulfamethoxazole	*Azulfidine*
	Trimethoprim	*Bethaprim*
	Oral Contraceptives	*Birth Control Pill*
	Oral Contraceptives	*Brevicon*
	Cimetidine	*Cimetidine*
	Clofibrate	*Clofibrate*
	Colchicine	*Colchicine*
	Trimethoprim	*Comoxol*
	Cycloserine	*Cycloserine*
	Oral Contraceptives	*Demulen*
	Tricyclic Antidepressants	*Desipramine*
	Tricyclic Antidepressants	*Doxepin*
	Erythromycin	*EES*
	Tricyclic Antidepressants	*Elavil*
	Erythromycin	*E-Mycin*
	Oral Contraceptives	*Enovid*
	Erythromycin	*Eryc Ery-Tab Erythromycin*
	Famotidine	*Famotidine*
	Sulfamethoxazole	*Gantanol*
	Oral Contraceptives	*Genora*
	Metformin	*Glucophage*
	Tetracycline	*Helidac (Tetracycline)*
	Erythromycin	*Ilosone*
	Tricyclic Antidepressants	*Imipramine*
	Isoniazid	*INH*
	Isoniazid	*Isoniazid*
	Isoniazid	*Laniazid*
	Lansoprazole	*Lansoprazole*
	Oral Contraceptives	*Levlen*
	Oral Contraceptives	*Loestrin*
	Omeprazole	*Losec*
	Metformin	*Metformin*
	Methyldopa	*Methyldopa*
	Oral Contraceptives	*Micronor*
	Oral Contraceptives	*Modicon*

Supplement	Drug with Interaction	Generic or Trade Name(s)
Vitamin B$_{12}$	Neomycin	Neomycin
	Nitrous Oxide	Nitrous Oxide
	Nizatidine	Nizatidine
	Oral Contraceptives	Nordette
	Oral Contraceptives	Norinyl
	Tricyclic Antidepressants	Norpramin
	Omeprazole	Omeprazole
	Oral Contraceptives	Oral Contraceptives
	Oral Contraceptives	Ortho-Novum
	Oral Contraceptives	Ovcon
	Oral Contraceptives	Ovral
	Oral Contraceptives	Ovrette
	Famotidine	Pepcid
	Famotidine	Pepcid AC
	Lansoprazole	Prevacid
	Omeprazole	Prilosec
	Trimethoprim	Proloprim
	Ranitidine	Ranitidine
	AZT	Retrovir
	Isoniazid	Rifamate
	Isoniazid	Rimactane
	Cycloserine	Seromycin
	Tricyclic Antidepressants	Sinequan
	Sulfamethoxazole	Sulfamethoxazole
	Tetracycline	Sumycin
	Cimetidine	Tagamet
	Cimetidine	Tagamet HB
	Tetracycline	Tetracycline
	Tricyclic Antidepressants	Tofranil
	Tricyclic Antidepressants	Tricyclic Antidepressants
	Trimethoprim	Trimethoprim
	Trimethoprim	Trimpex
	Oral Contraceptives	Triphasil
	Ranitidine	Zantac
	Ranitidine	Zantac 75
	AZT	Zidovudine
Vitamin B$_2$ (Riboflavin)	Tetracycline	Achromycin
	Doxorubicin	Adriamycin
	Tricyclic Antidepressants	Amitriptyline
	Oral Contraceptives	Birth Control Pill
	Oral Contraceptives	Brevicon
	Oral Contraceptives	Demulen
	Tricyclic Antidepressants	Desipramine
	Tricyclic Antidepressants	Doxepin
	Doxorubicin	Doxorubicin
	Tricyclic Antidepressants	Elavil
	Oral Contraceptives	Enovid

Supplement	Drug with Interaction	Generic or Trade Name(s)
Vitamin B₂	Oral Contraceptives	Genora
	Tetracycline	Helidac (Tetracycline)
	Tricyclic Antidepressants	Imipramine
	Oral Contraceptives	Levlen
	Oral Contraceptives	Loestrin
	Oral Contraceptives	Micronor
	Oral Contraceptives	Modicon
	Oral Contraceptives	Nordette
	Oral Contraceptives	Norinyl
	Tricyclic Antidepressants	Norpramin
	Oral Contraceptives	Oral Contraceptives
	Oral Contraceptives	Ortho-Novum
	Oral Contraceptives	Ovcon
	Oral Contraceptives	Ovral
	Oral Contraceptives	Ovrette
	Tricyclic Antidepressants	Sinequan
	Tetracycline	Sumycin
	Tetracycline	Tetracycline
	Tricyclic Antidepressants	Tofranil
	Tricyclic Antidepressants	Tricyclic Antidepressants
	Oral Contraceptives	Triphasil
Vitamin B₃ (Niacin, Niacinamide)	Tricyclic Antidepressants	Amitriptyline
	Atorvastatin	Atorvastatin
	Oral Contraceptives	Birth Control Pill
	Oral Contraceptives	Brevicon
	Oral Contraceptives	Demulen
	Tricyclic Antidepressants	Desipramine
	Tricyclic Antidepressants	Doxepin
	Tricyclic Antidepressants	Elavil
	Oral Contraceptives	Enovid
	Fluvastatin	Fluvastatin
	Oral Contraceptives	Genora
	Tricyclic Antidepressants	Imipramine
	Isoniazid	INH
	Isoniazid	Isoniazid
	Isoniazid	Laniazid
	Fluvastatin	Lescol
	Oral Contraceptives	Levlen
	Atorvastatin	Lipitor
	Oral Contraceptives	Loestrin
	Lovastatin	Lovastatin
	Lovastatin	Mevacor
	Oral Contraceptives	Micronor
	Oral Contraceptives	Modicon
	Oral Contraceptives	Nordette
	Oral Contraceptives	Norinyl
	Tricyclic Antidepressants	Norpramin

Drug Interactions

Supplement	Drug with Interaction	Generic or Trade Name(s)
Vitamin B$_3$	*Oral Contraceptives*	*Oral Contraceptives*
	Oral Contraceptives	*Ortho-Novum*
	Oral Contraceptives	*Ovcon*
	Oral Contraceptives	*Ovral*
	Oral Contraceptives	*Ovrette*
	Pravastatin	*Pravachol*
	Pravastatin	*Pravastatin*
	Isoniazid	*Rifamate*
	Isoniazid	*Rimactane*
	Simvastatin	*Simvastatin*
	Tricyclic Antidepressants	*Sinequan*
	Tricyclic Antidepressants	*Tofranil*
	Tricyclic Antidepressants	*Tricyclic Antidepressants*
	Oral Contraceptives	*Triphasil*
	Simvastatin	*Zocor*
Pantothenic Acid (Vitamin B$_5$)	*Tricyclic Antidepressants*	*Amitriptyline*
	Tricyclic Antidepressants	*Desipramine*
	Tricyclic Antidepressants	*Doxepin*
	Tricyclic Antidepressants	*Elavil*
	Tricyclic Antidepressants	*Imipramine*
	Tricyclic Antidepressants	*Norpramin*
	Tricyclic Antidepressants	*Sinequan*
	Tricyclic Antidepressants	*Tofranil*
	Tricyclic Antidepressants	*Tricyclic Antidepressants*
Vitamin B$_6$ (Pyridoxine)	*Tetracycline*	*Achromycin*
	Fluorouracil	*Adrucil*
	Corticosteroids	*AeroBid*
	Theophylline	*Aminophylline*
	Tricyclic Antidepressants	*Amitriptyline*
	Anticonvulsants	*Anticonvulsants*
	Hydralazine	*Apresazide (Hydralazine)*
	Hydralazine	*Apresoline*
	Corticosteroids	*Aristocort*
	Corticosteroids	*Azmacort*
	Sulfamethoxazole	*Azulfidine*
	Corticosteroids	*Beclomethasone*
	Corticosteroids	*Beclovent*
	Corticosteroids	*Beconase*
	Trimethoprim	*Bethaprim*
	Oral Contraceptives	*Birth Control Pill*
	Oral Contraceptives	*Brevicon*
	Corticosteroids	*Budesonide*
	Anticonvulsants	*Carbamazepine*
	Carbidopa Levodopa	*Carbidopa/Levodopa*
	Trimethoprim	*Comoxol*
	Conjugated Estrogens	*Conjugated Estrogens*
	Corticosteroids	*Cortef*

Supplement	Drug with Interaction	Generic or Trade Name(s)
Vitamin B_6	Corticosteroids	Corticosteroids
	Corticosteroids	Cortisone-like drugs
	Penicillamine	Cuprimine
	Corticosteroids	Cutivate
	Cycloserine	Cycloserine
	Corticosteroids	Decadron
	Corticosteroids	Decadron Phosphate Turbinaire
	Corticosteroids	Delta-Cortef
	Corticosteroids	Deltasone
	Oral Contraceptives	Demulen
	Penicillamine	Depen
	Tricyclic Antidepressants	Desipramine
	Corticosteroids	Dexamethasone
	Anticonvulsants	Dilantin
	Docetaxel	Docetaxel
	Levodopa	Dopar
	Tricyclic Antidepressants	Doxepin
	Erythromycin	EES
	Fluorouracil	Efudex
	Tricyclic Antidepressants	Elavil
	Corticosteroids	Elocon
	Erythromycin	E-Mycin
	Oral Contraceptives	Enovid
	Erythromycin	Eryc Ery-Tab Erythromycin
	Fluorouracil	5-FU
	Corticosteroids	Flonase
	Fluorouracil	Fluoroplex
	Fluorouracil	Fluorouracil
	Corticosteroids	Flunisolide
	Corticosteroids	Fluticasone
	Sulfamethoxazole	Gantanol
	Gentamicin	Garamycin
	Oral Contraceptives	Genora
	Gentamicin	Gentamicin
	Tetracycline	Helidac (Tetracycline)
	Hydralazine	Hydralazine
	Corticosteroids	Hydrocortisone
	Corticosteroids	Hytone
	Erythromycin	Ilosone
	Tricyclic Antidepressants	Imipramine
	Isoniazid	INH
	Isoniazid	Isoniazid
	Isoniazid	Laniazid
	Levodopa	Larodapa
	Levodopa	L-dopa
	Oral Contraceptives	Levlen
	Levodopa	Levodopa

Supplement	Drug with Interaction	Generic or Trade Name(s)
Vitamin B$_6$	Oral Contraceptives	Loestrin
	Corticosteroids	Medrol
	Corticosteroids	Methylprednisolone
	Oral Contraceptives	Micronor
	Oral Contraceptives	Modicon
	Corticosteroids	Mometasone
	Anticonvulsants	Mysoline
	Phenelzine	Nardil
	Corticosteroids	Nasacort
	Corticosteroids	Nasalide
	Neomycin	Neomycin
	Oral Contraceptives	Nordette
	Oral Contraceptives	Norinyl
	Tricyclic Antidepressants	Norpramin
	Oral Contraceptives	Oral Contraceptives
	Corticosteroids	Orasone
	Oral Contraceptives	Ortho-Novum
	Oral Contraceptives	Ovcon
	Oral Contraceptives	Ovral
	Oral Contraceptives	Ovrette
	Corticosteroids	Pediapred
	Penicillamine	Penicillamine
	Phenelzine	Phenelzine
	Anticonvulsants	Phenobarbital
	Anticonvulsants	Phenytoin
	Theophylline	Phyllocontin
	Corticosteroids	Prednisolone
	Corticosteroids	Prednisone
	Conjugated Estrogens	Premarin
	Conjugated Estrogens	Prempro (Conjugated estrogens)
	Theophylline	Primatene Dual Action (Theophylline)
	Anticonvulsants	Primidone
	Trimethoprim	Proloprim
	Corticosteroids	Pulmicort
	Corticosteroids	Rhinocort
	Isoniazid	Rifamate
	Isoniazid	Rimactane
	Cycloserine	Seromycin
	Carbidopa Levodopa	Sinemet
	Tricyclic Antidepressants	Sinequan
	Theophylline	Slo-Bid
	Theophylline	Slo-Phyllin
	Corticosteroids	Steroids (Prednisone)
	Sulfamethoxazole	Sulfamethoxazole
	Tetracycline	Sumycin

Supplement	Drug with Interaction	Generic or Trade Name(s)
Vitamin B₆	Docetaxel	Taxotere
	Anticonvulsants	Tegretol
	Tetracycline	Tetracycline
	Theophylline	Theo-Dur
	Theophylline	Theolair
	Theophylline	Theophylline
	Corticosteroids	Tobradex (Dexamthasone)
	Tricyclic Antidepressants	Tofranil
	Corticosteroids	Triamcinolone
	Tricyclic Antidepressants	Tricyclic Antidepressants
	Trimethoprim	Trimethoprim
	Trimethoprim	Trimpex
	Oral Contraceptives	Triphasil
	Theophylline	Truphylline
	Theophylline	Uniphyl
	Corticosteroids	Vancenase
	Corticosteroids	Vanceril
Vitamin C (Ascorbic Acid)	Acetaminophen	Acetaminophen
	Aspirin	Acetylsalicylic Acid
	Tetracycline	Achromycin
	Phenylpropanolamine	Acutrim
	Ephedrine	Adrenaline
	Doxorubicin	Adriamycin
	Corticosteroids	AeroBid
	Ephedrine	Afrin
	Aspirin	Alka-Seltzer (Aspirin)
	Acetaminophen	Alka-Seltzer Plus (Aceta-minophen)
	Ephedrine	Alka-Seltzer Plus (Pseu-doephedrine)
	Aspirin	Anacin (Aspirin)
	Antibiotics	Antibiotics
	Warfarin	Anticoagulant (Warfarin)
	Acetaminophen	APAP
	Multi Vitamin	Appedrine (Multiple vitamins and minerals)
	Phenylpropanolamine	Appedrine (Phenyl-propanolamine)
	Corticosteroids	Aristocort
	Aspirin	ASA
	Aspirin	Aspirin
	Corticosteroids	Azmacort
	Corticosteroids	Beclomethasone
	Corticosteroids	Beclovent
	Corticosteroids	Beconase
	Oral Contraceptives	Birth Control Pill
	Oral Contraceptives	Brevicon

Supplement	Drug with Interaction	Generic or Trade Name(s)
Vitamin C (continued)	*Epinephrine*	*Bronkaid Mist*
	Epinephrine	*Brontin Mist*
	Corticosteroids	*Budesonide*
	Chemotherapy	*Cancer Chemotherapy*
	Chemotherapy	*Chemotherapy*
	Ephedrine	*Chlor-Trimeton 12 Hour (Pseudoephedrine)*
	Ephedrine	*Claritin-D (Pseudoephedrine)*
	Phenylpropanolamine	*Contac 12 Hour (Phenylpropanolamine)*
	Corticosteroids	*Cortef*
	Corticosteroids	*Corticosteroids*
	Corticosteroids	*Cortisone-like drugs*
	Warfarin	*Coumadin*
	Corticosteroids	*Cutivate*
	Cyclophosphamide	*Cyclophosphamide*
	Cyclophosphamide	*Cytoxan*
	Dapsone	*Dapsone*
	Acetaminophen	*Darvocet (Acetaminophen)*
	Acetaminophen	*Darvocet N (Acetaminophen)*
	Aspirin	*Darvon Compound (Aspirin)*
	Phenylpropanolamine	*DayQuil Allergy Relief (Phenylpropanolamine)*
	Corticosteroids	*Decadron*
	Corticosteroids	*Decadron Phosphate Turbinaire*
	Corticosteroids	*Delta-Cortef*
	Corticosteroids	*Deltasone*
	Oral Contraceptives	*Demulen*
	Phenylpropanolamine	*Dex-A-Diet*
	Phenylpropanolamine	*Dex-A-Diet Plus Vitamin C (Phenylpropanolamine)*
	Corticosteroids	*Dexamethasone*
	Phenylpropanolamine	*Dexatrim*
	Phenylpropanolamine	*Dexatrim Plus Vitamin C (Phenylpropanolamine)*
	Phenylpropanolamine	*Diadex Grapefruit Diet Plan (Phenylpropanolamine)*
	Phenylpropanolamine	*Dimetapp (Phenylpropanolamine)*
	Doxorubicin	*Doxorubicin*
	Corticosteroids	*Elocon*
	Aspirin	*Empirin with Codeine (Aspirin)*
	Oral Contraceptives	*Enovid*
	Phenylpropanolamine	*Entex LA (Phenylpropanolamine)*
	Ephedrine	*Ephedrine*
	Epinephrine	*Epinephrine*

Supplement	Drug with Interaction	Generic or Trade Name(s)
Vitamin C (continued)	*Acetaminophen*	*Excedrin PM (Acetaminophen)*
	Corticosteroids	*Flonase*
	Corticosteroids	*Flunisolide*
	Corticosteroids	*Fluticasone*
	Oral Contraceptives	*Genora*
	Tetracycline	*Helidac (Tetracycline)*
	Corticosteroids	*Hydrocortisone*
	Corticosteroids	*Hytone*
	Isosorbide Mononitrate	*Imdur*
	Indomethacin	*Indocin*
	Indomethacin	*Indomethacin*
	Isosorbide Mononitrate	*ISMO*
	Isosorbide Mononitrate	*Isosorbide Mononitrate*
	Oral Contraceptives	*Levlen*
	Oral Contraceptives	*Loestrin*
	Acetaminophen	*Lortab (Acetaminophen)*
	Corticosteroids	*Medrol*
	Corticosteroids	*Methylprednisolone*
	Oral Contraceptives	*Micronor*
	Oral Contraceptives	*Modicon*
	Corticosteroids	*Mometasone*
	Isosorbide Mononitrate	*Monoket*
	Corticosteroids	*Nasacort*
	Corticosteroids	*Nasalide*
	Cyclophosphamide	*Neosar*
	Oral Contraceptives	*Nordette*
	Oral Contraceptives	*Norinyl*
	Acetaminophen	*Nyquil (Acetaminophen)*
	Ephedrine	*Nyquil (Pseudoephedrine)*
	Acetaminophen	*Nyquil Hot Therapy Powder (Acetaminophen)*
	Ephedrine	*Nyquil Hot Therapy Powder (Pseudoephedrine)*
	Oral Contraceptives	*Oral Contraceptives*
	Corticosteroids	*Orasone*
	Oral Contraceptives	*Ortho-Novum*
	Oral Contraceptives	*Ovcon*
	Oral Contraceptives	*Ovral*
	Oral Contraceptives	*Ovrette*
	Acetaminophen	*Paracetemol*
	Corticosteroids	*Pediapred*
	Acetaminophen	*Percocet (Acetaminophen)*
	Aspirin	*Percodan (Aspirin)*
	Phenylpropanolamine	*Phenylpropanolamine*
	Phenylpropanolamine	*PPA*
	Corticosteroids	*Prednisolone*
	Corticosteroids	*Prednisone*

Supplement	Drug with Interaction	Generic or Trade Name(s)
Vitamin C (continued)	Ephedrine	Pretz-D
	Ephedrine	Primatene Dual Action (Ephedrine)
	Epinephrine	Primatene Mist
	Phenylpropanolamine	Propagest
	Ephedrine	Pseudoephedrine
	Corticosteroids	Pulmicort
	Phenylpropanolamine	Rhindecon
	Corticosteroids	Rhinocort
	Phenylpropanolamine	Robitussin CF (Phenylpropanolamine)
	Acetaminophen	Roxicet (Acetaminophen)
	Aspirin	Roxiprin (Aspirin)
	Aspirin	Soma Compound (Aspirin)
	Aspirin	Soma Compound with Codeine (Aspirin)
	Corticosteroids	Steroids (Prednisone)
	Ephedrine	Sudafed
	Tetracycline	Sumycin
	Phenylpropanolamine	Tavist-D (Phenylpropanolamine)
	Tetracycline	Tetracycline
	Acetaminophen	Theraflu (Acetaminophen)
	Ephedrine	Theraflu (Pseudoephedrine)
	Acetaminophen	Theraflu Flu and Cold (Acetaminophen)
	Ephedrine	Theraflu Flu and Cold (Pseudoephedrine)
	Corticosteroids	Tobradex (Dexamthasone)
	Corticosteroids	Triamcinolone
	Phenylpropanolamine	Triaminic-12 (Phenylpropanolamine)
	Oral Contraceptives	Triphasil
	Acetaminophen	Tylenol
	Acetaminophen	Tylenol Allergy Sinus (Acetaminophen)
	Ephedrine	Tylenol Allergy Sinus (Pseudoephedrine)
	Acetaminophen	Tylenol Cold (Acetaminophen)
	Ephedrine	Tylenol Cold (Pseudoephedrine)
	Acetaminophen	Tylenol Flu NightTime Maximum Strength Powder (Acetaminophen)
	Ephedrine	Tylenol Flu NightTime Maximum Strength Powder (Pseudoephedrine)
	Acetaminophen	Tylenol Multi-Symptom Hot Medication (Acetaminophen)

Drug Interactions

Supplement	Drug with Interaction	Generic or Trade Name(s)
Vitamin C (continued)	*Ephedrine*	*Tylenol Multi-Symptom Hot Medication (Pseudoephedrine)*
	Acetaminophen	*Tylenol PM (Acetaminophen)*
	Acetaminophen	*Tylenol PM Extra Strength (Acetaminophen)*
	Acetaminophen	*Tylenol Sinus (Acetaminophen)*
	Ephedrine	*Tylenol Sinus (Pseudoephedrine)*
	Acetaminophen	*Tylenol with Codeine (Acetaminophen)*
	Acetaminophen	*Tylenol Allergy Sinus*
	Phenylpropanolamine	*Unitrol*
	Corticosteroids	*Vancenase*
	Corticosteroids	*Vanceril*
	Ephedrine	*Vick Vatronol*
	Acetaminophen	*Vicodin (Acetaminophen)*
	Warfarin	*Warfarin*
	Acetaminophen	*Wygesic (Acetaminophen)*
Vitamin D (Colecalciferol)	*Corticosteroids*	*AeroBid*
	Thiazide Diuretics	*Aldactazide (Hydrochlorothiazide)*
	Thiazide Diuretics	*Aldoclor (Chlorothiazide)*
	Thiazide Diuretics	*Aldoril (Hydrochlorothiazide)*
	Estradiol	*Alora*
	Heparin	*Anticoagulant (Heparin)*
	Warfarin	*Anticoagulant (Warfarin)*
	Anticonvulsants	*Anticonvulsants*
	Multi Vitamin	*Appedrine (Multiple vitamins and minerals)*
	Thiazide Diuretics	*Apresazide (Hydrochlorothiazide)*
	Corticosteroids	*Aristocort*
	Corticosteroids	*Azmacort*
	Corticosteroids	*Beclomethasone*
	Corticosteroids	*Beclovent*
	Corticosteroids	*Beconase*
	Bile Acid Sequestrants	*Bile Acid Sequestrants*
	Corticosteroids	*Budesonide*
	Verapamil	*Calan*
	Thiazide Diuretics	*Captozide (Hydrochlorothiazide)*
	Anticonvulsants	*Carbamazepine*
	Thiazide Diuretics	*Chlorothiazide*
	Thiazide Diuretics	*Chlorothiazide/Methyldopa*
	Thiazide Diuretics	*Chlorthalidone*
	Bile Acid Sequestrants	*Cholestyramine*
	Cimetidine	*Cimetidine*

Supplement	Drug with Interaction	Generic or Trade Name(s)
Vitamin D (continued)	Estradiol	Climara
	Colestipol	Colestid
	Colestipol	Colestipol
	Thiazide Diuretics	Combipres (Chlorthalidone)
	Conjugated Estrogens	Conjugated Estrogens
	Corticosteroids	Cortef
	Corticosteroids	Corticosteroids
	Corticosteroids	Cortisone-like drugs
	Warfarin	Coumadin
	Corticosteroids	Cutivate
	Medroxyprogesterone	Cycrin
	Corticosteroids	Decadron
	Corticosteroids	Decadron Phosphate Turbinaire
	Corticosteroids	Delta-Cortef
	Corticosteroids	Deltasone
	Medroxyprogesterone	Depo-Provera
	Corticosteroids	Dexamethasone
	Anticonvulsants	Dilantin
	Thiazide Diuretics	Diuril
	Thiazide Diuretics	Dyazide (Hydrochlorothiazide)
	Corticosteroids	Elocon
	Estradiol	Esclim
	Thiazide Diuretics	Esidrix
	Estradiol	Estrace Estraderm Estradiol
	Estradiol	FemPatch
	Corticosteroids	Flonase
	Corticosteroids	Flunisolide
	Corticosteroids	Fluticasone
	Thiazide Diuretics	HCTZ
	Heparin	Heparin
	Thiazide Diuretics	Hydrochlorothiazide
	Corticosteroids	Hydrocortisone
	Thiazide Diuretics	HydroDIURIL
	Thiazide Diuretics	Hygroton
	Corticosteroids	Hytone
	Thiazide Diuretics	Inderide (Hydrochlorothiazide)
	Isoniazid	INH
	Isoniazid	Isoniazid
	Verapamil	Isoptin
	Isoniazid	Laniazid
	Thiazide Diuretics	Lopressor HCT (Hydrochlorothiazide)
	Thiazide Diuretics	Maxzide (Hydrochlorothiazide)
	Corticosteroids	Medrol
	Medroxyprogesterone	Medroxyprogesterone
	Corticosteroids	Methylprednisolone
	Thiazide Diuretics	Metolazone

Supplement	Drug with Interaction	Generic or Trade Name(s)
Vitamin D (continued)	*Mineral Oil*	*Mineral Oil*
	Thiazide Diuretics	*Moduretic (Hydrochloroth-iazide)*
	Corticosteroids	*Mometasone*
	Thiazide Diuretics	*Mykros*
	Anticonvulsants	*Mysoline*
	Corticosteroids	*Nasacort*
	Corticosteroids	*Nasalide*
	Neomycin	*Neomycin*
	Corticosteroids	*Orasone*
	Thiazide Diuretics	*Oretic*
	Corticosteroids	*Pediapred*
	Anticonvulsants	*Phenobarbital*
	Anticonvulsants	*Phenytoin*
	Corticosteroids	*Prednisolone*
	Corticosteroids	*Prednisone*
	Conjugated Estrogens	*Premarin*
	Conjugated Estrogens	*Prempro (Conjugated estrogens)*
	Medroxyprogesterone	*Prempro (Medroxyproges-terone)*
	Anticonvulsants	*Primidone*
	Thiazide Diuretics	*Prinizide (Hydrochlorothiazide)*
	Medroxyprogesterone	*Provera*
	Corticosteroids	*Pulmicort*
	Bile Acid Sequestrants	*Questran*
	Corticosteroids	*Rhinocort*
	Isoniazid	*Rifamate*
	Isoniazid	*Rimactane*
	Corticosteroids	*Steroids (Prednisone)*
	Cimetidine	*Tagamet*
	Cimetidine	*Tagamet HB*
	Anticonvulsants	*Tegretol*
	Thiazide Diuretics	*Tenoretic (Chlorthalidone)*
	Thiazide Diuretics	*Thiazide Diuretics*
	Thiazide Diuretics	*Timolide (Hydrochlorothiazide)*
	Corticosteroids	*Tobradex (Dexamthasone)*
	Corticosteroids	*Triamcinolone*
	Corticosteroids	*Vancenase*
	Corticosteroids	*Vanceril*
	Thiazide Diuretics	*Vaseretic (Hydrochlorothiazide)*
	Verapamil	*Verapamil*
	Verapamil	*Verelan*
	Estradiol	*Vivelle*
	Warfarin	*Warfarin*
	Thiazide Diuretics	*Zaroxolyn*
	Thiazide Diuretics	*Zestoretic (Hydrochloroth-iazide)*

Drug Interactions

Drug Interactions

Supplement	Drug with Interaction	Generic or Trade Name(s)
Vitamin D (continued)	*Thiazide Diuretics*	*Ziac (Hydrochlorothiazide)*
Vitamin E (Tocopherol)	*Aspirin*	*Acetylsalicylic Acid*
	Doxorubicin	*Adriamycin*
	Aspirin	*Alka-Seltzer (Aspirin)*
	Amiodarone	*Amiodarone*
	Aspirin	*Anacin (Aspirin)*
	Insulin	*Animal-Source Insulin*
	Anthralin	*Anthralin*
	Warfarin	*Anticoagulant (Warfarin)*
	Gemfibrozil	*Apo-Gemfibrozil*
	Multi Vitamin	*Appedrine (Multiple vitamins and minerals)*
	Aspirin	*ASA*
	Aspirin	*Aspirin*
	AZT	*Azidothymidine*
	AZT	*AZT*
	Bile Acid Sequestrants	*Bile Acid Sequestrants*
	Chemotherapy	*Cancer Chemotherapy*
	Chemotherapy	*Chemotherapy*
	Bile Acid Sequestrants	*Cholestyramine*
	Colestipol	*Colestid*
	Colestipol	*Colestipol*
	Amiodarone	*Cordarone*
	Warfarin	*Coumadin*
	Cyclophosphamide	*Cyclophosphamide*
	Cyclosporine	*Cyclosporine*
	Cyclophosphamide	*Cytoxan*
	Dapsone	*Dapsone*
	Aspirin	*Darvon Compound (Aspirin)*
	Valproic Acid	*Depakene Syrup*
	Valproic Acid	*Depakene*
	Valproic Acid	*Depakote*
	Vitamin C	*Dex-A-Diet Plus Vitamin C (Vitamin C)*
	Vitamin C	*Dexatrim Plus Vitamin C (Vitamin C)*
	Glyburide	*Diabeta*
	Anthralin	*Dithranol*
	Valproic Acid	*Divalproex sodium*
	Doxorubicin	*Doxorubicin*
	Anthralin	*Drithocreme*
	Aspirin	*Empirin with Codeine (Aspirin)*
	Griseofulvin	*Fluvicin*
	Gemfibrozil	*Gemfibrozil*
	Griseofulvin	*Gifulvin V*
	Glyburide	*Glibenclamide*
	Glyburide	*Glyburide*

Supplement	Drug with Interaction	Generic or Trade Name(s)
Vitamin E (continued)	Griseofulvin	Grifulvin
	Griseofulvin	Griseofulvin
	Griseofulvin	Gris-PEG
	Griseofulvin	Gristatin
	Haloperidol	Haldol
	Haloperidol	Haloperidol
	Insulin	Human Analog Insulin
	Insulin	Human Insulin
	Insulin	Humanlog
	Insulin	Humulin
	Insulin	Iletin
	Isoniazid	INH
	Insulin	Insulin
	Isoniazid	Isoniazid
	Isoniazid	Laniazid
	Gemfibrozil	Lopid
	Anthralin	Micanol Cream
	Glyburide	Micronase
	Mineral Oil	Mineral Oil
	Cyclosporine	Neoral
	Cyclophosphamide	Neosar
	Gemfibrozil	Novo-Gemfibrozil
	Insulin	Novolin
	Aspirin	Percodan (Aspirin)
	Glyburide	Pres Tab
	Bile Acid Sequestrants	Questran
	AZT	Retrovir
	Isoniazid	Rifamate
	Isoniazid	Rimactane
	Aspirin	Roxiprin (Aspirin)
	Cyclosporine	Sandimmune
	Simvastatin	Simvastatin
	Valproic Acid	Sodium Valproate
	Aspirin	Soma Compound (Aspirin)
	Aspirin	Soma Compound with Codeine (Aspirin)
	Valproic Acid	Valproic Acid
	Warfarin	Warfarin
	AZT	Zidovudine
	Simvastatin	Zocor
Vitamin K$_1$ (Phylloquinone)	Tetracycline	Achromycin
	Corticosteroids	AeroBid
	Tobramycin	AKTob
	Antibiotics	Antibiotics
	Warfarin	Anticoagulant (Warfarin)
	Anticonvulsants	Anticonvulsants
	Corticosteroids	Aristocort

Supplement	Drug with Interaction	Generic or Trade Name(s)
Vitamin K₁ (continued)	Corticosteroids	Azmacort
	Sulfamethoxazole	Azulfidine
	Corticosteroids	Beclomethasone
	Corticosteroids	Beclovent
	Corticosteroids	Beconase
	Trimethoprim	Bethaprim
	Bile Acid Sequestrants	Bile Acid Sequestrants
	Corticosteroids	Budesonide
	Anticonvulsants	Carbamazepine
	Cephalosporins	Ceclor
	Cephalosporins	Cefanex
	Cephalosporins	Cefixime
	Cephalosporins	Cefpodoxime
	Cephalosporins	Ceftin
	Cephalosporins	Ceftriaxone
	Cephalosporins	Cefuroxime
	Cephalosporins	Cephaclor
	Cephalosporins	Cephadroxil
	Cephalosporins	Cephalexin
	Cephalosporins	Cephalosporins
	Bile Acid Sequestrants	Cholestyramine
	Colestipol	Colestid
	Colestipol	Colestipol
	Trimethoprim	Comoxol
	Corticosteroids	Cortef
	Corticosteroids	Corticosteroids
	Corticosteroids	Cortisone-like drugs
	Warfarin	Coumadin
	Corticosteroids	Cutivate
	Cycloserine	Cycloserine
	Corticosteroids	Decadron
	Corticosteroids	Decadron Phosphate Turbinaire
	Corticosteroids	Delta-Cortef
	Corticosteroids	Deltasone
	Corticosteroids	Dexamethasone
	Anticonvulsants	Dilantin
	Doxycycline	Doxycycline
	Cephalosporins	Duricef
	Corticosteroids	Elocon
	Corticosteroids	Flonase
	Ofloxacin	Floxin
	Corticosteroids	Flunisolide
	Corticosteroids	Fluticasone
	Sulfamethoxazole	Gantanol
	Tetracycline	Helidac (Tetracycline)
	Corticosteroids	Hydrocortisone
	Corticosteroids	Hytone

Supplement	Drug with Interaction	Generic or Trade Name(s)
Vitamin K₁ (continued)	*Isoniazid*	*INH*
	Isoniazid	*Isoniazid*
	Cephalosporins	*Keflet*
	Cephalosporins	*Keflex*
	Cephalosporins	*Keftab*
	Isoniazid	*Laniazid*
	Corticosteroids	*Medrol*
	Corticosteroids	*Methylprednisolone*
	Mineral Oil	*Mineral Oil*
	Corticosteroids	*Mometasone*
	Anticonvulsants	*Mysoline*
	Corticosteroids	*Nasacort*
	Corticosteroids	*Nasalide*
	Tobramycin	*Nebicin*
	Neomycin	*Neomycin*
	Ofloxacin	*Oculflox Ofloxacin*
	Corticosteroids	*Orasone*
	Corticosteroids	*Pediapred*
	Anticonvulsants	*Phenobarbital*
	Anticonvulsants	*Phenytoin*
	Corticosteroids	*Prednisolone*
	Corticosteroids	*Prednisone*
	Anticonvulsants	*Primidone*
	Trimethoprim	*Proloprim*
	Corticosteroids	*Pulmicort*
	Bile Acid Sequestrants	*Questran*
	Corticosteroids	*Rhinocort*
	Isoniazid	*Rifamate*
	Isoniazid	*Rimactane*
	Cephalosporins	*Rocephin*
	Cycloserine	*Seromycin*
	Corticosteroids	*Steroids (Prednisone)*
	Sulfamethoxazole	*Sulfamethoxazole*
	Tetracycline	*Sumycin*
	Cephalosporins	*Suprax*
	Anticonvulsants	*Tegretol*
	Tetracycline	*Tetracycline*
	Tobramycin	*TOBI*
	Corticosteroids	*Tobradex (Dexamthasone)*
	Tobramycin	*Tobradex (Tobramycin)*
	Tobramycin	*Tobramycin*
	Tobramycin	*Tobrex*
	Corticosteroids	*Triamcinolone*
	Trimethoprim	*Trimethoprim*
	Trimethoprim	*Trimpex*
	Cephalosporins	*Ulracef*
	Corticosteroids	*Vancenase*

Drug Interactions

Supplement	Drug with Interaction	Generic or Trade Name(s)
Vitamin K₁ (continued)	*Corticosteroids*	*Vanceril*
	Cephalosporins	*Vantin*
	Doxycycline	*Vibramycin*
	Warfarin	*Warfarin*
Whey Protein	*(none)*	*(none)*
Zinc	*Quinapril*	*Accupril*
	ACE Inhibitors	*ACE Inhibitors*
	Aspirin	*Acetylsalicylic Acid*
	Tetracycline	*Achromycin*
	Corticosteroids	*AeroBid*
	Thiazide Diuretics	*Aldactazide (Hydrochloroth-iazide)*
	Thiazide Diuretics	*Aldoclor (Chlorothiazide)*
	Thiazide Diuretics	*Aldoril (Hydrochlorothiazide)*
	Aspirin	*Alka-Seltzer (Aspirin)*
	Ramipril	*Altace*
	Aspirin	*Anacin (Aspirin)*
	ACE Inhibitors	*Angiotensin Converting Enzyme Inhibitors*
	Warfarin	*Anticoagulant (Warfarin)*
	Multi Vitamin	*Appedrine (Multiple vitamins and minerals)*
	Thiazide Diuretics	*Apresazide (Hydrochloroth-iazide)*
	Corticosteroids	*Aristocort*
	Aspirin	*ASA*
	Aspirin	*Aspirin*
	AZT	*Azidothymidine*
	Corticosteroids	*Azmacort*
	AZT	*AZT*
	Corticosteroids	*Beclomethasone*
	Corticosteroids	*Beclovent*
	Corticosteroids	*Beconase*
	Benazepril	*Benazepril*
	Bile Acid Sequestrants	*Bile Acid Sequestrants*
	Oral Contraceptives	*Birth Control Pill*
	Oral Contraceptives	*Brevicon*
	Corticosteroids	*Budesonide*
	Captopril	*Capoten*
	Captopril	*Captopril*
	Captopril	*Captozide (Captopril)*
	Thiazide Diuretics	*Captozide (Hydrochloroth-iazide)*
	Thiazide Diuretics	*Chlorothiazide*
	Thiazide Diuretics	*Chlorothiazide/Methyldopa*
	Thiazide Diuretics	*Chlorthalidone*
	Bile Acid Sequestrants	*Cholestyramine*

Supplement	Drug with Interaction	Generic or Trade Name(s)
Zinc (continued)	Ciprofloxacin	Cipro
	Ciprofloxacin	Ciprofloxacin
	Thiazide Diuretics	Combipres (Chlorthalidone)
	Conjugated Estrogens	Conjugated Estrogens
	Corticosteroids	Cortef
	Corticosteroids	Corticosteroids
	Corticosteroids	Cortisone-like drugs
	Warfarin	Coumadin
	Penicillamine	Cuprimine
	Corticosteroids	Cutivate
	Medroxyprogesterone	Cycrin
	Aspirin	Darvon Compound (Aspirin)
	Corticosteroids	Decadron
	Corticosteroids	Decadron Phosphate Turbinaire
	Corticosteroids	Delta-Cortef
	Corticosteroids	Deltasone
	Oral Contraceptives	Demulen
	Valproic Acid	Depakene Syrup
	Valproic Acid	Depakene
	Valproic Acid	Depakote
	Penicillamine	Depen
	Medroxyprogesterone	Depo-Provera
	Corticosteroids	Dexamethasone
	Thiazide Diuretics	Diuril
	Valproic Acid	Divalproex sodium
	Doxycycline	Doxycycline
	Thiazide Diuretics	Dyazide (Hydrochlorothiazide)
	Corticosteroids	Elocon
	Aspirin	Empirin with Codeine (Aspirin)
	Oral Contraceptives	Enovid
	Thiazide Diuretics	Esidrix
	Corticosteroids	Flonase
	Ofloxacin	Floxin
	Corticosteroids	Flunisolide
	Corticosteroids	Fluticasone
	Oral Contraceptives	Genora
	Thiazide Diuretics	HCTZ
	Tetracycline	Helidac (Tetracycline)
	Thiazide Diuretics	Hydrochlorothiazide
	Corticosteroids	Hydrocortisone
	Thiazide Diuretics	HydroDIURIL
	Thiazide Diuretics	Hygroton
	Corticosteroids	Hytone
	Thiazide Diuretics	Inderide (Hydrochlorothiazide)
	Oral Contraceptives	Levlen
	Lisinopril	Lisinopril
	Oral Contraceptives	Loestrin

Drug Interactions

Drug Interactions

Supplement	Drug with Interaction	Generic or Trade Name(s)
Zinc (continued)	Thiazide Diuretics	Lopressor HCT (Hydrochlorothiazide)
	Benazepril	Lotensin
	Thiazide Diuretics	Maxzide (Hydrochlorothiazide)
	Corticosteroids	Medrol
	Medroxyprogesterone	Medroxyprogesterone
	Corticosteroids	Methylprednisolone
	Thiazide Diuretics	Metolazone
	Oral Contraceptives	Micronor
	Oral Contraceptives	Modicon
	Thiazide Diuretics	Moduretic (Hydrochlorothiazide)
	Corticosteroids	Mometasone
	Thiazide Diuretics	Mykros
	Corticosteroids	Nasacort
	Corticosteroids	Nasalide
	Oral Contraceptives	Nordette
	Oral Contraceptives	Norinyl
	Ofloxacin	Oculflox Ofloxacin
	Oral Contraceptives	Oral Contraceptives
	Corticosteroids	Orasone
	Thiazide Diuretics	Oretic
	Oral Contraceptives	Ortho-Novum
	Oral Contraceptives	Ovcon
	Oral Contraceptives	Ovral
	Oral Contraceptives	Ovrette
	Corticosteroids	Pediapred
	Penicillamine	Penicillamine
	Aspirin	Percodan (Aspirin)
	Corticosteroids	Prednisolone
	Corticosteroids	Prednisone
	Conjugated Estrogens	Premarin
	Conjugated Estrogens	Prempro (Conjugated estrogens)
	Medroxyprogesterone	Prempro (Medroxyprogesterone)
	Lisinopril	Prinivil
	Thiazide Diuretics	Prinizide (Hydrochlorothiazide)
	Lisinopril	Prinizide (Lisinopril)
	Medroxyprogesterone	Provera
	Corticosteroids	Pulmicort
	Bile Acid Sequestrants	Questran
	Quinapril	Quinapril
	Ramipril	Ramipril
	AZT	Retrovir
	Corticosteroids	Rhinocort
	Aspirin	Roxiprin (Aspirin)

Supplement	Drug with Interaction	Generic or Trade Name(s)
Zinc (continued)	*Valproic Acid*	*Sodium Valproate*
	Aspirin	*Soma Compound (Aspirin)*
	Aspirin	*Soma Compound with Codeine (Aspirin)*
	Corticosteroids	*Steroids (Prednisone)*
	Tetracycline	*Sumycin*
	Thiazide Diuretics	*Tenoretic (Chlorthalidone)*
	Tetracycline	*Tetracycline*
	Thiazide Diuretics	*Thiazide Diuretics*
	Thiazide Diuretics	*Timolide (Hydrochlorothiazide)*
	Corticosteroids	*Tobradex (Dexamthasone)*
	Corticosteroids	*Triamcinolone*
	Oral Contraceptives	*Triphasil*
	Valproic Acid	*Valproic Acid*
	Corticosteroids	*Vancenase*
	Corticosteroids	*Vanceril*
	Thiazide Diuretics	*Vaseretic (Hydrochlorothiazide)*
	Doxycycline	*Vibramycin*
	Warfarin	*Warfarin*
	Thiazide Diuretics	*Zaroxolyn*
	Thiazide Diuretics	*Zestoretic (Hydrochlorothiazide)*
	Lisinopril	*Zestoretic (Lisinopril)*
	Thiazide Diuretics	*Ziac (Hydrochlorothiazide)*
	AZT	*Zidovudine*

Drug Interactions

Appendix 3

DRUGS BY PHARMACIST CLASSIFICATION

a. **Atropine** (page 22)
b. **Ipratropium Bromide** (page 118)
C. Sympathomimetic (Adrenergic) agents
1. **Albuterol** (proventil) (page 4)
2. **Ephedrine and Pseudoephedrine** (page 83)
3. **Epinephrine** (page 85)
4. **Phenylpropanolamine** (page 172)
D. Sympatholytic (Adrenergic blocking) agents
E. Skeletal muscle relaxants
1. **Carisoprodol** (page 38, 59)
2. **Cyclobenzaprine** (page 63)
F. Miscellaneous autonomic drugs
1. **Dicyclomine** (page 70)
2. **Phentermine** (page 171)
5. Blood Formation and Coagulation
A. Antianemia drugs
1. Iron preparations
2. Liver and stomach preparations
B. Coagulants and anticoagulants
1. Anticoagulants
a. **Heparin** (page 107)
b. **Warfarin** (page 108, 224)
2. Antiheparin agents
3. Coagulants
4. Hemostatics
C. Hematopoietic agents
1. **Deferoxamine** (page 69)
D. Hemorrheologic agents
1. Pentoxifylline
E. Thrombolytic agents
F. Antiplatelet
1. **Ticlopidine** (page 207)
6. Cardiovascular Drugs
A. Cardiac drugs
1. **ACE Inhibitors** (page 1)
2. **Amiodarone** (page 9)
3. **Amlodipine** (page 9)
4. **Atenolol** (page 20)
5. **Captopril** (page 1, 35)
6. **Digoxin** (page 1, 71)
7. **Enalapril** (page 1, 82)
8. **Isosorbide Mononitrate** (page 120)
9. **Lisinopril** (page 126)
10. **Metoprolol** (page 143)
11. **Nifedipine** (page 152)
12. **Propranolol** (page 180)
13. **Quinapril** (page 181)

Drugs by Pharmacist Classification

Drugs by Pharmacist Classification

Drugs by Pharmacist Classification

8. Contraceptives
   A. **Oral Contraceptives** (page 160)
9. Antitussives, Expectorants, and Mucolytic Agents
   A. Antitussives
      1. **Codeine** (page 54)
      2. **Dextromethorphan** (page 70)
      3. **Hydrocodone/Acetaminophen** (page 110)
   B. Expectorants
      1. **Guaifenesin** (page 105)
   C. Mucolytic agents
10. Eye, Ear, Nose, and Throat (EENT) Preparations
    A. Antiallergic agents
       1. **Cetirizine** (page 39)
       2. **Fexofenadine** (page 92)
    B. Anti-infectives
       1. **Antibiotics** (page 14)
       2. Antifungals
       3. Antivirals
       4. Sulfonamides
       5. Miscellaneous anti-infectives
    C. Anti-inflammatory agents
    D. Carbonic anhydrase inhibitors
       1. **Dorzolamide** (page 78)
    E. Contact lens solutions
    F. Local anesthetics
    G. Miotics
    H. Mydriatics
    I. Mouthwashes and gargles
    J. Vasoconstrictors
    K. Miscellaneous EENT drugs
11. Gastrointestinal Drugs
    A. Antacids and absorbents
       1. **Aluminum Hydroxide** (page 6, 135, 136, 189)
       2. **Magnesium Hydroxide** (page 135, 189)
    B. Antidiarrheal agents
       1. **Bismuth Subsalicylate** (page 30)
       2. **Loperamide** (page 131)
       3. **Simethicone** (page 189)
    C. Antiflatulents
    D. Cathartics and laxatives
       1. **Bisacodyl** (page 29)
       2. **Psyllium** (page 128, 181)
       3. **Senna** (page 72, 186)
    E. Cholelitholytic agents
    F. Digestants
    G. Emetics
    H. Antiemetics

1. **Dimenhydrinate** (page 74)
I. Lipotropic agents
J. Miscellaneous GI drugs
   1. **Cimetidine** (page 46)
   2. **Cisapride** (page 49)
   3. **Famotidine** (page 91)
   4. **Lansoprazole** (page 123)
   5. **Methylcellulose** (page 141)
   6. Metoclorpropamide
   7. **Nizatidine** (page 156)
   8. **Omeprazole** (page 159)
   9. **Ranitidine** (page 184)
   10. **Sulfasalazine** (page 195)
12. Hormones and Synthetic Substitutes
A. Adrenals
   1. **Corticosteroids** (page 59)
B. Androgens
   1. **Stanozolol** (page 193)
C. Contraceptives
   1. **Oral Contraceptives** (page 160)
D. Estrogens
   1. Estrogens
      a. **Estradiol** (page 88)
      b. **Conjugated Estrogens** (page 57, 137)
   2. Antiestrogens
   3. Estrogen agonist-antagonist
E. Gonadotropins
F. Antidiabetic agents
   1. **Insulins** (page 115)
   2. Sulfonylureas
      a. **Glipizide** (page 102)
      b. **Glyburide** (page 103)
   3. Miscellaneous antidiabetic agents
      a. **Metformin** (page 138)
G. Parathyroid
H. Pituitary
I. Progestins
   1. **Medroxyprogesterone** (page 57, 137)
J. Other corpus luteum hormones
K. Thyroid and antithyroid agents
   1. **Thyroid agents** (page 205)
   2. Antithyroid agents
L. Hormones and synthetic substitutes
   1. **Alendronate** (page 5)
13. Skin and Mucous Membrane Agents
Anthralin (page 13)
Econazole (page 82)

Drugs by Pharmacist Classification

Drugs by Pharmacist Classification

References

DRUGS

Angiotensin-Converting Enzyme (ACE) Inhibitors

1. Good CB, McDermott L, McCloskey B. Diet and serum potassium in patients on ACE inhibitors. *JAMA* 1995;274:538.

2. Golik A, Modai D, Averbukh Z, et al. Zinc metabolism in patients treated with captopril versus enalapril. *Metabolism* 1990;39:665–67.

3. Golik A, Zaidenstein R, Dishi V, et al. Effects of captopril and enalapril on zinc metabolism in hypertensive patients. *J Am Coll Nutr* 1998;17:75–80.

Acetaminophen

1. Vale JA, Proudfoot AT. Paracetamol (acetaminophen) poisoning. *Lancet* 1995;346:547–52.

2. Houston JB, Levy G. Drug biotransformation interactions in man. VI: Acetaminophen and ascorbic acid. *J Pharm Sci* 1976;65:121–21.

3. Valenzuela A, Aspillaga M, Vial S, Guerra R. Selectivity of silymarin on the increase of the glutathione content in different tissues of the rat. *Planta Med* 1989;55:420–22.

4. Threlkeld DS, ed. Central Nervous System Drugs, Acetaminophen. In *Facts and Comparisons Drug Information*. St. Louis, MO: Facts and Comparisons, Mar 1997, 247–247f.

5. Campos R, Garrido A, Guerra R, Valenzuela A. Silybin dihemisuccinate protects against glutathione depletion and lipid peroxidation induced by acetaminophen on rat liver. *Planta Med* 1989;55:417–19.

6. Yamada S, Murawaki Y, Kawasaki H. Preventive effect of gomisin A, a lignan component of schizandra fruits, on acetaminophen-induced hepatotoxicity in rats. *Biochem Pharmacol* 1993;46:1081–85.

7. Holt GA. *Food & Drug Interactions.* Chicago: Precept Press, 1998, 2.

8. Threlkeld DS, ed. Central Nervous System Drugs, Acetaminophen. In *Facts and Comparisons Drug Information.* St. Louis, MO: Facts and Comparisons, Mar 1997, 247–247f.

Albuterol

1. Phillips PJ, Vedig AE, Jones PL, et al. Metabolic and cardiovascular side effects of the beta 2-adrenoceptor agonists salbutamol and rimiterol. *Br J Clin Pharmacol* 1980;9:483–91.

2. Edner M, Jogestrand T. Oral salbutamol decreases serum digoxin concentration. *Eur J Clin Pharmacol* 1990;38:195–97.

3. Spector SL. Adverse reactions associated with parenteral beta agonists: serum potassium changes. *N Engl Reg Allergy Proc* 1987;8:317–22.

4. Edner M, Jogestrand T. Oral salbutamol decreases serum digoxin concentration. *Eur J Clin Pharmacol* 1990;38:195–97.

5. Threlkeld DS, ed. Respiratory Drugs, Bronchodilators, Sympathomimetics. In *Facts and Comparisons Drug Information.* St. Louis, MO: Facts and Comparisons, May 1994, 174a–175.

Alendronate

1. Threlkeld DS, ed. Hormones, Bisphosphonates. In *Facts and Comparisons Drug Information.* St. Louis, MO: Facts and Comparisons, Jul 1998, 134r.

2. Adami S. Bisphosphonates in prostate carcinoma. *Cancer* 1997;80:1674–79.

3. Threlkeld DS, ed. Hormones, Bisphosphonates. In *Facts and Comparisons Drug Information.* St. Louis, MO: Facts and Comparisons, Jul 1998, 134r.

4. Gertz BJ, Holland SD, Kline WF, et al. Studies of the oral bioavailability of alendronate. *Clin Pharmacol Ther* 1995;58:288–98.

5. Threlkeld DS, ed. Hormones, Bisphosphonates. In *Facts and Comparisons Drug Information.* St. Louis, MO: Facts and Comparisons, Jul 1998, 134r.

6. Threlkeld DS, ed. Hormones, Bisphosphonates. In *Facts and Comparisons Drug Information.* St. Louis, MO: Facts and Comparisons, Jul 1998, 134r.

Aluminum Hydroxide

1. McHardy G. A multicentric, randomized clinical trial of Gaviscon in reflux esophagitis. *South Med J* 1978;71(suppl 1):16–21.

2. Graham DY, Lanza F, Dorsch ER. Symptomatic reflux esophagitis: A double-blind controlled comparison of antacids and alginate. *Curr Ther Res* 1977;22:653–58.

3. Spencer H, Kramer L. Antacid-induced calcium loss. *Arch Intern Med* 1983;143:657–58 [editorial].

4. Anonymous. Is aluminum harmless? *Nutr Rev* 1980;38:242–43 [review].

5. Gaby AR. Aluminum: The ubiquitous poison. *Nutr Healing* 1997;4:3,4,11.

6. Walker JA, Sherman RA, Cody RP. The effect of oral bases on enteral aluminum absorption. *Arch Intern Med* 1990;150:2037–39.

7. Weberg R, Berstad A. Gastrointestinal absorption of aluminum from single doses of aluminum containing antacids in man. *Eur J Clin Invest* 1986;16:42–32.

8. Fairweather-Tait S, Hickson K, McGaw B, Redi M. Orange juice enhances aluminum absorption from antacid preparation. *Eur J Clin Nutr* 1994;48:71–73.

9. Nolan CR, Califano JR, Butzin CA. Influence of calcium acetate or calcium citrate on intestinal aluminum absorption. *Kidney Int* 1990;38:937–41.

10. Anonymous. Preliminary findings suggest calcium citrate supplements may raise aluminum levels in blood, urine. *Family Practice News* 1992;22:74–75.

11. Fairweather-Tait S, Hickson K, McGaw B, Redi M. Orange juice enhances aluminum absorption from antacid preparation. *Eur J Clin Nutr* 1994;48:71–73.

12. Nolan CR, Califano JR, Butzin CA. Influence of calcium acetate or calcium citrate on intestinal aluminum absorption. *Kidney Int* 1990;38:937–41.

13. Walker JA, Sherman RA, Cody RP. The effect of oral bases on enteral aluminum absorption. *Arch Intern Med* 1990;150:2037–39.

Amiloride
Amiloride/Hydrochlorothiazide

1. Devane J, Ryan MP. The effects of amiloride and triamterene on urinary magnesium excretion in conscious saline-loaded rats. *Br J Pharmacol* 1981;72:285–89.

Amiodarone

1. Kachel DL et al. Amiodarone-induced injury of human pulmonary artery endothelial cells: Protection by alpha-tocopherol. *J Pharmacol Exp Ther* 1990;254:1107–12.

Amlodipine

1. Bailey DG, Arnold MO, Strong HA, Munoz C, Spence JD, et al. Effect of grapefruit juice and naringin on nisoldipine pharmacokinetics. *Clin Pharmacol Ther* 1993;54:589–94.

2. Faulkner JK, Hayden ML, Chasseaud LF, Taylor T. Absorption of amlodipine unaffected by food. Solid dose equivalent to solution dose. *Arzneimittelforschung* 1989;39:799–801.

Amoxicillin

1. Tinozzi S, Venegoni A. Effect of bromelain on serum and tissue levels of amoxicillin. *Drugs Exp Clin Res* 1978;4:39–44.

2. Luerti M, Vignali M. Influence of bromelain on penetration of antibiotics in uterus, salpinx and ovary. *Drugs Exp Clin Res* 1978;4:45–48.

3. Neubauer RA. A plant protease for potentiation of and possible replacement of antibiotics. *Exp Med Surg* 1961;19:143–60.

4. Surawicz CM, Elmer GW, Speelman P, et al. Prevention of antibiotic-associated diarrhea by *Saccharomyces boulardii*: A prospective study. *Gastroenterol* 1989;96:981–88.

5. McFarland LV, Surawicz CM, Greenberg RN, et al. Prevention of beta-lactam-associated diarrhea by *Saccharomyces boulardii* compared with placebo. *Am J Gastroenterol* 1995;90:439–48.

6. Tankanow RM, Ross MB, Ertel IJ, et al. A double-blind, placebo-controlled study of the efficacy of Lactinex in the prophylaxis of amoxicillin-induced diarrhea. *DICP Ann Pharmacother* 1990;24:382–84.

Amphotericin B

1. McLean R. Magnesium and its therapeutic uses: A review. *Am J Med* 1994;96: 63–76.

Anesthetics, Major

1. Phillips S, Ruggier R, Hutchinson SE. *Zingiber officinale* (ginger)—an antiemetic for day case surgery. *Anaesthesia* 1993;48:715–17.

2. Bone ME, Wilkinson DJ, Young JR, et al. Ginger root—a new antiemetic: The effect of ginger root on postoperative nausea and vomiting after major gynaecological surgery. *Anaesthesia* 1990;45:669–71.

Antacids

1. Russell RM, Dutta SK, Oaks EV, et al. Impairment of folic acid absorption by oral pancreatic extracts. *Dig Dis Sci* 1980;25(5):369–73.

2. Werbach MR. *Foundations of Nutritional Medicine.* Tarzana, CA: Third Line Press, 1997, 206 [review].

3. Russel RM, Golner BB, Krasinski SC, et al. Effect of antacid and H2 receptor antagonists on the intestinal absorption of folic acid. *J Lab Clin Sci* 1988;112:458–63.

Anthralin

1. Finnen MJ, Lawrence CM, Shuster S. Inhibition of dithranol inflammation by free-radical scavengers. *Lancet* 1984;ii:1129–30.

Antibiotics

1. Fuller R. Probiotics in human medicine. *Gut* 1991;32:439–42 [review].

2. Elmer GW, Surawicz CM, McFarland LV. Biotherapeutic agents. A neglected modality for the treatment and prevention of selected intestinal and vaginal infections. *JAMA* 1996;275:870–76.

3. Surawicz CM, Elmer GW, Speelman P, et al. Prevention of antibiotic-associated diarrhea by *Saccharomyces boulardii*: A prospective study. *Gastroenterol* 1989;96:981–88.

4. Surawicz CM, McFarland LV, Elmer G, Chinn J. Treatment of recurrent *Clostridium difficile* colitis with vancomycin and *Saccharomyces boulardii*. *Am J Gastroenterol* 1989;84:1285–87.

5. Schellenberg D, Bonington A, Champion CM, et al. Treatment of *Clostridium difficile* diarrhoea with brewer's yeast. *Lancet* 1994;343:171–72.

6. Freinberg N, Lite T. Adjunctive ascorbic acid administration in antibiotic therapy. *J Dental Res* 1957;36:260–62.

7. Rawal BD, McKay G, Blackhall MI. Inhibition of *Pseudomonas aeruginosa* by ascorbic acid acting singly and in combination with antimicrobials: In-vitro and in-vivo studies. *Med J Austral* 1974;1:164–74.

Anticonvulsants

1. Mock DM, Dyken ME. Biotin catabolism is accelerated in adults receiving long-term therapy with anticonvulsants. *Neurology* 1997;49:1444–47.

2. Mock DM, Mock NI, Nelson RP, Lombard KA. Disturbances in biotin metabolism in children undergoing long-term anticonvulsant therapy. *J Pediatr Gastroenterol Nutr* 1998;26:245–50.

3. Chung S, Cho J, Hyun T, et al. Alterations in the carnitine metabolism in epileptic children treated with valproic acid. *J Korean Med Soc* 1997;12:553–58.

4. Van Wouwe JP. Carnitine deficiency during valproic acid treatment. *Int J Vit Nutr Res* 1995;65:211–14.

5. Freeman JM, Vining EPG, Cost S, Singhi P. Does carnitine administration improve the symptoms attributed to anticonvulsant medications?: A double-blinded, crossover study. *Pediatrics* 1994;93:893–95.

6. Van Wouwe JP. Carnitine deficiency during valproic acid treatment. *Int J Vit Nutr Res* 1995;65:211–14.

7. Murphy JV, Marquardt KM, Shug AL. Valproic acid associated abnormalities of carnitine metabolism. *Lancet* 1985;1:820–21.

8. Hendel J et al. The effects of carbamazepine and valproate on folate metabolism. *Acta Neurol Scand* 1984;69:226–31.

9. Berg MJ, Stumbo PH, Chenard CA, et al. Folic acid improves phenytoin pharmacokinetics. *J Am Dietet Assoc* 1995;95:352–56.

10. Roe DA. *Drug-Induced Nutritional Deficiencies*, 2d ed. Westport, CT: ARI Publishing, 1985, 249 [review].

11. Schwaninger M, Ringleb P, Winter R, et al. Elevated plasma concentrations of homocysteine in antiepileptic drug treatment. *Epilepsia* 1999;40:345–50.

12. Biale Y, Lewenthan H. Effect of folic acid supplementation on congenital malformations due to anticonvulsive drugs. *Eur J Obstet Gynecol Reprod Biol* 1984;18:211–16.

13. Berg MJ, Stumbo PH, Chenard CA, et al. Folic acid improves phenytoin pharmacokinetics. *J Am Dietet Assoc* 1995;95:352–56.

14. Reynolds EH. Effects of folic acid on the mental state and fit frequency of drug treated epileptic patients. *Lancet* 1967;1:1086.

15. Francetti L, Maggiore E, Marchesi A, et al. Oral hygiene in subjects treated with diphenylhydantoin: effects of a professional program. *Prev Assist Dent* 1991;17(30):40–43 [Italian].

16. Fitchie JG, Comer RW, Hanes PJ, Reeves GW. The reduction of phenytoin-induced gingival overgrowth in a severely disabled patient: a case report. *Compendium* 1989;10(6):314.

17. Steinberg SC, Steinberg AD. Phenytoin-induced gingival overgrowth control in severely retarded children. *J Periodontol* 1982; 53(7)429–33.

18. Drew HJ et al. Effect of folate on phenytoin hyperplasia. *J Clin Periodontol* 1987;14:350.

19. Monteleone P, Tortorella A, Borriello R, et al. Suppression of nocturnal plasma melatonin levels by evening administration of sodium valproate in healthy humans. *Biol Psychiatry* 1997;41:336–41.

20. D'Erasmo E, Ragno A, Raejntroph N, Pisanti D. Drug-induced osteomalacia. *Recenti Prog Med* 1998;89:529–33 [review, in Italian].

21. Williams C, Netzloff M, Folkerts L, et al. Vitamin D metabolism and anticonvulsant therapy: effect of sunshine on incidence of osteomalacia. *Southern Med J* 1984;77:834.

22. Cornelissen M, Steegers-Theunissen R, Kollee, L, et al. Increased incidence of neonatal vitamin K deficiency resulting from maternal anticonvulsant therapy. *Am J Obstet Gynecol* 1993;168:923–28.

23. Cornelissen M, Steegers-Theunissen R, Kollee L, et al. Supplementation of vitamin K in pregnant women receiving anticonvulsant therapy prevents neonatal vitamin K deficiency. *Am J Obstet Gynecol* 1993;168:884–88.

Aspirin

1. Buist RA. Drug-nutrient interactions—an overview. *Intl Clin Nutr Rev* 1984;4(3):114 [review].

2. Alter HJ, Zvaifler MJ, Rath CE. Interrelationship of rheumatoid arthritis, folic acid and aspirin. *Blood* 1971;38:405–16.

3. Coffey G, Wilson CWM. Ascorbic acid deficiency and aspirin-induced haematemesis. *BMJ* 1975;I:208.

4. Kim JM, White RH. Effect of vitamin E on the anticoagulant response to warfarin. *Am J Cardiol* 1996;77:545–46.

5. Liede KE, Haukka JK, Saxén LM, Heinon OP. Increased tendency towards gingival bleeding caused by joint effect of alpha-tocopherol supplementation and acetylsalicylic acid. *Ann Med* 1998;30:542–46.

6. Ambanelli U, Ferraccioli GF, Serventi G, Vaona GL. Changes in serum and urinary zinc induced by ASA and indomethacin. *Scand J Rheumatol* 1982;11:63–64.

7. Abdel Salam OME, Mószik G, Szolcsányi J. Studies on the effect of intragastric capsaicin on gastric ulcer and on the prostacyclin-induced cytoprotection in rats. *Pharmacol Res* 1995;32:209–15.

8. Holzer P, Pabst MA, Lippe IT. Intragastric capsaicin protects against aspirin-induced lesion formation and bleeding in the rat gastric mucosa. *Gastroenterol* 1989;96:1425–33.

9. Yeoh KG, Kang JY, Yap I, et al. Chili protects against aspirin-induced gastroduodenal mucosal injury in humans. *Dig Dis Sci* 1995;40:580–83.

10. Rees WDW, Rhodes J, Wright JE, et al. Effect of deglycyrrhizinated liquorice on gastric mucosal damage by aspirin. *Scand J Gastroenterol* 1979;14:605–7.

11. Morgan AG, McAdam WAF, Pascoo C, Darnborough A. Comparison between cimetidine and Caved-S in the treatment of gastric ulceration, and subsequent maintenance therapy. *Gut* 1982;23:545–51.

12. Bennett A, Clark-Wibberley T, et al. Aspirin-induced gastric mucosal damage in rats: Cimetidine and deglycyrrhizinated liquorice together give greater protection than low doses of either drug alone. *J Pharm Pharmacol* 1980;32:151.

Atenolol

Atenolol/Chlorthalidone

1. Threlkeld DS, ed. Diuretics and Cardiovasculars, Beta-Adrenergic Blocking Agents. In *Facts and Comparisons Drug Information*. St. Louis, MO: Facts and Comparisons, Feb 1993, 158L.

2. Threlkeld DS, ed. Diuretics and Cardiovasculars, Beta-Adrenergic Blocking Agents. In *Facts and Comparisons Drug Information*. St. Louis, MO: Facts and Comparisons, Feb 1993, 158L.

3. Deanfield J, Wright C, Krikler S, et al. Cigarette smoking and the treatment of angina with propranolol, atenolol, and nifedipine. *N Engl J Med* 1984;310:951–54.

Atorvastatin

1. Mortensen SA, Leth A, Agner E, Rohde M. Dose-related decrease of serum coenzyme Q10 during treatment with HMG-CoA reductase inhibitors. *Mol Aspects Med* 1997;18(suppl):S137–44.

2. Bargossi AM, Grossi G, Fiorella PL, et al. Exogenous CoQ10 supplementation prevents plasma ubiquinone reduction induced by HMG-CoA reductase inhibitors. *Molec Aspects Med* 1994;15(suppl):s187–93.

3. Threlkeld DS, ed. Diuretics and Cardiovasculars, Antihyperlipidemic Agents, HMG-CoA Reductase Inhibitors. In *Facts and Comparisons Drug Information*. St. Louis, MO: Facts and Comparisons, Sep 1998, 172a.

4. Garnett WR. Interactions with hydroxymethylglutaryl-coenzyme A reductase inhibitors. *Am J Health Syst Pharm* 1995;52:1639–45.

5. Yee HS, Fong NT. Atorvastatin in the treatment of primary hypercholesterolemia and mixed dyslipidemias. *Ann Pharmacother* 1998;32:1030–43.

6. Jacobson TA, Amorosa LF. Combination therapy with fluvastatin and niacin in hypercholesterolemia: a preliminary report on safety. *Am J Cardiol* 1994;73:25D–29D.

7. Jokubaitis LA. Fluvastatin in combination with other lipid-lowering agents. *Br J Pract Suppl* 1996;77A:28–32.

8. Davignon J, Roederer G, Montigny M, et al. Comparative efficacy and safety of *pravastatin, nicotinic acid* and the two combined in patients with hypercholesterolemia. *Am J Cardiol* 1994;73:339–45.

9. Jacobson TA, Jokubaitis LA, Amorosa LF. Fluvastatin and niacin in hypercholesterolemia: a preliminary report on gender differences in efficacy. *Am J Med* 1994;96(suppl 6A):64S–68S.

10. Muggeo M, Zenti MG, Travia D, et al. Serum retinol levels throughout 2 years of cholesterol-lowering therapy. *Metabolism* 1995;44:398–403.

11. Radulovic LL, Cilla DD, Posvar EL, et al. Effect of food on the bioavailability of atorvastatin, an HMG-CoA reductase inhibitor. *J Clin Pharmacol* 1995;35:990–94.

12. Cilla DD Jr, Gibson DM, Whitfield LR, Sedman AJ. Pharmacodynamic effects and pharmacokinetics of atorvastatin after administration to normocholesterolemic subjects in the morning and evening. *J Clin Pharmacol* 1996;36:604–9.

13. Radulovic LL, Cilla DD, Posvar EL, et al. Effect of food on the bioavailability of atorvastatin, an HMG-CoA reductase inhibitor. *J Clin Pharmacol* 1995;35:990–94.

Atropine

1. Brinker F. *Herb Contraindications and Drug Interactions.* Sandy, OR: Eclectic Institute, 1997, 100.

Azithromycin

1. Foulds G, Hilligoss DM, Henry EB, Gerber N. The effects of an antacid or cimetidine on the serum concentrations of azithromycin. *J Clin Pharmacol* 1991; 31:164–67.

2. Bizjak ED, Mauro VF. Digoxin-macrolide drug interaction. *Ann Pharmacother* 1997;31:1077–79.

3. Threlkeld DS, ed. Systemic Anti-Infectives, Macrolides. In *Facts and Comparisons Drug Information.* St. Louis, MO: Facts and Comparisons, Oct 1998, 343–343b.

4. Threlkeld DS, ed. Systemic Anti-Infectives, Macrolides. In *Facts and Comparisons Drug Information.* St. Louis, MO: Facts and Comparisons, Oct 1998, 343–343b.

AZT

1. Werbach MR. *Foundations of Nutritional Medicine.* Tarzana, CA: Third Line Press, 1997, 248–49.

2. Dalakas MC, Leon-Monzon ME, Bernardini I, et al. Zidovudine-induced mitochondrial myopathy is associated with muscle carnitine deficiency and lipid storage. *Ann Neurol* 1994;35:482–87.

3. Paltiel O, Falutz J, Veilleux M, et al. Clinical correlates of subnormal vitamin B12 levels in patients infected with the human immunodeficiency virus. *Am J Hematol* 1995;49:318–22.

4. Richman DD, Fischl MA, Griego MH, et al. The toxicity of azidothymidine (AZT) in the treatment of patients with AIDS and AIDS-related complex. *New Engl J Med* 1987;317:192–97.

5. Goldstein G, Conant MA, Beall G, et al. Safety and efficacy of thymopentin in zidovudine (AZT)-treated asymptomatic HIV-infected subjects with 200–500 CD4 cells/mm3: A double-blind placebo-controlled trial. *J Acq Imm Def Syn Human Retrovirol* 1995;8:279–88.

6. Mocchegiani E, Veccia S, Ancarani F, et al. Benefit of oral zinc supplementation as an adjunct to zidovudine (AZT) therapy against opportunistic infections in AIDS. *Int J Immunopharmacol* 1995;17:719–27.

Benazepril

1. Good CB, McDermott L, McCloskey B. Diet and serum potassium in patients on ACE inhibitors. *JAMA* 1995;274:538.

2. Golik A, Zaidenstein R, Dishi V, et al. Effects of captopril and enalapril on zinc metabolism in hypertensive patients. *J Am Coll Nutr* 1998;17:75–78.

3. Gengo FM, Brady E. The pharmacokinetics of benazepril relative to other ACE inhibitors. *Clin Cardiol* 1991;14(8 suppl 4):IV44–50 [review].

Benzodiazepines

1. Ferini-Strambi L, Zucconi M, Biella G, et al. Effect of melatonin on sleep microstructure: Preliminary results in healthy subjects. *Sleep* 1993;16:744–47.

2. Davies LP, Drew CA, Duffield P, et al. Kava pyrones and resin: Studies on GABAA, GABAB and benzodiazepine binding sites in rodent brain. *Pharm Toxicol* 1992;71:120–26.

3. Holm E, Staedt U, Heep J, et al. Studies on the profile of the neurophysiological effects of D,L-kavain: Cerebral sites of action and sleep-wakefulness rhythm in animals. *Arzneim Forsch* 1991;41:673–83.

4. Almeida JC. Coma from the health food store: Interaction between kava and alprazolam. *Ann Intern Med* 1996;125:940–41.

Bile Acid Sequestrants

1. Werbach MR. *Foundations of Nutritional Medicine.* Tarzana, CA: Third Line Press, 1997, 221–22 [review].

2. Threlkeld DS, ed. Diuretics and Cardiovasculars, Antihyperlipidemic Agents, Bile Acid Sequestrants. In *Facts and Comparisons Drug Information.* St. Louis, MO: Facts and Comparisons, Feb 1997, 171i–171l.

3. Threlkeld DS, ed. Diuretics and Cardiovasculars, Antihyperlipidemic Agents, Bile Acid Sequestrants. In *Facts and Comparisons Drug Information.* St. Louis, MO: Facts and Comparisons, Feb 1997, 171i–171l.

4. Watkins DW, Cassidy MM, Khalafi R, Vahouny GV. Calcium and zinc balances in rats chronically fed the bile salt-sequestrant cholestyramine (Questran). *Fed Proc* 1983;42:819.

5. Probstfield JL, Lin T, Peters J, Hunninghake DB. Carotenoids and vitamin A: The effect of hypocholesterolemic agents on serum levels. *Metabolism* 1985;34:88–91.

6. Threlkeld DS, ed. Diuretics and Cardiovasculars, Antihyperlipidemic Agents, Bile Acid Sequestrants. In *Facts and Comparisons Drug Information.* St. Louis, MO: Facts and Comparisons, Feb 1997, 171i–171l.

Bisacodyl

1. Fleming BJ, Genuth SM, Gould AB, Kaminokowski MD. Laxative induced hypokalemia, sodium depletion, and hyperreninemia. Effects of potassium and sodium replacement on the rennin angiotensin system. *Ann Intern Med* 1975;83:60–62.

2. Threlkeld DS, ed. Gastrointestinal Drugs, Laxatives. In *Facts and Comparisons Drug Information.* St. Louis, MO: Facts and Comparisons, May 1991, 319a.

3. Threlkeld DS, ed. Gastrointestinal Drugs, Laxatives. In *Facts and Comparisons Drug Information.* St. Louis, MO: Facts and Comparisons, May 1991, 319a.

4. Holt GA. *Food & Drug Interactions.* Chicago: Precept Press, 1998, 49.

Bismuth Subsalicylate

1. Wichtl M, Bisset NG, eds. *Herbal Drugs and Phytopharmaceuticals.* Stuttgart: Medpharm GmBH Scientific Publishers.

2. Janssen PL, Katan MB, van Staveren WA, et al. Acetylsalicylate and salicylates in foods. *Cancer Lett* 1997:114(1–2):163–64.

3. McGuffin M, Hobbs C, Upton R, Goldberg A, eds. (1997) *American Herbal Product Association's Botanical Safety Handbook.* Boca Raton, FL: CRC Press, 1997, 154–55.

Bisoprolol
Bisoprolol/Hydrochlorothiazide

1. Leopold G, Pabst J, Ungethum W, Buhring KU. Basic pharmacokinetics of bisoprolol, a new highly beta 1-selective adrenoceptor antagonist. *J Clin Pharmacol* 1986;26:616–21.

2. Threlkeld DS, ed. Diuretics and Cardiovasculars, Beta-Adrenergic Blocking Agents. In *Facts and Comparisons Drug Information.* St. Louis, MO: Facts and Comparisons, Feb 1993, 158o.

Brompheniramine
Brompheniramine/Phenylpropanolamine

1. Blumenthal M, Busse WR, Goldberg A, et al. (eds). *The Complete Commission E Monographs: Therapeutic Guide to Herbal Medicines.* Boston, MA: Integrative Medicine Communications, 1998, 146.

2. Threlkeld DS, ed. Respiratory Drugs, Antihistamines. In *Facts and Comparisons Drug Information.* St. Louis, MO: Facts and Comparisons, May 1998, 192a.

3. Threlkeld DS, ed. Respiratory Drugs, Antihistamines. In *Facts and Comparisons Drug Information.* St. Louis, MO, Facts and Comparisons, May 1998, 192a.

Buspirone

1. Gammans RE, Mayol RF, LaBudde JA. Metabolism and disposition of buspirone. *Am J Med* 1986;80:41–51.

2. Threlkeld DS, ed. Central Nervous System Drugs, Antianxiety Agents, Miscellaneous Agents. In *Facts and Comparisons Drug Information.* St. Louis, MO: Facts and Comparisons, May 1990, 262–262c.

Caffeine
Caffeine/Aspirin

1. Harris SS, Dawson-Hughes B. Caffeine and bone loss in healthy postmenopausal women. *Am J Clin Nutr* 1994;60:573–78.

2. Barrett-Connor E, Chang JC, Edelstein SL. Coffee-associated osteoporosis offset by daily milk consumption. The Rancho Bernardo Study. *JAMA* 1994;271:280–83.

3. Lloyd T, Rollings N, Eggli DF, et al. Dietary caffeine intake and bone status of postmenopausal women. *Am J Clin Nutr* 1997;65:1826–30.

4. Tyler VE. *Herbs of Choice: The Therapeutic Use of Phytomedicinals.* New York, Pharmaceutical Press, 1994, 88–89.

5. Joeres R, Klinker H, Heusler H, et al. Influence of smoking on caffeine elimination in healthy volunteers and in patients with alcoholic liver cirrhosis. *Hepatology* 1988;8:575–79.

Captopril

1. Good CB, McDermott L, McCloskey B. Diet and serum potassium in patients on ACE inhibitors. *JAMA* 1995;274:538.

2. Golik A, Modai D, Averbukh Z, et al. Zinc metabolism in patients treated with captopril versus enalapril. *Metabolism* 1990;39:665–67.

3. Golik A, Zaidenstein R, Dishi V, et al. Effects of captopril and enalapril on zinc metabolism in hypertensive patients. *J Am Coll Nutr* 1998;17:75–80.

Carbidopa
Carbidopa/Levodopa

1. Campbell NR, Hasinoff BB. Iron supplements: A common cause of drug interactions. *Brit J Clin Pharmacol* 1991;31:251–55 [review].

2. Van Woert MH, Rosenbaum D, Howieson J, Bowers MB Jr. Long-term therapy of myoclonus and other neurologic disorders with L-5-hydroxytryptophan and carbidopa. *N Engl J Med* 1977;296:70–75.

3. Magnussen I, Dupont E, Engbaek F, de Fine Olivarius B. Post-hypoxic intention myoclonus treated with 5-hydroxytryptophan and an extracerebral decarboxylase inhibitor. *Acta Neurol Scand* 1978;57:289–94.

4. Growdon JH, Young RR, Shahani BT. L-5-hydroxytryptophan in treatment of several different syndromes in which myoclonus is prominent. *Neurology* 1976;26:1135–40.

5. Sternberg EM, Van Woert MH, Young SN, et al. Development of a scleroderma-like illness during therapy with L-5-hydroxytryptophan and carbidopa. *New Engl J Med* 1980;303:782–87.

6. Joly P, Lampert A, Thromine E, Lauret P. Development of pseudobullous morphea and scleroderma-like illness during therapy with L-5-hydroxytryptophan and carbidopa. *J Am Acad Dermatol* 1991;25:332–33.

7. Auffranc JC, Berbis P, Fabre JF, et al. Sclerodermiform and poikilodermal syndrome observed during treatment with carbidopa and 5-hydroxytryptophan. *Ann Dermatol Verereol* 1985;112:691–92.

Carbidopa/Levodopa

1. Trovato A et al. Drug-nutrient interactions. *Am Family Phys* 1991;44:1651–58.

2. Campbell NR, Hasinoff BB. Iron supplements: a common cause of drug interactions. *Brit J Clin Pharmacol* 1991;31:251–55 [review].

3. Van Woert MH, Rosenbaum D, Howieson J, Bowers MB Jr. Long-term therapy of myoclonus and other neurologic disorders with L-5-hydroxytryptophan and carbidopa. *N Engl J Med* 1977;296:70–75.

4. Magnussen I, Dupont E, Engbaek F, de Fine Olivarius B. Post-hypoxic intention myoclonus treated with 5-hydroxytryptophan and an extracerebral decarboxylase inhibitor. *Acta Neurol Scand* 1978;57:289–94.

5. Growdon JH, Young RR, Shahani BT. L-5-hydroxytryptophan in treatment of several different syndromes in which myoclonus is prominent. *Neurology* 1976;26:1135–40.

6. Sternberg EM, Van Woert MH, Young SN, et al. Development of a scleroderma-like illness during therapy with L-5-hydroxytryptophan and carbidopa. *New Engl J Med* 1980;303:782–87.

7. Joly P, Lampert A, Thromine E, Lauret P. Development of pseudobullous morphea and scleroderma-like illness during therapy with L-5-hydroxytryptophan and carbidopa. *J Am Acad Dermatol* 1991;25:332–33.

8. Auffranc JC, Berbis P, Fabre JF, et al. Sclerodermiform and poikilodermal syndrome observed during treatment with carbidopa and 5-hydroxytryptophan. *Ann Dermatol Verereol* 1985;112:691–92.

9. Threlkeld DS, ed. Central Nervous System Drugs, Antiparkinson Agents, Levodopa. In *Facts and Comparison Drug Information*. St. Louis, MO: Facts and Comparisons Drug Information, Apr 1998, 289p–290a.

10. Threlkeld DS, ed. Central Nervous System Drugs, Antiparkinson Agents, Levodopa. In *Facts and Comparison Drug Information*. St. Louis, MO: Facts and Comparisons Drug Information, Apr 1998, 289p–290a.

Carisoprodol
Carisoprodol/Aspirin
Carisoprodol/Aspirin/Codeine

1. Threlkeld DS, ed. Central Nervous System Drugs, Skeletal Muscle Relaxants, Centrally Acting, Carisoprodol. In *Facts and Comparisons Drug Information*. St. Louis, MO: Facts and Comparisons, Nov 1993, 287f–287g.

2. Threlkeld DS, ed. Central Nervous System Drugs, Skeletal Muscle Relaxants, Centrally Acting, Carisoprodol. In *Facts and Comparisons Drug Information*. St. Louis, MO: Facts and Comparisons, Nov 1993, 287f–287g.

Cephalosporins

1. Anonymous. New examples of vitamin K-drug interaction. *Nutr Rev* 1984;42(4):161–63 [review].

Cetirizine

1. Threlkeld DS, ed. Respiratory Drugs, Antihistamines. In *Facts and Comparisons Drug Information*. St. Louis, MO: Facts and Comparisons, May 1998, 194c.

2. Threlkeld DS, ed. Respiratory Drugs, Antihistamines. In *Facts and Comparisons Drug Information*. St. Louis, MO: Facts and Comparisons, May 1998, 194c.

Chemotherapy

1. De Blasio F et al. N-acetyl cysteine (NAC) in preventing nausea and vomiting induced by chemotherapy in patients suffering from inoperable non small cell lung cancer (NSCLC). *Chest* 1996;110(4, Suppl):103S.

2. Meyer K, Schwartz J, Crater D, Keyes B. *Zingiber officinale* (ginger) used to prevent 8-Mop associated nausea. *Dermatol Nurs* 1995;7:242–44.

3. Pace JC. Oral ingestion of encapsulated ginger and reported self care actions for the relief of chemotherapy-associated nausea and vomiting. *Dissertaion Abstr Internat* 1987;8:3297.

4. Mills EED. The modifying effect of beta-carotene on radiation and chemotherapy induced oral mucositis. *Brit J Cancer* 1988;57:416–17.

5. Wadleigh RG, Redman RS, Graham ML, et al. Vitamin E in the treatment of chemotherapy-induced mucositis. *Am J Med* 1992;92:481–84.

6. Lopez I, Goudou C, Ribrag V, et al. Treatment of mucositis with vitamin E during administration of neutropenic antineoplastic agents. *Ann Med Intern* [Paris] 1994;145:405–8.

7. Lopez I, Goudou C, Ribrag V, et al. Traitement des mucites par la vitamine E lors de l'administration d'anti-neoplasiques neutropeniants. *Ann Med Interne* 1994;145:405–8.

8. Legha SS, Wang YM, Mackay B, et al. Clinical and pharmacologic investigation of the effects of alpha-tocopherol on Adriamycin cardiotoxicity. *Ann NY Acad Sci* 1982;393:411–18.

9. Mattes RD. Prevention of food aversions in cancer patients during treatment. *Nutr Cancer* 1994;21:13–24.

10. Israel L, Hajji O, Grefft-Alami A, et al. Agumentation par la vitamine A des effets de la chimiotherapie dans les cancers du sein metastases apres la menopause. *Ann Med Interne* 1985;136:551–54.

11. Witenberg B, Kalir HH, Raviv Z, et al. Inhibition by ascorbic acid of apoptosis induced by oxidative stress in HL-60 myeloid leukemia cells. *Biochem Pharmacol* 1999;57:823–32.

12. Sacks PG, Harris D, Chou T-C. Modulation of growth and proliferation in squamous cell carcinoma by retinoic acid: A rationale for combination therapy with chemotherapeutic agents. *Int J Cancer* 1995;61:409–15.

13. Taper HS et al. Non-toxic potentiation of cancer chemotherapy by combined C and K3 vitamin pre-treatment. *Int J Cancer* 1987;40:575–79.

14. Kurbacher CM, Wagner U, Kolster B, et al. Ascorbic acid (vitamin C) improves the antineoplastic activity of doxorubicin, cisplatin, and paclitaxel in human breast carcinoma cells in vitro. *Cancer Letters* 1996:103–19.

15. Wagdi P, Fluri M, Aeschbacher B, et al. Cardioprotection in patients undergoing chemo- and/or radiotherapy for neoplastic disease. *Jpn Heart J* 1996;37:353–59.

16. Weijl NI, Cleton FJ, Osanto S. Free radicals and antioxidants in chemotherapy-induced toxicity. *Cancer Treatment Rev* 1997;23:209–40 [review].

17. Bozzetti F, Biganzoli L, Gavazzi C, et al. Glutamine supplementation in cancer patients receiving chemotherapy: A double-blind randomized study *Nutr* 1997;13:748–51.

18. van Zaanen HCT, van der Lelie H, Timmer JG, et al. Parenteral glutamine dipeptide supplementation does not ameliorate chemotherapy-induced toxicity. *Cancer* 1994;74:2879–84.

19. Klimberg VS, McClellan JL. Glutamine, cancer, and its therapy. *Am J Surg* 1996;172:418–424.

20. Souba WW. Glutamine and cancer. *Ann Surg* 1993;218:715–28 [review].

21. Skubitz KM, Anderson PM. Oral glutamine to prevent chemotherapy induced stomatitis: a pilot study. *J Lab Clin Med* 1996;127:223–8.

22. Anderson PM, Schroeder G, Skubitz KM. Oral glutamine reduces the duration and severity of stomatitis after cytotoxic cancer chemotherapy. *Cancer* 1998;83:1433–9.

23. Muscaritoli M, Micozzi A, Conversano L, et al. Oral glutamine in the prevention of chemotherapy-induced gastrointestinal toxicity *Eur J Cancer* 1997;33:319–20.

24. Bozzetti F, Biganzoli L, Gavazzi C, et al. Glutamine supplementation in cancer patients receiving chemotherapy: A double-blind randomized study *Nutr* 1997;13:748–51.

25. Van Zaanen HCT, van der Lelie H, Timmer JG, et al. Parenteral glutamine dipeptide supplementation does not ameliorate chemotherapy-induced toxicity. *Cancer* 1994;74:2879–84.

26. MacBurney M, Young LS, Ziegler TR, Wilmore DW. A cost-evaluation of Glutamine-supplemented parenteral nutrition in adult bone marrow transplant patients. *J Am Dietet Assoc* 1994;94:1263–6.

27. Holoya PY, Duelge J, Hansen RM, et al. Prophylaxis of ifosfamide toxicity with oral acetylcysteine. *Sem Oncol* 1983;10(suppl 1):66–71.

28. Slavik M, Saiers JH. Phase I clinical study of acetylcysteine's preventing ifosfamide-induced hematuria. *Sem Oncol* 1983;10(suppl 1):62–65.

29. Loehrer PJ, Williams SD, Einhorn LH. N-Acetylcysteine and ifosfamide in the treatment of unresectable pancreatic adenocarcinoma and refractory testicular cancer. *Sem Oncol* 1983;10(suppl 1):72–75.

30. Morgan LR, Donley PJ, Harrison EF. The control of ifosfamide induced hematuria with N-acetylcysteine. *Proc Am Assoc Cancer Res* 1981;22:190.

31. Lissoni P, Cazzaniga M, Tancini G, et al. Reversal of clinical resistance to LHRH analogue in metastatic prostate cancer by the pineal hormone melatonin: Efficacy of LHRH analogue plus melatonin in patients progressing on LHRH analogue alone. *Eur Urol* 1997;31:178–81.

32. Dreizen S et al. Nutritional deficiencies in patients receiving cancer chemotherapy. *Postgrad Med* 1990;87(1):163–70.

33. Desai TK, Maliakkal J, Kinzie JL, et al. Taurine deficiency after intensive chemotherapy and/or radiation. *Am J Clin Nutr* 1992;55:708–11.

34. Toi M, Hattori T, Akagi M, et al. Randomized adjuvant trial to evaluate the addition of tamoxifen and PSK to chemotherapy in patients with primary breast cancer. *Cancer* 1992;70:2475–83.

35. Iino Y, Yokoe T, Maemura M, et al. Immunochemotherapies *versus* chemotherapy as adjuvant treatment after curative resection of operable breast cancer. *Anticancer Res* 1995;15:2907–12.

36. Mitomi T, Tsuchiya S, Iijima N, et al. Randomized, controlled study on adjuvant immunochemotherapy with PSK in curatively resected colorectal concer. The Cooperative Study Group of Surgical Adjuvant Immunochemotherapy for Cancer of Colon and Rectum (Kanagawa). *Dis Colon Rectum* 1992;35:123–30.

37. Lersch C, Zeuner M, Bauer A, et al. Nonspecific immunostimulation with low doses of cyclophosphamide (LDCY), thymostimulin, and *Echinacea purpurea* extracts (Echinacin) in patients with far advanced colorectal cancers: Preliminary results. *Cancer Invest* 1992;10:343–48.

38. Scambia G, De Vincenzo R, Ranelletti FO, et al. Antiproliferative effect of silybin on gynaecological malignancies: Synergism with cisplatin and doxorubicin. *Eur J Cancer* 1996;32A:877–82.

39. Gaedeke J, Fels LM, Bokemeyer C, Mengs U, et al. Cisplatin nephrotoxicity and protection by silibinin. *Nephrol Dial Transplant* 1996;11:55–62.

40. Invernizzi R, Bernuzzi S, Ciani D, Ascari E. Silymarine during maintenance therapy of acute promyelocytic leukemia. *Haemotologia* 1993;78:340–41.

41. Kupin VJ. *Eleutherococcus and Other Biologically Active Modifiers in Oncology.* Moscow: Medexport, 1984, 21.

42. Kupin VI, Polevaya YB, Sorokin AM. Eleutherococcus extract treatment for immunostimulation in cancer patients. *Vopr Onkol* 1986;32:21–26 [in Russian].

43. Cohen MH, Chretien PB, Ihde DC, et al. Thymosin fraction V and intensive combination chemotherapy. Prolonging the survival of patients with small-cell lung cancer. *JAMA* 1979;241:1813–15.

44. Macchiarini P, Danesi R, Del Tacca M, Angeletti CA. Effects of thymostimulin on chemotherapy-induced toxicity and long-term survival in small cell lung cancer patients. *Anticancer Res* 1989;9:193–6.

45. Shoham J, Theodor E, Brenner HJ, et al. Enhancement of the immune system of chemotherapy-treated cancer patients by simultaneous treatment with thymic extract, TP-1. *Cancer Immunol Immunother* 1980;9:173–80.

Chlorpheniramine

1. Blumenthal M, ed. *The Complete German Commission E Monographs.* Austin, TX: American Botanical Council, 1998, 146.

2. Threlkeld DS, ed. Respiratory Drugs, Antihistamines. In *Facts and Comparisons Drug Information*. St. Louis, MO: Facts and Comparisons, May 1998, 192.

3. Threlkeld DS, ed. Respiratory Drugs, Antihistamines. In *Facts and Comparisons Drug Information*. St. Louis, MO: Facts and Comparisons, May 1998, 192.

Cimetidine

1. Aymard JP, Aymard B, Netter P, et al. Haematological adverse effects of histamine H2-receptor antagonists. *Med Toxicol Adverse Drug Exp* 1988;3:430–48.

2. Bachmann KA, Sullivan TJ, Jauregui L, et al. Drug interactions of H2-receptor antagonists. *Scand J Gastroenterol Suppl* 1994;206:14–19.

3. Salom IL, Silvis SE, Doscherholmen A. Effect of cimetidine on the absorption of vitamin B12. *Scand J Gastroenterol* 1982;17:129–31.

4. Anonymous. Cimetidine inhibits the hepatic hydroxylation of vitamin D. *Nutr Rev* 1985;43:184–85 [review].

5. Threlkeld DS, ed. Central Nervous System Drugs, Analeptics, Caffeine. In *Facts and Comparisons Drug Information*. St. Louis, MO: Facts and Comparisons, Feb 1998, 230–230d.

Ciprofloxacin

1. Campbell NR, Hasinoff BB. Iron supplements: A common cause of drug interactions. *Brit J Clin Pharmacol* 1991;31:251–55.

2. Lim D, McKay M. Food-drug interactions. *Drug Information Bull* 1995;15(2) [review].

3. Threlkeld DS, ed. Systemic Anti-Infectives, Fluoroquinolones. In *Facts and Comparisons Drug Information*. St. Louis, MO: Facts and Comparisons, Feb 1994, 340n–340o.

4. Holt GA. *Food & Drug Interactions*. Chicago: Precept Press, 1998, 74.

5. Threlkeld DS, ed. Systemic Anti-Infectives, Fluoroquinolones. In *Facts and Comparisons Drug Information*. St. Louis, MO: Facts and Comparisons, Feb 1994, 340n–340o.

6. Ledergerber B, Bettex JD, Joos B, et al. Effect of standard breakfast on drug absorption and multiple-dose pharmacokinetics of ciprofloxacin. *Antimicrob Agents Chemother* 1985;27:350–352.

7. Threlkeld DS, ed. Systemic Anti-Infectives, Fluoroquinolones. In *Facts and Comparisons Drug Information*. St. Louis, MO: Facts and Comparisons, Feb 1994, 340n–340o.

8. Threlkeld DS, ed. Systemic Anti-Infectives, Fluoroquinolones. In *Facts and Comparisons Drug Information*. St. Louis, MO: Facts and Comparisons, Feb 1994, 340n–340o.

Cisapride

1. Sigmund CJ, McNally EF. The action of a carminative on the lower esophageal sphincter. *Gastroenterol* 1969;56:13–18.

2. Threlkeld DS, ed. Gastrointestinal Drugs, GI Stimulants, Cisapride. In *Facts and Comparisons Drug Information*. St. Louis, MO: Facts and Comparisons, Nov 1998, 308b–308c.

3. Threlkeld DS, ed. Gastrointestinal Drugs, GI Stimulants, Cisapride. In *Facts and Comparisons Drug Information*. St. Louis, MO: Facts and Comparisons, Nov 1998, 308b–308c.

4. Threlkeld DS, ed. Gastrointestinal Drugs, GI Stimulants, Cisapride. In *Facts and Comparisons Drug Information*. St. Louis, MO: Facts and Comparisons, Nov 1998, 308b–308c.

Cisplatin

1. Threlkeld DS, ed. Antineoplastics, alkylating agents, cisplatin (CDDP). In *Facts and Comparisons Drug Information*. St. Louis, MO: Facts and Comparisons, Feb 1999, 652a–652d.

2. Cascinu S, Cordella L, Del Ferro E, et al. Neuroprotective effect of reduced glutathione on cisplatin-based chemotherapy in advanced gastric cancer: A randomized double-blind placebo-controlled trial. *J Clin Oncol* 1995;13:26–32.

3. Smyth JF, Bowman A, Perren T, et al. Glutathione reduces the toxicity and improves quality of life of women diagnosed with ovarian cancer treated with cisplatin: Results of a double-blind, randomised trial. *Ann Oncol* 1997;8:569–73.

4. Buckley JE et al. Hypomagnesemia after cisplatin combination chemotherapy. *Arch Intern Med* 1984;144:2347.

5. Threlkeld DS, ed. Antineoplastics, Alkylating Agents, Cisplatin (CDDP). In *Facts and Comparisons Drug Information*. St. Louis, MO: Facts and Comparisons, Feb 1999, 652a–652d.

6. Rodriguez M et al. Refractory potassium repletion due to cisplatin-induced magnesium depletion. *Arch Intern Med* 1989;149:2592–94.

7. Whang R, Whang DD, Ryan MP. Refractory potassium repletion. A consequence of magnesium deficiency. *Arch Intern Med* 1992;152(1):40–45.

8. Hu Y-J, Chen Y, Zhang Y-Q, Zhou M-Z, Song X-M, Zhang B-Z, et al. The protective role of selenium on the toxicity of cisplatin-contained chemotherapy regimen in cancer patients. *Biol Trace Elem Res* 1997;56:331–41.

9. Threlkeld DS, ed. Antineoplastics, Alkylating Agents, Cisplatin (CDDP). In *Facts and Comparisons Drug Information*. St. Louis, MO: Facts and Comparisons, Feb 1999, 652a–652d.

Clarithromycin

1. Bizjak ED, Mauro VF. Digoxin-macrolide drug interaction. *Ann Pharmacother* 1997; 31:1077–79.

2. Threlkeld DS, ed. Systemic Anti-Infectives, Macrolides. In *Facts and Comparisons Drug Information*. St. Louis, MO: Facts and Comparisons, Oct 1998, 342r–343.

3. Threlkeld DS, ed. Systemic Anti-Infectives, Macrolides. In *Facts and Comparisons Drug Information*. St. Louis, MO: Facts and Comparisons, Oct 1998, 342r–343.

Clemastine
Clemastine/Phenylpropanolamine

1. Blumenthal M, ed. *The Complete German Commission E Monographs*. Austin, TX: American Botanical Council, 1998, 146.

2. Threlkeld DS, ed. Respiratory Drugs, Antihistamines. In *Facts and Comparisons Drug Information*. St. Louis, MO: Facts and Comparisons, May 1998, 191c.

3. Threlkeld DS, ed. Respiratory Drugs, Antihistamines. In *Facts and Comparisons Drug Information*. St. Louis, MO: Facts and Comparisons, May 1998, 191c.

Clofibrate

1. Robinson C, Weigly E. *Basic Nutrition and Diet Therapy*. New York: Macmillan, 1984, 46–54.

Clonidine
Clonidine/Chlorthalidone

1. Threlkeld DS, ed. Central Nervous System Drugs, Central Analgesics, Clonidine HCl. In *Facts and Comparisons Drug Information*. St. Louis, MO: Facts and Comparisons, Mar 1997, 246g–246k.

Codeine

1. Brinker F. Interactions of pharmaceutical and botanical medicines. *J Naturopathic Med* 1997;7(2):14–20.

2. Threlkeld DS, ed. Central Nervous System Drugs, Narcotic Agonist Analgesics. In *Facts and Comparisons Drug Information*. St. Louis, MO: Facts and Comparisons, Feb 1990, 243d.

Colchicine

1. Palopoli JJ, Waxman J. Colchicine neuropathy or vitamin B12 deficiency neuropathy? *N Engl J Med* 1987;317:1290 [letter].

2. Kuncl RW et al. Colchicine neuropathy or vitamin B12 deficiency neuropathy? *N Engl J Med* 1987;317:1290–91 [letter].

3. Werbach MR. *Foundations of Nutritional Medicine*. Tarzana, CA: Third Line Press, 1997, 223–24 [review].

Colestipol (Colestid)

1. Werbach MR. *Foundations of Nutritional Medicine*. Tarzana, CA: Third Line Press, 1997, 224 [review].

2. Threlkeld DS, ed. Cardiovascular Drugs, Antihyperlipidemic Agents, Bile Acid Sequestrants. In *Facts and Comparisons Drug Information*. St. Louis, MO: Facts and Comparisons, Feb 1999, 171L.

References

3. Threlkeld DS(ed). Cardiovascular Drugs, Antihyperlipidemic Agents, Bile Acid Sequestrants. In *Facts and Comparisons Drug Information*. St. Louis, MO: Facts and Comparisons, Feb 1999, 171L.

Conjugated Estrogens
Conjugated Estrogens/Medroxyprogesterone

1. Lobo RA, Roy S, Shoupe D, et al. Estrogen and progestin effects on urinary calcium and calciotropic hormones in surgically-induced postmenopausal women. *Horm Metab Res* 1985;17:370–73.

2. Gallagher JC, Riggs BL, DeLuca HF. Effect of estrogen on calcium absorption and serum vitamin D metabolites in postmenopausal osteoporosis. *J Clin Endocrinol Metab* 1980;51:1359–64.

3. Gambacciani M, Ciaponi M, Cappagli B, et al. Effects of combined low dose of the isoflavone derivative ipriflavone and estrogen replacement on bone mineral density and metabolism in postmenopausal women. *Maturitas* 1997;28:75–81.

4. Melis GB, Paoletti AM, Bartolini R, et al. Ipriflavone and low doses of estrogens in the prevention of bone mineral loss in climacterium. *Bone Miner* Oct 1992;19(suppl 1):S49–56.

5. Herzberg M, Lusky A, Blonder J, et al. The effect of estrogen replacement therapy on zinc in serum and urine. *Obstet Gynecol* 1996;87:1035–40.

6. Haspels AA, Bennink HJ, Schreurs WH. Disturbance of tryptophan metabolism and its correction during oestrogen treatment in postmenopausal women. *Maturitas* 1978;1:15–20.

7. Lubby AL, Brin M, Gordon M, et al. Vitamin B6 metabolism in users of oral contraceptive agents. I. Abnormal urinary xanthurenic acid excretion and its correction by pyridoxine. *Am J Clin Nutr* 1971;24:684–93.

8. Adams PW, Rose DP, Folkard J, et al. Effect of pyridoxine hydrochloride (vitamin B6) upon depression associated with oral contraception. *Lancet* 1973;1:897–904.

9. Massé PG, van den Berg H, Duguay C, et al. Early effect of a low dose (30 mcg) ethinyl estradiol-containing Triphasil on vitamin B6 status. *Int J Vit Nutr Res* 1996;66:46–54.

10. Lobo RA, Roy S, Shoupe D, et al. Estrogen and progestin effects on urinary calcium and calciotropic hormones in surgically-induced postmenopausal women. *Horm Metab Res* 1985;17:370–73.

11. Gallagher JC, Riggs BL, DeLuca HF. Effect of estrogen on calcium absorption and serum vitamin D metabolites in postmenopausal osteoporosis. *J Clin Endocrinol Metab* 1980;51:1359–64.

12. Tuppurainen MT, Komulainen M, Kröger H, et al. Does vitamin D strengthen the increase in femoral neck BMD in osteoporotic women treated with estrogen? *Osteoporosis Int* 1998;7:32–38.

13. Collins BM, McLachlan JA, Arnold SF. The estrogenic and antiestrogenic activities of phytochemicals with the human estrogen receptor expressed in yeast. *Steroids* 1997;62:365–72.

14. Hulley S, Grady D, Bush T, et al. Randomized trial of estrogen plus progestin for secondary prevention of coronary heart disease in postmenopausal women. *JAMA* 1998;280:605–13.

15. Krauss RM, Perlman JA, Ray R, Petitti D. Effects of estrogen dose and smoking on lipid and lipoprotein levels in postmenopausal women. *Am J Obstet Gynecol* 1988;158:1606–11.

Corticosteroids

1. Holt GA. *Food & Drug Interactions.* Chicago: Precept Press, 1998, 83.

2. Behr J, Maier K, Degenkolb B, et al. Antioxidative and clinical effects of high-dose N-acetylcysteine in fibrosing alveolitis. Adjunctive therapy to maintenance immunosuppresion. *Am J Respir Crit Care Med* 1997;156:1897–901.

3. Thelkeld DS, ed. Hormones, Adrenal Cortical Steroids, Glucocorticoids. In *Facts and Comparisons Drug Information.* St. Louis, MO: Facts and Comparisons, Apr 1991, 128b.

4. Hunt TK, Ehrlich HP, Garcia JA, Dunphy JE. Effect of vitamin A on reversing the inhibitory effect of cortisone on healing of open wounds in animals and man. *Ann Surg* 1969;170:633–40

5. Holt GA. *Food & Drug Interactions.* Chicago: Precept Press, 1998, 83.

6. Sur S, Camara M, Buchmeier A, et al. Double-blind trial of pyridoxine (vitamin B6) in the treatment of steroid-dependent asthma. *Ann Allergy* 1993;70:147–52.

7. Trovato A et al. Drug-nutrient interactions. *Am Family Phys* 1991;44:1651–58 [review].

8. Chesney RW et al. Reduction of serum-1,25-dihydroxyvitamin-D, in children receiving glucocorticoids. *Lancet* 1978;ii:1123–25.

9. Buckley LM, Leib ES, Cartularo KS, et al. Calcium and vitamin D3 supplementation prevents bone loss in the spine secondary to low-dose corticosteroids in patients with rheumatoid arthritis. A randomized, double-blind, placebo-controlled trial. *Ann Intern Med* 1996;125:961–68.

10. Smith BJ, Buxton JR, Dickeson J, Heller RF. Does beclomethasone dipropionate suppress dehydroepiandrosterone sulphate in postmenopausal women? *Austral NZ J Med* 1994;24:396–401.

11. Demisch L, Demisch K, Nickelsen T. Influence of dexamethasone on nocturnal melatonin production in healthy adult subjects. *J Pineal Res* 1987;5:317–22.

12. Buist RA. Drug-nutrient interactions—an overview. *Intl Clin Nutr Rev* 1984;4(3):114 [review].

13. Davis RH, Parker WL, Murdoch DP. *Aloe vera* as a biologically active vehicle for hydrocortisone acetate. *J Am Podiatric Med Assoc* 1991;81:1–9.

14. Threlkeld DS, ed. Hormones, Adrenal Cortical Steroids, Glucocorticoids. In *Facts and Comparisons Drug Information.* St. Louis, MO: Facts and Comparisons, Apr 1991, 128b.

15. Jubiz W, Meikle AW. Alterations of glucocorticoid actions by other drugs and disease states. *Drugs* 1979;18:113–21.

16. Tamura Y, Nishikawa T, Yamada K, et al. Effects of glycyrrhetinic acid and its derivatives on delta-4-5-alpha- and 5-beta-reductase in rat liver. *Arzneim Forsch* 1979;29:647–49.

17. Chen MF, Shimada F, Kato H, et al. Effect of glycyrrhizin on the pharmacokinetics of prednisolone following low dosage of prednisolone hemisuccinate. *Endocrinol Japon* 1990;37:331–41.

18. Kumagai A, Nanaboshi M, Asanuma Y, et al. Effects of glycyrrhizin on thymolytic and immunosupressive action of cortisone. *Endocrinol Japon* 1967;14:39–42.

19. Teelucksingh S, Mackie ADR, Burt D, et al. Potentiation of hydrocortisone activity in skin by glycyrrhetinic acid. *Lancet* 1990;335:1060–63.

20. Chen MF, Shimada F, Kato H, et al. Effect of glycyrrhizin on the pharmacokinetics of prednisolone following low dosage of prednisolone hemisuccinate. *Endocrinol Japon* 1990;37:331–41.

21. Threlkeld DS, ed. Hormones, Adrenal Cortical Steroids, Glucocorticoids. In *Facts and Comparisons Drug Information*. St. Louis, MO: Facts and Comparisons, Apr 1991, 128b.

22. Trovato A et al. Drug–nutrient interactions. *Am Family Phys* 1991;44:1651–58 [review].

23. Holt GA. *Food & Drug Interactions*. Chicago: Precept Press, 1998, 82.

Cyclobenzaprine

1. Threlkeld DS, ed. Central Nervous System Drugs, Skeletal Muscle Relaxants, Centrally Acting, Cyclobenzaprine. In *Facts and Comparisons Drug Information*. St. Louis, MO: Facts and Comparisons, Nov 1993, 287l–287n.

Cyclophosphamide

1. Ghosh J, Das S. Role of vitamin A in prevention and treatment of sarcoma 180 in mice. *Chemotherapy* 1987;33:211–18.

2. Taper HS, de Gerlache J, Lans M, Roberfroid M. Non-toxic potentiation of cancer chemotherapy by combined C and K3 vitamin pre-treatment. *Int J Cancer* 1987;40:575–79.

3. Jaakkola K, Lahteenmaki P, Laakso J, et al. Treatment with antioxidant and other nutrients in combination with chemotherapy and irradiation in patients with small-cell lung cancer. *Anticancer Res* 1992;12:599–606.

4. Threlkeld DS, ed. Antineoplastics, Alkylating Agents, Nitrogen Mustards, Cyclophosphamide. In *Facts and Comparisons Drug Information*. St. Louis, MO: Facts and Comparisons, Aug 1997, 647–647d.

Cycloserine

1. Holt GA. *Food & Drug Interactions*. Chicago: Precept Press, 1998, 86.

2. Roe D, Campbell T, eds. *Drugs and Nutrients: The Interactive Effects.* New York: Marcel Decker, 1984, 288–89, 505–23.

3. Holt GA. *Food & Drug Interactions.* Chicago: Precept Press, 1998, 86.

4. Holt GA. *Food & Drug Interactions.* Chicago: Precept Press, 1998, 86.

5. Threlkeld DS, ed. Anti-Infectives, Antituberculosis Drugs, Cycloserine. In *Facts and Comparisons Drug Information.* St. Louis, MO: Facts and Comparisons, Mar 1990, 394–395.

6. Holt GA. *Food & Drug Interactions.* Chicago: Precept Press, 1998, 85.

Cyclosporine

1. June CH, Thompson CB, Kennedy MS, et al. Profound hypomagnesemia and renal magnesium wasting associated with the use of cyclosporine for marrow transplantation. *Transplantation* 1985;39:620–24.

2. Thompson CB et al. Association between cyclosporine neurotoxicity and hypomagnesemia. *Lancet* 1984;ii:1116.

3. June CH, Thompson CB, Kennedy MS, et al. Correlation of hypomagnesemia with the onset of cyclosporine-associated hypertension in marrow transplant patients. *Transplantation* 1986;41:47–51.

4. Ventura HO, Milani RV, Lavie CJ, et al. Cyclosporine-induced hypertension. Efficacy of omega-3 fatty acids in patients after cardiac transplantation. *Circulation* 1993;88(5 Pt 2):II281–85.

5. Andreassen AK, Harmann A, Offstad J, et al. Hypertension prophylaxis with omega-3 fatty acids in heart transplant recipients. *J Am Coll Cardiol* 1997;29:1324–31.

6. Homan van der Heide JJ, Bilo HJ, Tegzess AM, Donker AJ. The effects of dietary supplementation with fish oil on renal function in cyclosporine-treated renal transplant recipients. *Transplantation* 1990;49:523–27.

7. Kooijmans-Coutinho MF, Rischen-Vos J, Hermans J, et al. Dietary fish oil in renal transplant recipients treated with cyclosporine-A: No beneficial effects shown. *J Am Soc Nephrol* 1996;7:513–18.

8. Pan SH, Lopez RR Jr, Sher LS, et al. Enhanced oral cyclosporine absorption with water-soluble vitamin E early after liver transplantation. *Pharmacotherapy* 1996;16:59–65.

9. Barth SA, Inselmann G, Engemann R, Heidemann HT. Influences of *Ginkgo biloba* on cyclosporine A included lipid peroxidation in human liver microsomes in comparison to vitamin E, glutathione and N-acetylcysteine. *Biochem Pharmacol* 1991;41:1521–26.

10. Bagnis C, Deray G, Dubois M, Pirotzky E, et al. Prevention of cyclosporine nephrotoxicity with a platelet-activating factor (PAF) antagonist. *Nephrol Dial Transplant* 1996;11:507–13.

11. Holt GA. *Food & Drug Interactions.* Chicago: Precept Press, 1998, 87.

12. Ioannides-Demos LL, Christophidis N, Ryan P, et al. Dosing implication of a clinical interaction between grapefruit juice and cyclosporine and metabolite concentrations in patients with autoimmune diseases. *J Rheumatol* 1997;24:49–54.

13. Threlkeld DS, ed. Miscellaneous Products, Immunosuppressive Drugs, Cyclosporine. In *Facts and Comparisons Drug Information*. St. Louis, MO: Facts and Comparisons, Apr 1998, 738a–738k.

14. Threlkeld DS, ed. Miscellaneous Products, Immunosuppressive Drugs, Cyclosporine. In *Facts and Comparisons Drug Information*. St. Louis, MO: Facts and Comparisons, Apr 1998, 738a–738k.

Dapsone

1. Holt GA. *Food & Drug Interactions*. Chicago: Precept Press, 1998, 88.

2. Prussick R, Ali MAMA, Rosenthal D, Guyatt G. The protective effect of vitamin E on the hemolysis associated with Dapsone treatment in patients with dermatitis herpetiformis. *Arch Dermatol* 1992;128:210–13.

Didanosine

1. Gordon M, Guralnik M, Kaneko Y, et al. A phase II controlled study of a combination of the immune modulator, lentinan, with didanosine (ddI) in HIV patients with CD4 cells of 200–500/mm3. *J Med* 1995;26:193–207.

2. Threlkeld DS, ed. News, Keeping Up, December 1994, Lentinan. In *Facts and Comparisons Drug Information*. St. Louis, MO: Facts and Comparisons, Dec 1997, 805.

3. Threlkeld DS, ed. Anti-Infectives, Antiviral Agents, Didanosine. In *Facts and Comparisons Drug Information*. St. Louis, MO: Facts and Comparisons, Mar 1993, 406k–406t.

Digoxin

1. Whang R, Oei TO, Watanabe A. Frequency of hypomagnesiumia in hospitalized patients receiving digitalis. *Arch Intern Med* 1985;145:655–56.

2. Holt GA. *Food & Drug Interactions*. Chicago: Precept Press, 1998, 94.

3. Landauer RA. Magnesium deficiency and digitalis toxicity. *JAMA* 1984;251:730 [letter/review].

4. Cohen L, Kitzes R. Letter. *JAMA* 1984;251:730.

5. Blumenthal M, ed. *The Complete German Commission E Monographs*. Austin, TX: American Botanical Council, 1998, 143.

6. Tyler VE. *The Honest Herbal*, 3rd ed. New York: Pharmaceutical Products Press, 1993, 198.

7. Wang DJ, Chu KM, Chen JD, et al. Drug interaction between digoxin and bisacodyl. *J Formes Med Assoc* 1990;89:913, 915–19 [in Chinese].

8. Botzler R, Ritter U. Effect of laxative measures on the serum concentration of digoxin in the human. *Leber Magen Darm* Nov 1982; 12(6):255–57 [in German].

9. Newall CA, Anderson LA, Phillipson JD. *Herbal Medicines: A Guide for Healthcare Professionals.* London: Pharmaceutical Press, 1996, 244.

10. McRae S. Elevated serum digoxin levels in a patient taking digoxin and Siberian ginseng. *Can Med Assoc J* 1996;155:293–95.

11. Holt GA. *Food & Drug Interactions.* Chicago: Precept Press, 1998, 93.

Diltiazem

1. Du Souich P, Lery N, Lery L, et al. Influence of food on the bioavailability of diltiazem and two of its metabolites following the administration of conventional tablets and slow-release capsules. *Biopharm Drug Dispos* 1990;11:137–47.

2. Threlkeld DS, ed. Diuretics and Cardiovasculars, Calcium Channel Blocking Agents. In *Facts and Comparisons Drug Information.* St. Louis, MO: Facts and Comparisons, Mar 1996, 149r–149t.

Dimenhydrinate

1. Blumenthal M, ed. *The Complete German Commission E Monographs.* Austin, TX: American Botanical Council, 1998, 146.

2. Threlkeld DS, ed. Respiratory Drugs, Antihistamines. In *Facts and Comparisons Drug Information.* St. Louis, MO: Facts and Comparisons, May 1989, 188–194c.

3. Threlkeld DS, ed. Respiratory Drugs, Antihistamines. In *Facts and Comparisons Drug Information.* St. Louis, MO: Facts and Comparisons, May 1989, 188–194c.

Diphenhydramine

1. Blumenthal M, ed. *The Complete German Commission E Monographs.* Austin, TX: American Botanical Council, 1998, 146.

2. Threlkeld DS, ed. Respiratory Drugs, Antihistamines. In *Facts and Comparisons Drug Information.* St. Louis, MO: Facts and Comparisons, May 1998, 191a–191b.

3. Threlkeld DS, ed. Respiratory Drugs, Antihistamines. In *Facts and Comparisons Drug Information.* St. Louis, MO: Facts and Comparisons, May 1998, 191a–191b.

Docetaxel

1. Vukelja SJ, Baker WJ, Burris HA, et al. Pyridoxine therapy for palmar-plantar erythrodysesthesia associated with Taxotere. *J Natl Cancer Inst* 1993;85:432 [letter].

Doxorubicin

1. Alberts DS, Peng Y-M, Moon TE, Bressler R. Carnitine prevention of Adriamycin toxicity in mice. *Biomedicine* 1978;29:265–68.

2. Judy WV, Hall JH, Dugan W, et al. Coenzyme Q10 reduction of Adriamycin cardiotoxicity. In *Biomedical and Clinical Aspects of Coenzyme Q*, vol. 4, ed. K Folkers, Y Yamamura. Amsterdam: Elsevier/North Holland Biomedical Press, 1984, 231–41.

3. Ogura R, Toyama H, Shimada T, Murakami M. The role of ubiquinone (coenzyme Q10) in preventing Adriamycin-induced mitochondrial disorders in rat heart. *J Appl Biochem* 1979;1:325.

4. Doroshow JH, Locker GY, Ifrim I, et al. Prevention of doxorubicin cardiac toxicity in the mouse by N-acetylcysteine. *J Clin Invest* 1981;68:1053–64.

5. Meyers C, Bonow R, Palmeri S, et al. A randomized controlled trial assessing the prevention of doxorubicin cardiomyopathy by N-acetylcysteine. *Semin Oncol* 1983;10:53–55.

6. Pinto J, Raiczyk GB, Huang YP, Rivlin RS. New approaches to the possible prevention of side effects of chemotherapy by nutrition. *Cancer* 1986;58:1911–14.

7. Fujita K, Shinpo K, Yamada K, et al. Reduction of Adriamycin toxicity by ascorbate in mice and guinea pigs. *Cancer Res* 1982;42:309–16.

8. Myers C, McQuire W, Young R. Adriamycin amelioration of toxicity by alpha-tocopherol. *Cancer Treat Rep* 1976;60:961–62.

9. Sonneveld P. Effect of alpha-tocopherol on the cardiotoxicity of Adriamycin in the rat. *Cancer* 1978;62:1033–36.

10. Ripoll EAP, Rama BN, Webber MM. Vitamin E enhances the chemotherapeutic effects of Adriamycin on human prostatic carcinoma cells in vitro. *J Urol* 1986;136:529–31.

11. Weijl NI, Cleton FJ, Osanto S. Free radicals and antioxidants in chemotherapy-induced toxicity. *Cancer Treatment Rev* 1997;23:209–40 [review].

12. Wood LA. Possible prevention of Adriamycin-induced allopecia by tocopherol. *N Engl J Med* 1985;312:1060 [letter].

13. Weijl NI, Cleton FJ, Osanto S. Free radicals and antioxidants in chemotherapy-induced toxicity. *Cancer Treatment Rev* 1997;23:209–40 [review].

Doxycycline

1. Threlkeld DS, ed. Anti-Infectives, Tetracyclines. In *Facts and Comparisons Drug Information*. St. Louis, MO: Facts and Comparisons, Dec 1989, 342b–342d.

2. Ceccaldi B, Coutant G, Lecoules S, Algayres JP, Daly JP. Hypovitaminosis K during treatment with doxycycline. *Presse Med* Mar 28 1998;27(12):571 [French].

3. Khin-Maung-U, Myo-Khin, Nyunt-Nyunt-Wai, et al. Clinical trial of berberine in acute watery diarrhoea. *BMJ* 1985;291:160–65.

4. Rabbani GH, Butler T, Knight J, et al. Randomized controlled trial of berberine sulfate therapy for diarrhea due to enterotoxigenic *Escherichia coli* and *Vibrio cholerae*. *J Infect Dis* 1987;155:979–84.

5. Threlkeld DS, ed. Anti-Infectives, Tetracyclines. In *Facts and Comparisons Drug Information.* St. Louis, MO: Facts and Comparisons, Dec 1989, 342b–342d.

6. Meyer FP, Specht H, Quednow B, Walther H. Influence of milk on the bioavailability of doxycycline—new aspects. *Infection* 1989;17:245–46.

Doxylamine

1. Blumenthal M, ed. *The Complete German Commission E Monographs.* Austin, TX: American Botanical Council, 1998, 146.

2. Threlkeld DS, ed. Central Nervous System Drugs, Nonprescription Sleep Aids. In *Facts and Comparisons Drug Information.* St. Louis, MO: Facts and Comparisons, Dec 1993, 273e.

3. Threlkeld DS, ed. Central Nervous System Drugs, Nonprescription Sleep Aids. In *Facts and Comparisons Drug Information.* St. Louis, MO, Facts and Comparisons, Dec 1993, 273e.

Econazole

1. Coeugniet EG, Kuhnast R. Recurrent candidiasis: Adjuvant immunotherapy with different formulations of Echinacin. *Therapiewoche* 1986;36:3352–58.

Enalapril

1. Good CB, McDermott L, McCloskey B. Diet and serum potassium in patients on ACE inhibitors. *JAMA* 1995;274:538.

2. Ohaya Y, Ueno M, Takata Y, et al. Crossover comparison of the effects of enalapril and captopril on potassium homeostasis in patients with mild hypertension. *Int J Clin Pharmacol Ther* 1994;32:655–59.

3. Egan BM, Stepniakowski K. Effects of enalapril on the hyperinsulinemic response to severe salt restriction in obese young men with mild systemic hypertension. *Am J Cardiol* 1993;72:53–57.

4. Threlkeld DS, ed. Diuretics and Cardiovasculars, Antihypertensives, Angiotensin Converting Enzyme Inhibitors. In *Facts and Comparisons Drug Information.* St. Louis, MO: Facts and Comparisons, Apr 1998, 165o–165p.

Ephedrine and Pseudoephedrine

1. Brinker F. Interactions of pharmaceutical and botanical medicines. *J Naturopathic Med* 1997;7(2):14–20.

2. Holt GA. *Food & Drug Interactions.* Chicago: Precept Press, 1998, 105.

3. Holt GA. *Food & Drug Interactions.* Chicago: Precept Press,1998, 105–6.

Epinephrine

1. Cox BD, Clarkson AR, Whichelow MJ, et al. Effect of adrenaline on plasma vitamin C levels in normal subjects. *Horm Metab Res* 1974;6:234–37.

2. Raab W. Cardiotoxic effects of emotional, socioeconomic, and environmental stresses. In *Myocardiology*, vol I, ed. E Bajusz, G Rona. Baltimore: University Park Press 1970, 707–13.

3. Threlkeld DS, ed. Respiratory Drugs, Bronchodilators, Sympathomimetics. In *Facts and Comparisons Drug Information*. St. Louis, MO: Facts and Comparisons, May 1994, 177–177a.

4. Threlkeld DS, ed. Respiratory Drugs, Bronchodilators, Sympathomimetics. In *Facts and Comparisons Drug Information*. St. Louis, MO: Facts and Comparisons, May 1994, 177–177a.

5. Threlkeld DS, ed. Central Nervous System Drugs, Analeptics, Caffeine. In *Facts and Comparisons Drug Information*. St. Louis, MO: Facts and Comparisons, Feb 1998, 230–230d.

6. Brown NJ, Ryder D, Branch RA. A pharmacodynamic interaction between caffeine and phenylpropanolamine. *Clin Pharmacol Ther* 1991;50:363–71.

Erythromycin

1. Colombel JF, Cortot A, Neut, Romond C. Yoghurt with *Bifidobacterium longum* reduces erythromycin-induced gastrointestinal effects. *Lancet* 1987;ii:43 [letter].

2. Neubauer RA. A plant protease for potentiation of and possible replacement of antibiotics. *Exp Med Surg* 1961;19:143–60.

3. Holt GA. *Food and Drug Interactions*. Chicago: Precept Press, 1998, 107–8.

4. Bizjak ED, Mauro VF. Digoxin-macrolide drug interaction. *Ann Pharmacother* 1997;31:1077–79.

5. Threlkeld DS, ed. Systemic Anti-Infectives, Macrolides. In *Facts and Comparisons Drug Information*. St. Louis, MO: Facts and Comparisons, Oct 1998, 343c–344.

6. Threlkeld DS, ed. Systemic Anti-Infectives, Macrolides. In *Facts and Comparisons Drug Information*. St. Louis, MO: Facts and Comparisons, Oct 1998, 343c–344.

7. Holt GA. *Food and Drug Interactions*. Chicago: Precept Press, 1998, 106–7.

8. Threlkeld DS, ed. Systemic Anti-Infectives, Macrolides. In *Facts and Comparisons Drug Information*. St. Louis, MO: Facts and Comparisons, Oct 1998, 343c–344.

Estradiol

1. Schubert W, Cullberg G, Edgar B, Hedner T. Inhibition of 17 beta-estradiol metabolism by grapefruit juice in ovariectomized women. *Maturitas* 1994;20:155–63.

2. Weber A, Jager R, Borner A, et al. Can grapefruit juice influence ethinylestradiol bioavailability? *Contraception* 1996;53:41–47.

3. Schubert W, Eriksson U, Edgar B, et al. Flavonoids in grapefruit juice inhibit the in vitro hepatic metabolism of 17 beta-estradiol. *Eur J Drug Metab Pharmacokinet* 1995;3:219–24.

4. Kuiper GG, Lemmen JG, Carlsson B, et al. Interaction of estrogenic chemicals and phytoestrogens with estrogen receptor beta. *Endocrinology* 1998;139:4252–63

5. Komulainen M, Tuppurainen MT, Kroger H, et al. Vitamin D and HRT: no benefit additional to that of HRT alone in prevention of bone loss in early postmenopausal women. A 2.5-year randomized placebo-controlled study. *Osteoporosis Int* 1997;7:126–32.

6. Schubert W, Cullberg G, Edgar B, Hedner T. Inhibition of 17 beta-estradiol metabolism by grapefruit juice in ovariectomized women. *Maturitas* 1994;20:155–63.

7. Weber A, Jager R, Borner A, et al. Can grapefruit juice influence ethinylestradiol bioavailability? *Contraception* 1996;53:41–47.

Etodolac

1. Sorenson JRJ. Copper chelates as possible active forms of the antiarthritic agents. *J Medicinal Chem* 1976;19:135–48.

2. Bjarnason I, Macpherson AJ. Intestinal toxicity of non-steroidal anti-inflammatory drugs. *Pharmacol Ther* 1994;62:145–57.

3. Threlkeld DS, ed. Blood Modifiers, Iron-Containing Products. In *Facts and Comparisons Drug Information*. St. Louis, MO: Facts and Comparisons, Jun 1998, 62–69a.

4. Bailie GR. Acute renal failure. In *Applied Therapeutics: The Clinical Use of Drugs*, 6th ed. Vancouver, WA: Applied Therapeutics, 1995, 29–33.

5. Threlkeld DS, ed. Central Nervous System Drugs, Nonsteroidal Anti-Inflammatory Agents. In *Facts and Comparisons Drug Information*. St. Louis, MO: Facts and Comparisons, Mar 1993, 252c.

6. Rees WDW, Rhodes J, Wright JE, et al. Effect of deglycyrrhizinated liquorice on gastric mucosal damage by aspirin. *Scand J Gastroenterol* 1979;14:605–7.

7. Morgan AG, McAdam WAF, Pascoo C, Darnborough A. Comparison between cimetidine and Caved-S in the treatment of gastric ulceration, and subsequent maintenance therapy. *Gut* 1982;23:545–51.

8. Threlkeld DS, ed. Central Nervous System Drugs, Nonsteroidal Anti-Inflammatory Agents. In *Facts and Comparisons Drug Information*. St. Louis, MO: Facts and Comparisons, Feb 1992, 252c.

9. Threlkeld DS, ed. Central Nervous System Drugs, Nonsteroidal Anti-Inflammatory Agents. In *Facts and Comparisons Drug Information*. St. Louis, MO: Facts and Comparisons, Feb 1992, 252c.

Famotidine

1. Aymard JP, Aymard B, Netter P, et al. Haematological adverse effects of histamine H2-receptor antagonists. *Med Toxicol Adverse Drug Exp* 1988;3:430–48.

2. Bachmann KA, Sullivan TJ, Jauregui L, et al. Drug interactions of H2-receptor antagonists. *Scand J Gastroenterol Suppl* 1994;206:14–19.

3. Aymard JP, Aymard B, Netter P, et al. Haematological adverse effects of histamine H2-receptor antagonists. *Med Toxicol Adverse Drug Exp* 1988;3:430–48.

4. Russell RM, Krasinski SD, Samloff IM. Correction of impaired folic acid (Pte Glu) absorption by orally administered HCl in subjects with gastric atrophy. *Am J Clin Nutr* 1984;39:656.

5. Tompsett SL. Factors influencing the absorption of iron and copper from the alimentary tract. *Biochem J* 1940;34:961–69.

6. Lin JH, Chremos AN, Kanovsky SM, et al. Effects of antacids and food on absorption of famotidine. *Br J Clin Pharmacol* 1987;24:551–53.

7. Threlkeld DS, ed. Gastrointestinal Drugs, Histamine H2 Antagonists, Famotidine. In *Facts and Comparisons Drug Information*. St. Louis, MO: Facts and Comparisons, Sep 1995, 305f–305g.

8. Schurer-Maly CC, Varga L, Koelz HR, Halter F. Smoking and pH response to H2-receptor antagonists. *Scand J Gastroenterol* 1989;24:1172–78.

9. Reynolds JC, Schoen RE, Maislin G, Zangari GG. Risk factors for delayed healing of duodenal ulcers treated with famotidine and ranitidine. *Am J Gastroenterol* 1994;89:571–80.

Fexofenadine

1. Threlkeld DS, ed. Respiratory Drugs, Antihistamines. In *Facts and Comparisons Drug Information*. St. Louis, MO: Facts and Comparisons, May 1998, 194c.

Fluconazole

1. Zimmermann T, Yeates RA, Laufen H, et al. Influence of concomitant food intake on the oral absorption of two triazole antifungal agents, itraconazole and fluconazole. *Eur J Clin Pharmacol* 1994;46:147–50.

Fluorouracil

1.Vukelja SJ, Lombardo F, James WD, Weiss RB. Pyroxidine [sic] for the palmar-plantar erythrodysesthesia syndrome. *Ann Intern Med* 1989;111:688–89 [letter].

2. Molina R, Fabian C, Slavik M, Dahlberg S. Reversal of palmar-plantar erythrodysesthesia (PPE) by B6 without loss of response in colon cancer patients receiving 200/mg/m2/day continuous 5-FU. *Proc Am Soc Clin Oncol* 1987;6:90 [abstract].

Fluoxetine

1. Fava M, Borus JS, Alpert JE, et al. Folate, vitamin B12, and homocysteine in major depressive disorder. *Am J Psychiatry* 1997;154:426–28.

2. Childs PA, Rodin I, Martin NJ, et al. Effect of fluoxetine on melatonin in patients with seasonal affective disorder and matched controls. *Br J Psychiatry* 1995;166:196–98.

3. Threlkeld DS, ed. Central Nervous System Drugs, Antidepressants, Selective Serotonin Reuptake Inhibitors. In *Facts and Comparisons Drug Information*. St. Louis, MO: Facts and Comparisons, Apr 1997, 264r–264s.

4. Cohen AJ. Long term safety and efficacy of *Ginkgo biloba* extract in the treatment of anti-depressant-induced sexual dysfunction. *Psychiatry On-Line* http://www.priory.com/ginkgo.html.

5. Sohn M, Sikora R. *Ginkgo biloba* extract in the therapy of erectile dysfunction. *J Sex Educ Ther* 1991;17:53–61.

6. Demott K. St. John's wort tied to serotonin syndrome. *Clinical Psychiatry News* 1998;26:28.

7. Gordon JB. SSRIs and St. John's wort: possible toxicity? *Am Fam Physician* 1998;57:950.

8. Threlkeld DS, ed. Central Nervous System Drugs, Antidepressants, Selective Serotonin Reuptake Inhibitors. In *Facts and Comparisons Drug Information*. St. Louis, MO: Facts and Comparison, Apr 1997, 264r–264s.

9. Threlkeld DS, ed. Central Nervous System Drugs, Antidepressants, Selective Serotonin Reuptake Inhibitors. In *Facts and Comparisons Drug Information*. St. Louis, MO: Facts and Comparison, Apr 1997, 264r–264s.

10. Naranjo CA, Pouos CX, Bremner KE, Lanctot KL. Fluoxetine attenuates alcohol intake and desire to drink. *Int Clin Psychopharmacol* 1994;9:163–72.

Fluvastatin

1. Mortensen SA, Leth A, Agner E, Rohde M. Dose-related decrease of serum coenzyme Q10 during treatment with HMG-CoA reductase inhibitors. *Mol Aspects Med* 1997;18(suppl):S137–44.

2. Bargossi AM, Grossi G, Fiorella PL, et al. Exogenous CoQ10 supplementation prevents plasma ubiquinone reduction induced by HMG-CoA reductase inhibitors. *Molec Aspects Med* 1994;15(suppl):s187–93.

3. Jacobson TA, Chin MM, Fromell GJ, et al. Fluvastatin with and without niacin for hypercholesterolemia. *Am J Cardiol* 1994;74:149–54.

4. Garnett WR. Interactions with hydroxymethylglutaryl-coenzyme A reductase inhibitors. *Am J Health Syst Pharm* 1995;52:1639–45.

5. Yee HS, Fong NT. Atorvastatin in the treatment of primary hypercholesterolemia and mixed dyslipidemias. *Ann Pharmacother* 1998;32:1030–43.

6. Jacobson TA, Amorosa LF. Combination therapy with fluvastatin and niacin in hypercholesterolemia: a preliminary report on safety. *Am J Cardiol* 1994;73:25D–29D.

7. Jokubaitis LA. Fluvastatin in combination with other lipid-lowering agents. *Br J Pract Suppl* 1996;77A:28–32.

8. Muggeo M, Zenti MG, Travia D, et al. Serum retinol levels throughout 2 years of cholesterol-lowering therapy. *Metabolism* 1995;44:398–403.

9. Dujovne CA, Davidson MH. Fluvastatin administration at bedtime versus with the evening meal: a multicenter comparison of bioavailability, safety, and efficacy. *Am J Med* 1994;96:37S–40S.

10. Smit JW, Wijnne HJ, Schobben F, et al. Effects of alcohol and fluvastatin on lipid metabolism and hepatic function. *Ann Intern Med* 1995;122:678–80.

Fluvoxamine

1. Cohen AJ, Bartlik B. *Ginkgo biloba* for antidepressant-induced sexual dysfunction. *J Sex Marital Therapy* 1998;24:139–45.

2. Sohn M, Sikora R. *Ginkgo biloba* extract in the therapy of erectile dysfunction. *J Sex Educ Ther* 1991;17:53–61.

3. Demott K. St. John's wort tied to serotonin syndrome. *Clin Psychiatr News* 1998;26:28.

4. Gordon JB. SSRIs and St. John's wort: possible toxicity? *Am Fam Phys* 1998;57:950.

5. Threlkeld DS, ed. Central Nervous System Drugs, Antidepressants, Selective Serotonin Reuptake Inhibitors. In *Facts and Comparisons Drug Information*. St. Louis, MO: Facts and Comparisons, Apr 1997, 264s.

6. Spigset O, Carleborg L, Hedenmalm K, Dahlqvist R. Effect of cigarette smoking on fluvoxamine pharmacokinetics in humans. *Clin Pharmacol Ther* 1995;58:399–403.

Gabapentin

1. Threlkeld DS, ed. Central Nervous System Drugs, Anticonvulsants, Miscellaneous, Gabapentin. In *Facts and Comparisons Drug Information*. St. Louis, MO: Facts and Comparisons, Nov 1993, 284t–284xa.

Gemfibrozil

1. Aberg F, Appelkvist EL, Broijersen A, et al. Gemfibrozil-induced decrease in serum ubiquinone and alpha- and gamma-tocopherol levels in men with combined hyperlipidaemia. *Eur J Clin Invest* 1998;28:235–42.

2. Aberg F, Appelkvist EL, Broijersen A, et al. Gemfibrozil-induced decrease in serum ubiquinone and alpha- and gamma-tocopherol levels in men with combined hyperlipidaemia. *Eur J Clin Invest* 1998;28:235–42.

3. Garnett WR. Interactions with hydroxymethylglutaryl-coenzyme A reductase inhibitors. *Am J Health Syst Pharm* 1995;52:1639–45 [review].

4. Threlkeld DS, ed. Diuretics and Cardiovasculars, Antihyperlipidemic Agents, Gemfibrozil. In *Facts and Comparisons Drug Information*. St. Louis, MO, Facts and Comparisons, Feb 1997, 172h–172j.

5. Threlkeld DS, ed. Diuretics and Cardiovasculars, Antihyperlipidemic Agents, Gemfibrozil. In *Facts and Comparisons Drug Information*. St. Louis, MO: Facts and Comparisons, Feb 1997, 172h–172j.

Gentamicin

1. Kes P, Reiner Z. Symptomatic hypomagnesemia associated with gentamicin therapy. *Magnes Trace Elem* 1990;9:54–60.

2. Humes HD et al. Calcium is a competitive inhibitor of gentamicin-renal membrane binding interactions and dietary calcium supplementation protects against gentamicin nephrotoxicity. *J Clin Invest* 1984;73:134.

3. McLean R. Magnesium and its therapeutic uses: A review. *Am J Med* 1994;96:63–76.

4. Kes P, Reiner Z. Symptomatic hypomagnesemia associated with gentamicin therapy. *Magnes Trace Elem* 1990;9:54–60.

5. Kes P, Reiner Z. Symptomatic hypomagnesemia associated with gentamicin therapy. *Magnes Trace Elem* 1990;9:54–60.

6. Weir MR, Keniston RC, Enriquez JI Sr, McNamee GA. Depression of vitamin B6 levels due to gentamicin. *Vet Hum Toxicol* 1990;32:235–38.

Glipizide

1. McBain AM, Brown IR, Menzies DG, Campbell IW. Effects of improved glycaemic control on calcium and magnesium homeostasis in type II diabetes. *J Clin Pathol* 1988;41:933–35.

2. Kivisto KT, Neuvonen PJ. Enhancement of absorption and effect of glipizide by magnesium hydroxide. *Clin Pharmacol Ther* 1991;49:39–43.

3. Sharma RD, Raghuram TC, Sudhakar Rao N. Effect of fenugreek seeds on blood glucose and serum lipids in type 1 diabetes. *Eur J Clin Nutr* 1990;44:301–6.

4. Sharma RD, Sakar A, Hazra DK, et al. Use of fenugreek seed powder in the management of non-insulin dependent diabetes mellitus. *Nutr Res* 1996;16:1131–39.

5. Wahlin-Boll E, Melander A, Sartor G, Schersten B. Influence of food intake on the absorption and effect of glipizide in diabetics and in healthy subjects. *Eur J Clin Pharmacol* 1980;18:279–83.

Glyburide

1. Bunyapraphatsara N, Yongchaiyudha S, Rungpitarangsi V, Chokechaijaroenporn O. Antidiabetic activity of *Aloe vera* L. juice. II. Clinical trial in diabetes mellitus patients in combination with glibenclamide. *Phytomed* 1996;3:245–48.

2. Threlkeld DS, ed. Hormones, Antidiabetic Agents, Sulfonylureas. In *Facts and Comparisons Drug Information*. St. Louis, MO: Facts and Comparisons, Jun 1992, 130m.

3. Threlkeld DS, ed. Hormones, Antidiabetic Agents, Sulfonylureas. In *Facts and Comparisons Drug Information*. St. Louis, MO: Facts and Comparisons, Jun 1992, 130m.

4. Threlkeld DS, ed. Hormones, Antidiabetic Agents, Sulfonylureas. In *Facts and Comparisons Drug Information*. St. Louis, MO: Facts and Comparisons, Jun 1992, 130m.

Griseofulvin

1. Anonymous. Vitamin E boosts griseofulvin. *Mycol Observer* Nov/Dec 1990:8.

2. Holt GA. *Food & Drug Interactions*. Chicago: Precept Press, 1998, 124.

3. Holt GA. *Food & Drug Interactions*. Chicago: Precept Press, 1998, 123–24.

Haloperidol

1. Heresco-Levy U, Javitt DC, Ermilov M, et al. Double-blind, placebo-controlled, crossover trial of glycine adjuvant therapy for treatment-resistant schizophrenia. *Br J Psychiatry* 1996;169:610–17.

2. Javitt DC, Zylberman I, Zukin SR, et al. Amelioration of negative symptoms in schizophrenia by glycine. *Am J Psychiatry* 1994;151:1234–36.

3. Potkin SG, Costa J, Roy S, et al. Glycine in treatment of schizophrenia—theory and preliminary results. In: Meltzer HY (ed). *Novel Antipsychotic Drugs*. New York: Raven Press, 1990:179–88.

4. Heresco-Levy U, Javitt DC, Ermilov M, et al. Double-blind, placebo-controlled, crossover trial of glycine adjuvant therapy for treatment-resistant schizophrenia. *Br J Psychiatry* 1996;169:610–17.

5. Threlkeld DS, ed. Central Nervous System Drugs, Antipsychotic Agents. In *Facts and Comparisons Drug Information*. St. Louis, MO: Facts and Comparisons, May 1998, 266k–266m.

6. Threlkeld DS, ed. Central Nervous System Drugs, Antipsychotic Agents. In *Facts and Comparisons Drug Information*. St. Louis, MO: Facts and Comparisons, May 1998, 266k–266m.

7. Adler LA, Peselow E, Rotrosen J, et al. Vitamin E treatment of tardive dyskinesia. *Am J Psychiatry* 1993;150:1405–7.

8. Adler LA, Edson R, Lavori P, et al. Long-term treatment effects of vitamin E for tardive dyskinesia. *Biol Psychiatry* 1998;43:868–72.

9. Threlkeld DS, ed. Central Nervous System Drugs, Antipsychotic Agents. In *Facts and Comparisons Drug Information*. St. Louis, MO: Facts and Comparisons, May 1998, 266k–266m.

10. Palasciano G, Portincasa P, Palmieri V, et al. The effect of silymarin on plasma levels of malon-dialdehyde in patients receiving long-term treatment with psychotropic drugs. *Curr Ther Res* 1994;55:537–45.

11. Lasswell WL Jr, Weber SS, Wilkins JM. In vitro interaction of neuroleptics and tricylic antidepressants with coffee, tea, and gallotannic acid. *J Pharm Sci* 1984;73:1056–58.

12. Threlkeld DS, ed. Central Nervous System Drugs, Antipsychotic Agents. In *Facts and Comparisons Drug Information*. St. Louis, MO: Facts and Comparisons, May 1998, 266k–266m.

Heparin

1. Threlkeld DS, ed. Blood Modifiers, Anticoagulants, Heparin. In *Facts and Comparisons Drug Information.* St. Louis, MO: Facts and Comparisons, Jun 1997, 87a–87f.

2. Aarskog D, Aksens L, Markestad TK, et al. Heparin induced inhibition of 1,25-dihydroxyvitamin D formation. *Am J Obstet Gynecol* 1984;148:1141–42.

3. Majerus PW, Broze GJ Jr, Miletich JP, Tollefsen DM. Anticoagulant, thrombolytic, and antiplatelet drugs. In *Goodman and Gilman's The Pharmacological Basis of Therapeutics*, 9th ed. New York: McGraw-Hill 1996, 1346.

4. Wise PH, Hall AS. Heparin induced osteopenia in pregnancy. *BMJ* 1980;281:110–11.

5. Haram K, Hervig T, Thordarson H, Aksnes L. Osteopenia caused by heparin treatment in pregnancy. *Acta Obstet Gynecol Scand* 1993;72:674–75.

6. Threlkeld DS, ed. Blood Modifiers, Anticoagulants, Heparin. In *Facts and Comparisons Drug Information.* St. Louis, MO: Facts and Comparisons, Jun 1997, 87a–87f.

7. Newall CA, Anderson LA, Phillipson JD. *Herbal Medicines: A Guide for Health-Care Professionals.* London: The Pharmaceutical Press, 1996, 135–37.

8. Kleijnen J, Knipschild P. *Ginkgo biloba. Lancet* 1992;340:1136–39.

9. Rosenblatt M, Mindel J. Spontaneous hyphema associated with ingestion of *Ginkgo biloba* extract. *New Engl J Med* 1997;336:1108.

10. Rowin J, Lewis SL. Spontaneous bilateral subdural hematoma with chronic *Gingko biloba* ingestion. *Neurology* 1996;46:1775–76.

11. Mathews MK. Association of *Ginkgo biloba* with intracerebral hemorrhage. *Neurology* 1998;50:1934.

12. Miller LG, Murray WJ, eds. *Herbal Medicinals: A Clinician's Guide.* New York: Pharmaceutical Products Press, 1999, 313–15.

13. Holt GA. *Food & Drug Interactions.* Chicago: Precept Press, 1998, 127.

Hydralazine

1. Holt GA. *Food & Drug Interactions.* Chicago: Precept Press, 1998, 131–32.

2. Raskin NH, Rishman RA. Pyridoxine-deficiency neuropathy due to hydralazine. *N Engl J Med* 1965;273:1182–85.

3. Threlkeld DS, ed. Diuretics and Cardiovasculars, Antihypertensives, Vasodilators, Hydralazine. In *Facts and Comparisons Drug Information.* St. Louis, MO: Facts and Comparisons, Dec 1993, 163r–164b.

Hydrocodone/Acetaminophen

1. Threlkeld DS, ed. Central Nervous System Drugs, Narcotic Agonist Analgesics. In *Facts and Comparisons Drug Information.* St. Louis, MO: Facts and Comparisons, Feb 1990, 242–243v.

2. Threlkeld DS, ed. Central Nervous System Drugs, Narcotic Agonist Analgesics. In *Facts and Comparisons Drug Information.* St. Louis, MO: Facts and Comparisons, Feb 1990, 242–243v.

3. Threlkeld DS, ed. Central Nervous System Drugs, Narcotic Agonist Analgesics. In *Facts and Comparisons Drug Information.* St. Louis, MO: Facts and Comparisons, Feb 1990, 242–243v.

Ibuprofen

1. Sorenson JRJ. Copper chelates as possible active forms of the antiarthritic agents. *J Medicinal Chem* 1976;19:135–48.

2. Bjarnason I, Macpherson AJ. Intestinal toxicity of non-steroidal anti-inflammatory drugs. *Pharmacol Ther* 1994;62:145–57.

3. Threlkeld DS, ed. Blood Modifiers, Iron-Containing Products. In *Facts and Comparisons Drug Information.* St. Louis, MO: Facts and Comparisons, Jun 1998, 62–69a.

4. Bailie GR. Acute renal failure. In *Applied Therapeutics: The Clinical Use of Drugs,* 6th ed. Vancouver, WA: Applied Therapeutics, 1995, 29–33.

5. Threlkeld DS, ed. Central Nervous System Drugs, Nonsteroidal Anti-Inflammatory Agents. In *Facts and Comparisons Drug Information.* St. Louis, MO: Facts and Comparisons, Mar 1993, 251j–251l.

6. Rees WDW, Rhodes J, Wright JE, et al. Effect of deglycyrrhizinated liquorice on gastric mucosal damage by aspirin. *Scand J Gastroenterol* 1979;14:605–7.

7. Morgan AG, McAdam WAF, Pascoo C, Darnborough A. Comparison between cimetidine and Caved-S in the treatment of gastric ulceration, and subsequent maintenance therapy. *Gut* 1982;23:545–51.

8. Threlkeld DS, ed. Central Nervous System Drugs, Nonsteroidal Anti-Inflammatory Agents. In *Facts and Comparisons Drug Information.* St. Louis, MO: Facts and Comparisons, Feb 1992, 251j–251l.

9. Threlkeld DS, ed. Central Nervous System Drugs, Nonsteroidal Anti-Inflammatory Agents. In *Facts and Comparisons Drug Information.* St. Louis, MO: Facts and Comparisons, Feb 1992, 251j–251l.

Indomethacin

1. Holt GA. *Food & Drug Interactions.* Chicago: Precept Press, 1998, 139–40.

2. Tan SY, Shapiro R, Franco R, et al. Indomethacin-induced prostaglandin inhibition with hyper kalemia. *Ann Intern Med* 1979;90:783–85.

3. Goldszer RC, Coodley EL, Rosner MJ, et al. Hyperkalemia associated with indomethacin. *Arch Intern Med* 1981;141:802–4.

4. Threlkeld DS, ed. Central Nervous System Drugs, Nonsteroidal Anti-Inflammatory Agents. In *Facts and Comparisons Drug Information.* St. Louis, MO: Facts and Comparisons, Mar 1993, 252–252a.

5. Hodges R. *Nutrition in Medical Practice.* Philadelphia: W. B. Saunders, 1980, 323–31 [review].

6. Ogilry CS, DuBois AB, Douglas JS. Effects of ascorbic acid and indomethacin on the airways of healthy male subjects with and without induced bronchonstriction. *J Allerg Clin Immunol* 1981;67:363–69.

7. Holt GA. *Food & Drug Interactions.* Chicago, Precept Press, 1998, 138,140.

8. Smova L, Zaharieva S, Ivanova M. Humoral factors involved in the regulation of sodium-fluid balance in normal man. II. Effects of indomethacin on sodium concentration, renal prostaglandins, vasopressin and renin-angiotensin-aldosterone system. *Acta Physiol Pharmacol Bulg* 1984;10:29–33.

9. Threlkeld DS, ed. Central Nervous System Drugs, Nonsteroidal Anti-Inflammatory Agents. In *Facts and Comparisons Drug Information.* St. Louis, MO: Facts and Comparisons, Mar 1993, 252–252a.

10. Holt GA. *Food & Drug Interactions.* Chicago, Precept Press, 1998, 138–39.

11. Threlkeld DS, ed. Central Nervous System Drugs, Nonsteroidal Anti-Inflammatory Agents. In *Facts and Comparisons Drug Information.* St. Louis, MO: Facts and Comparisons, Mar 1993, 252–252a.

12. Holt GA. *Food & Drug Interactions.* Chicago, Precept Press, 1998, 137–38.

Influenza Virus Vaccine

1. Scaglione F, Cattaneo G, Alessandria M, Cogo R. Efficacy and safety of the standardized ginseng extract G 115 for potentiating vaccination against common cold and/or influenza syndrome. *Drugs Exptl Clin Res* 1996;22:65–72.

2. Zykov MP, Protasova SF. Prospects of immunostimulating vaccination against influenza including the use of *Eleutherococcus* and other preparations of plants. In *New Data on Eleutherococcus: Proceedings of the Second International Symposium on Eleutherococcus*, Moscow, 1984, 164–69.

Insulin

1. Sharma RD, Raghuram TC, Sudhakar Rao N. Effect of fenugreek seeds on blood glucose and serum lipids in type 1 diabetes. *Eur J Clin Nutr* 1990;44:301–6.

2. Sharma RD, Sakar A, Hazra DK, et al. Use of fenugreek seed powder in the management of non-insulin dependent diabetes mellitus. *Nutr Res* 1996;16:1131–39.

3. Shanmugasundaram ER, Rajeswari G, Baskaran K, et al. Use of *Gymnema sylvestre* leaf extract in the control of blood glucose in insulin-dependent diabetes mellitus. *J Ethnopharmacol* 1990;30:281–94.

4. Threlkeld DS, ed. Hormones, Antidiabetic Agents, Insulin. In *Facts and Comparisons Drug Information.* St. Louis, MO: Facts and Comparisons, Oct 1997, 129f–129j.

5. Threlkeld DS, ed. Hormones, Antidiabetic Agents, Insulin. In *Facts and Comparisons Drug Information.* St. Louis, MO: Facts and Comparisons, Oct 1997, 129f–129j.

Interferon

1. Beloqui O, Prieto J, Sua'rez B, et al. N-acetyl cysteine enhances the response to interferon-alpha in chronic hepatitis C: A pilot study. *J Interferon Res* 1993;13:279–82.

2. Farhat BA, Marinos G, Daniels HM, et al. Evaluation of efficacy and safety of thymus humoral factor-gamma 2 in the management of chronic hepatitis B. *J Hepatol* 1995;23:21–27.

3. Nakagawa A, Yamaguchi I, Takao T, Amano H. Five cases of drug-induced pneumonitis due to sho-saiko-to or interferon alpha or both. *Nippon Kyobu Shikkan Gakkai Zasshi* 1995;33:1361–66 [in Japanese].

4. Ishizaki T, Sasaki F, Ameshima S, et al. Pneumonitis during interferon and/or herbal drug therapy in patients with chronic active hepatitis. *Eur Respir J* 1996;9:2691–96.

5. Sugiyama H, Nagai M, Kotajima F, et al. A case of interstitial pneumonia with chronic hepatitis C following interferon-alpha and sho-saiko-to therapy. *Arerugi* 1995;44:711–14 [in Japanese].

6. Sato A, Toyoshima M, Kondo A, et al. Pneumonitis induced by the herbal medicine sho-saiko-to in Japan. *Nippon Kyobu Shikkan Gakkai Zasshi* 1997;35:391–95 [in Japanese].

7. Fujisawa K. Interferon therapy in hepatitis C virus (HCV) induced chronic hepatitis: Clinical significance of pretreatment with glycyrrhizine. *Trop Gastroenterol* 1991;12:176–79.

8. Abe Y, Ueda T, Kato T, et al. Effectiveness of interferon, glycyrrhizin combination therapy in patients with chronic hepatitis C. *Nippon Rinsho* 1994;52:1817–22 [in Japanese].

Ipratropium Bromide
Ipratropium Bromide/Albuterol

1. Threlkeld DS, ed. Respiratory Drugs, Respiratory Inhalant Products, Anticholinergies, Ipratropium Bromide. In *Facts and Comparisons Drug Information*. St. Louis, MO: Facts and Comparisons, Jun 1996, 182f–182g.

Isoniazid

1. Holt GA. *Food & Drug Interactions*. Chicago: Precept Press, 1998, 147.

2. Mandell GL, Petri WA Jr. Antimicrobial Agents: Drugs used in the chemotherapy of tuberculosis, *Mycobacterium avium* complex disease and leprosy. In *Goodman and Gilman's The Pharmacological Basis of Therapeutics*, 9th ed. New York: McGraw-Hill, 1996, 1158.

3. Brent J, Vo N, Kulig K, Rumack BH. Reversal of prolonged isoniazid-induced coma by pyridoxine. *Arch Intern Med* 1990;150:1751–53.

4. Holt GA. *Food & Drug Interactions*. Chicago: Precept Press, 1998, 147.

5. Werbach MR. *Foundations of Nutritional Medicine*. Tarzana, CA: Third Line Press, 1997, 231–32 [review].

6. Holt GA. *Food & Drug Interactions.* Chicago, Precept Press, 1998, 146–47.

7. Aoki K, Tokiwa T, Yamamoto T, Teramatsu T. Combined treatment of pulmonary tuberculosis with glycyrrhizin and INH. *Acta Tubercul Japon* 1963;13:32–39.

8. Threlkeld DS, ed. Systemic Anti-Infectives, Antituberculosis Drugs, Isoniazid. In *Facts and Comparisons Drug Information.* St. Louis, MO: Facts and Comparisons, Mar 1990, 382–385.

9. Threlkeld DS, ed. Systemic Anti-Infectives, Antituberculosis Drugs, Isoniazid. In *Facts and Comparisons Drug Information.* St. Louis, MO: Facts and Comparisons, Mar 1990, 382–385.

10. Holt GA. *Food & Drug Interactions.* Chicago: Precept Press, 1998, 146.

11. Threlkeld DS, ed. Systemic Anti-Infectives, Antituberculosis Drugs, Isoniazid. In *Facts and Comparisons Drug Information.* St. Louis, MO: Facts and Comparisons, Mar 1990, 382–385.

12. Threlkeld DS, ed. Systemic Anti-Infectives, Antituberculosis Drugs, Isoniazid. In *Facts and Comparisons Drug Information.* St. Louis, MO: Facts and Comparisons, Mar 1990, 382–385.

13. Holt GA. *Food & Drug Interactions.* Chicago: Precept Press, 1998, 144.

Isosorbide Mononitrate

1. Svendsen JH, Klarlund K, Aldershvile J, Waldorff S. N-acetylcysteine modifies the acute effects of isosorbide-5-mononitrate in angina pectoris patients evaluated by exercise testing. *J Cardiovasc Pharmacol* 1989;13:320–23.

2. Watanabe H, Kakihana M, Ohtsuka S, Sugishita Y. Randomized, double-blind, placebo-controlled study of the preventive effect of supplemental oral vitamin C on attentuation of development of nitrate tolerance. *J Am Coll Cardiol* 1998;31:1323–29.

3. Bassenge E, Fink N, Skatchkov M, Fink B. Dietary supplement with vitamin C prevents nitrate tolerance. *J Clin Invest* 1998;102:67–71.

4. Threlkeld DS, ed. Diuretics and Cardiovasculars, Antianginal Agents, Nitrates. In *Facts and Comparisons Drug Information.* St. Louis, MO: Facts and Comparisons, Apr 1992, 143e.

5. Kosoglou T, Kazierad DJ, Schentag JJ, et al. Effect of food on the oral bioavailability of isosorbide-5-mononitrate administered as an extended-release tablet. *J Clin Pharmacol* 1995;35:151–58.

6. Threlkeld DS, ed. Diuretics and Cardiovasculars, Antianginal Agents, Nitrates. In *Facts and Comparisons Drug Information.* St. Louis, MO: Facts and Comparisons, Apr 1992, 143e.

7. Threlkeld DS, ed. Diuretics and Cardiovasculars, Antianginal Agents, Nitrates. In *Facts and Comparisons Drug Information.* St. Louis, MO: Facts and Comparisons, Apr 1992, 143e.

Lansoprazole

1. Tang G, Serfaty-Lacronsniere C, Camilo ME, Russell RM. Gastric acidity influences the blood response to a beta-carotene dose in humans. *Am J Clin Nutr* 1996;64:622–26.

2. Marcuard SP, Albernaz L, Khazanie PG. Omeprazole therapy causes malabsorption of cyanocobalamin (Vitamin B12). *Ann Intern Med* 1994;120:211–15.

3. Termanini B, Gibril F, Sutliff VE, et al. Effect of long-term gastric acid suppressive therapy on serum vitamin B12 levels in patients with Zollinger-Ellison syndrome. *Am J Med* 1998;104:422–30.

4. Koop H, Bachem MG. Serum iron, ferritin, and vitamin B12 during prolonged omeprazole therapy. *J Clin Gastroenterol* 1992;14:288–92.

5. Schenk BE, Festen HP, Kuipers EJ, et al. Effect of short-and long-term treatment with omeprazole on the absorption and serum levels of cobalamin. *Aliment Pharmacol Ther* 1996;10:541–45.

6. Saltzman JR, Kemp JA, Golner BB, et al. Effect of hypochlorhydria due to omeprazole treatment or atrophic gastritis on protein-bound vitamin B12 absorption. *J Am Coll Nutr* 1994;13:584–91.

7. Saltzman JR, Kemp JA, Golner BB, et al. Effect of hypochlorhydria due to omeprazole treatment or atrophic gastritis on protein-bound vitamin B12 absorption. *J Am Coll Nutr* 1994;13:584–91.

8. Brummer RJ, Geerling BJ, Stockbrugger RW. Initial and chronic gastric acid inhibition by lansoprazole and omeprazole in relation to meal administration. *Dig Dis Sci* 1997;42:2132–37.

9. Threlkeld DS, ed. Gastrointestinal Drugs, Proton Pump Inhibitors. In *Facts and Comparisons Drug Information*. St. Louis, MO: Facts and Comparisons, Apr 1998, 305r.

Levodopa

Carbidopa/Levodopa

1. Long JW. *The Essential Guide to Prescription Drugs 1992*. New York: Harper Perennial, 1991.

2. Trovato A et al. Drug-nutrient interactions. *Am Family Phys* 1991;44:1651–58.

3. Threlkeld DS, ed. Central Nervous System Drugs, Antiparkinson Agents, Levodopa. In *Facts and Comparisons Drug Information*. St. Louis, MO: Facts and Comparisons, Sep 1991, 289p–290a.

4. Threlkeld DS, ed. Central Nervous System Drugs, Antiparkinson Agents, Levodopa. In *Facts and Comparisons Drug Information*. St. Louis, MO: Facts and Comparisons, Sep 1991, 289p–290a.

Lisinopril

1. Good CB, McDermott L, McCloskey B. Diet and serum potassium in patients on ACE inhibitors. *JAMA* 1995;274:538.

2. Golik A, Zaidenstein R, Dishi V, et al. Effects of captopril and enalapril on zinc metabolism in hypertensive patients. *J Am Coll Nutr* 1998;17:75–78.

3. Mojaverian P, Rocci ML Jr, Vlasses PH, et al. Effect of food on the bioavailability of lisinopril, a nonsulfhydryl angiotensin-converting enzyme inhibitor. *J Pharm Sci* 1986;75:395–97.

Lithium

1. Lieb J. Linoleic acid in the treatment of lithium toxicity and familial tremor. *Prostaglandins Med* 1980;4:275–9.

2. Coppen A, Abou-Saleh MT. Plasma folate and affective morbidity during long-term lithium therapy. *Br J Psychiatry* 1982;141:87–89.

3. Lee S, Chow CC, Shek CC, et al. Folate concentration in Chinese psychiatric outpatients on long-term lithium treatment. *J Affect Disorders* 1992;24:265–70.

4. Stern SL, Brandt JT, Hurley RS, et al. Serum and red cell folate concentrations in outpatients receiving lithium carbonate. *Int Clin Psychopharmacol* 1988;3:49–52.

5. Coppen A, Chaudhry S, Swade C. Folic acid enhances lithium prophylaxis. *J Affect Disorders* 1986;10:9–13.

6. Brewerton TD, Reus VI. Lithium carbonate and L-tryptophan in the treatment of bipolar and schizoaffective disorders. *Am J Psychiatry* 1983;140:757–60.

7. Threlkeld DS, ed. Central Nervous System Drugs, Antipsychotic Agents, Antimanic Agents, Lithium. In *Facts and Comparisons Drug Information*. St. Louis, MO: Facts and Comparisons, May 1998, 268a–268f.

8. Holt GA. *Food & Drug Interactions*. Chicago: Precept Press, 1998, 158.

9. Perlman BB. Interaction between lithium salt and ispaghula husk. *Lancet* 1990;335:416.

10. Threlkeld DS, ed. Central Nervous System Drugs, Antipsychotic Agents, Antimanic Agents, Lithium. In *Facts and Comparisons Drug Information*. St. Louis, MO: Facts and Comparisons, May 1998, 268a–268f.

11. Holt GA. *Food & Drug Interactions*. Chicago: Precept Press, 1998, 157.

12. Jefferson JW. Lithium tremor and caffeine intake: two cases of drinking less and shaking more. *J Clin Psychiatry* 1988;49:72–73.

13. Mester R, Toren P, Mizrachi I, et al. Caffeine withdrawal increases lithium blood levels. *Biol Psychiatry* 1995;37:348–50.

Loop Diuretics

1. Martin B, Milligan K. Diuretic-associated hypomagnesiumia in the elderly. *Arch Intern Med* 1987;147:1768–71.

2. Kroenke K, Wood DR, Hanley JF. The value of serum magnesium determination in hypertensive patients receiving diuretics. *Arch Intern Med* 1987;147:1553–56.

3. Whang R, Whang DD, Ryan MP. Refractory potassium repletion—a consequence of magnesium deficiency. *Arch Intern Med* 1992;152:40–45.

4. Brady JA, Rock CL, Horneffer MR. Thiamin status, diuretic medications, and the management of congestive heart failure. *J Am Dietet Assoc* 1995;95:541–44.

5. Seligman H, Halkin H, Rauchfleisch S, et al. Thiamine deficiency in patients with congestive heart failure receiving long-term furosemide therapy: A pilot study. *Am J Med* 1991;91:151–55.

6. Shimon I, Almog S, Vered Z, et al. Improved left ventricular function after thiamine supplementation in patients with congestive heart failure receiving long-term furosemide therapy. *Am J Med* 1995;98:485–90.

7. Brinker F. *Herb Contraindications and Drug Interactions.* Sandy, OR: Eclectic Institute, 1997, 102–3.

8. Threlkeld DS, ed. Diuretics and Cardiovasculars, Thiazides and Related Diuretics. In *Facts and Comparisons Drug Information.* St. Louis, MO: Facts and Comparisons Drug Information, Apr 1993, 135a–137c.

9. Shintani S, Murase H, Tsukagoshi H, Shiigai T. Glycyrrhizin (licorice)-induced hypokalemic myopathy. Report of two cases and review of the literature. *Eur Neurol* 1992;32:44–51.

10. Threlkeld DS, ed. Diuretics and Cardiovasculars, Loop Diuretics. In *Facts and Comparisons Drug Information.* St. Louis, MO: Facts and Comparisons, Apr 1994, 137d–138.

11. Threlkeld DS, ed. Diuretics and Cardiovasculars, Loop Diuretics. In *Facts and Comparisons Drug Information.* St. Louis, MO: Facts and Comparisons, Apr 1994, 137d–138.

12. Threlkeld DS, ed. Diuretics and Cardiovasculars, Loop Diuretics. In *Facts and Comparisons Drug Information.* St. Louis, MO: Facts and Comparisons, Apr 1994, 137d–138.

Loperamide

1. Threlkeld DS, ed. Gastrointestinal Drugs, Antidiarrheals, Loperamide HCl.I In *Facts and Comparisons Drug Information.* St. Louis, MO: Facts and Comparisons, Aug 1993, 324b–324c.

Loratadine

Loratadine/Pseudoephedrine

1. Threlkeld DS, ed. Respiratory Drugs, Antihistamines. In *Facts and Comparisons Drug Information.* St. Louis, MO: Facts and Comparisons, May 1998, 194b.

2. Threlkeld DS, ed. Respiratory Drugs, Antihistamines. In *Facts and Comparisons Drug Information.* St. Louis, MO: Facts and Comparisons, May 1998, 194b.

3. Threlkeld DS, ed. Respiratory Drugs, Antihistamines. In *Facts and Comparisons Drug Information*. St. Louis, MO: Facts and Comparisons, May 1998, 194b.

Losartan

1. Burnier M, Rutschmann B, Nussberger J, et al. Salt-dependent renal effects of an angiotensin II antagonist in healthy subjects. *Hypertension* 1993;22:339–47.

2. Threlkeld DS, ed. Diuretics and Cardiovasculars, Antihypertensives, Angiotensin II Receptor Antagonists. In *Facts and Comparisons Drug Information*. St. Louis, MO: Facts and Comparisons, Sep 1998, 165w–165x.

Lovastatin

1. Mortensen SA, Leth A, Agner E, Rohde M. Dose-related decrease of serum coenzyme Q10 during treatment with HMG-CoA reductase inhibitors. *Mol Aspects Med* 1997;18(suppl):S137–44.

2. Bargossi AM, Grossi G, Fiorella PL, et al. Exogenous CoQ10 supplementation prevents plasma ubiquinone reduction induced by HMG-CoA reductase inhibitors. *Molec Aspects Med* 1994;15(suppl):s187–93.

3. Paloma'ki A, Malminiemi K, Solakivi T, Malminiemi O. Ubiquinone supplementation during lovastatin treatment: Effect of LDL oxidation ex vivo. *J Lipid Res* 1998;39:1430–37.

4. Richter W, Jacob B, Schwandt P. Interaction between fibre and lovastatin. *Lancet* 1991;338:706 [letter].

5. Garnett WR. Interactions with hydroxymethylglutaryl-coenzyme A reductase inhibitors. *Am J Health Syst Pharm* 1995;52:1639–45.

6. Malloy MJ, Kane JP, Kunitake ST, Tun P. Complimentarity of colestipol, niacin, and lovastatin in treatment of severe familial hypercholesterolemia. *Ann Intern Med* 1987;107:616–23.

7. Gardner SF, Schneider EF, Granberry MG, Carter IR. Combination therapy with low-dose lovastatin and niacin is as effective as higher-dose lovastatin. *Pharmacotherapy* 1996;16:419–23.

8. Muggeo M, Zenti MG, Travia D, et al. Serum retinol levels throughout two years of cholesterol-lowering therapy. *Metabolism* 1995;44:398–403.

9. Heber D, Yip I, Ashley JM, et al. Cholesterol-lowering effects of a proprietary Chinese red-yeast-rice dietary supplement. *Am J Clin Nutr* 1999;69:231–36.

10. Threlkeld DS, ed. Diuretics and Cardiovasculars, Antihyperlipidemic Agents, HMG-CoA Reductase Inhibitors. In *Facts and Comparisons Drug Information*. St. Louis, MO: Facts and Comparisons, Sep 1998, 171v.

11. Threlkeld DS, ed. Diuretics and Cardiovasculars, Antihyperlipidemic Agents, HMG-CoA Reductase Inhibitors. In *Facts and Comparisons Drug Information*. St. Louis, MO: Facts and Comparisons, Sep 1998, 171v.

12. Kantola T, Kivisto KT, Neuvonen PJ. Grapefruit juice greatly increases serum concentrations of lovastatin and lovastatin acid. *Clin Pharmacol Ther* 1998;63:396–402.

Magnesium Hydroxide

1. O'Neil-Cutting MA, Crosby WH. The effect of antacids on the absorption of simultaneously ingested iron. *JAMA* 1986;255:1468–70.

2. Dyckner T, Wester PO. Ventricular extrasystoles and intracellular electrolytes before and after potassium and magnesium infusions in patients on diuretic treatment. *Am Heart J* 1979;97:12–18.

Medroxyprogesterone
Medroxyprogesterone/Conjugated Estrogens

1. Herzberg M, Lusky A, Blonder J, Frenkel. The effect of estrogen replacement therapy on zinc in serum and urine. *Obstet Gynecol* 1996;87:1035–40.

2. Joshi UM, Virkar KD, Amatayakul K, et al. Impact of hormonal contraceptives vis-a-vis non-hormonal factors on the vitamin status of malnourished women in India and Thailand. World Health Organization: Special Programme of Research, Development and Research Training in Human Reproduction. Task Force on Oral Contraceptives. *Hum Nutr Clin Nutr* 1986;40:205–20.

3. Bikle DD, Halloran BP, Harris ST, Portale AA. Progestin antagonism of estrogen stimulated 1,25-dihydroxyvitamin D levels. *J Clin Endocrinol Metab* 1992;75:519–23.

4. Komulainen M, Tuppurainen MT, Kroger H, et al. Vitamin D and HRT: no benefit additional to that of HRT alone in prevention of bone loss in early postmenopausal women. A 2.5-year randomized placebo-controlled study. *Osteoporosis Int* 1997;7:126–32.

Metformin

1. Carpentier JL, Bury J, Luyckx A, Lefebvre P. Vitamin B 12 and folic acid serum levels in diabetics under various therapeutic regimens. *Diabete Metab* 1976;2:187–90.

2. Carlsen SM, Folling I, Grill V, et al. Metformin increases total serum homocysteine levels in non-diabetic male patients with coronary heart disease. *Scand J Clin Lab Invest* 1997;57:521–27.

3. McBain AM, Brown IR, Menzies DG, Campbell IW. Effects of improved glycaemic control on calcium and magnesium homeostasis in type II diabetes. *J Clin Pathol* 1988;41:933–35.

4. Gin H, Orgerie MB, Aubertin J. The influence of guar gum on absorption of metformin from the gut in healthy volunteers. *Horm Metab Res* 1989;21:81–83.

5. Cardot JM, Saffar F, Aiache JM. Influence of food on glycemia, insulin, C-peptide and glucagon levels in diabetic patients treated with antidiabetic metformin at steady-state. *Methods Find Exp Clin Pharmacol* 1997;19:715–21.

6. Sambol NC, Brookes LG, Chiang J, et al. Food intake and dosage level, but not tablet vs solution dosage form, affect the absorption of metformin HCl in man. *Br J Clin Pharmacol* 1996;42:510–12.

7. Threlkeld DS, ed. Hormones, Antidiabetic Agents, Biguanides, Metformin HCl. In *Facts and Comparisons Drug Information*. St. Louis, MO: Facts and Comparisons, May 1995, 130n–130u.

Methotrexate

1. Threlkeld DS, ed. Antineoplastics, Antimetabolites, Methotrexate. In *Facts and Comparisons Drug Information*. St. Louis, MO: Facts and Comparisons, Aug 1990.

2. Morgan SL, Baggott JE, Vaughn WH, et al. Supplementation with folic acid during methotrexate therapy for rheumatoid arthritis. A double-blind, placebo-controlled trial. *Ann Intern Med* 1994;121:833–41.

3. Shiroky JB, Neville C, Esdaile JM, et al. Low-dose methotrexate with leucovorin (folinic acid) in the management of rheumatoid arthritis. Results of a multicenter randomized, double-blind, placebo-controlled trial. *Arthrit Rheum* 1993;36:795.

4. Duhra P. Treatment of gastrointestinal symptoms associated with methotrexate therapy for psoriasis. *J Am Acad Dermatol* 1993;28:466–69.

5. Holt GA. *Food & Drug Interactions*. Chicago: Precept Press, 1998, 170.

6. Threlkeld DS, ed. Antineoplastics, Antimetabolites, Methotrexate. In *Facts and Comparisons Drug Information*. St. Louis, MO: Facts and Comparisons, Aug 1990, 653–654.

7. Threlkeld DS, ed. Antineoplastics, Antimetabolites, Methotrexate. In *Facts and Comparisons Drug Information*. St. Louis, MO: Facts and Comparisons, Aug 1990, 653–654.

Methyldopa

1. Campbell NR, Hasinoff BB. Iron supplements: A common cause of drug interactions. *Brit J Clin Pharmacol* 1991;31:251–55.

2. Campbell N, Paddock V, Sundaram R. Alteration of methyldopa absorption, metabolism, and blood pressure control caused by ferrous sulfate and gluconate. *Clin Pharmacol Ther* 1988;43:381–86.

3. Holt GA. *Food & Drug Interactions*. Chicago: Precept Press, 1998, 74.

4. Holt GA. *Food & Drug Interactions*. Chicago: Precept Press, 1998, 171–72.

5. Holt GA. *Food & Drug Interactions*. Chicago: Precept Press, 1998, 170–71.

Methylphenidate

1. Threlkeld DS, ed. Central Nervous System Drugs, Miscellaneous Psychotherapeutic Agents, Methylphenidate HCl. In *Facts and Compar-*

isons Drug Information. St. Louis, MO: Facts and Comparisons, Feb 1997, 268t–268v.

2. Chan YP, Swanson JM, Soldin SS, et al. Methylphenidate hydrochloride given with or before breakfast: II. Effects on plasma concentration of methylphenidate and ritalinic acid. *Pediatrics* 1983;72:56–59.

3. Swanson JM, Sandman CA, Deutsch C, Baren M. Methylphenidate hydrochloride given with or before breakfast: I. Behavioral, cognitive, and electrophysiologic effects. *Pediatrics* 1983;72:49–55.

4. Threlkeld DS, ed. Central Nervous System Drugs, Miscellaneous Psychotherapeutic Agents, Methylphenidate HCl. In *Facts and Comparisons Drug Information.* St. Louis, MO: Facts and Comparisons, Feb 1997, 268t–268v.

5. Threlkeld DS, ed. Central Nervous System Drugs, Miscellaneous Psychotherapeutic Agents, Methylphenidate HCl. In *Facts and Comparisons Drug Information.* St. Louis, MO: Facts and Comparisons, Feb 1997, 268t–268v.

Metoprolol

Metoprolol/Hydrochlorothiazide

1. Melander A, Danielson K, Schersten B, Wahlin E. Enhancement of the bioavailability of propranolol and metoprolol by food. *Clin Pharmacol Ther* 1977;22:108–12.

2.Threlkeld DS, ed. Diuretics and Cardiovasculars, Beta-Adrenergic Blocking Agents. In *Facts and Comparisons Drug Information.* St. Louis, MO: Facts and Comparisons, Oct 1992, 158p–158q.

3. Threlkeld DS, ed. Diuretics and Cardiovasculars, Beta-Adrenergic Blocking Agents. In *Facts and Comparisons Drug Information.* St. Louis, MO: Facts and Comparisons, Feb 1993, 158p–158q.

Metronidazole

Metronidazole/Bismuth Subsalicylate/Tetracycline

1. Morazzoni P, Bombardelli E. *Silybum marianum* (*Carduus marianus*). *Fitoterapia* 1995;66:3–42 [review].

2. Threlkeld DS, ed. Systemic Anti-Infectives, Metronidazole. In *Facts and Comparisons Drug Information.* St. Louis, MO: Facts and Comparisons, Nov 1992, 353a–353e.

Mineral Oil

1. Holt GA. *Food & Drug Interactions.* Chicago: Precept Press, 1998, 176.

2. Clark JH, Russell GJ, Fitzgerald JF, Nagamori KE. Serum beta-carotene, retinol, and alpha-tocopherol levels during mineral oil therapy for constipation. *Am J Dis Child* 1987;141:1210–12.

Nabumetone

1. Sorenson JRJ. Copper chelates as possible active forms of the antiarthritic agents. *J Medicinal Chem* 1976;19:135–48.

2. Bjarnason I, Macpherson AJ. Intestinal toxicity of non-steroidal anti-inflammatory drugs. *Pharmacol Ther* 1994;62:145–57.

3. Threlkeld DS, ed. Blood Modifiers, Iron-Containing Products. In *Facts and Comparisons Drug Information*. St. Louis, MO: Facts and Comparisons, Jun 1998, 62–69a.

4. Bailie GR. Acute renal failure. In *Applied Therapeutics: The Clinical Use of Drugs*, 6th ed. Vancouver, WA: Applied Therapeutics, 1995, 29–33.

5. Threlkeld DS, ed. Central Nervous System Drugs, Nonsteroidal Anti-Inflammatory Agents. In *Facts and Comparisons Drug Information*. St. Louis, MO: Facts and Comparisons, Mar 1993, 251i.

6. Rees WDW, Rhodes J, Wright JE, et al. Effect of deglycyrrhizinated liquorice on gastric mucosal damage by aspirin. *Scand J Gastroenterol* 1979;14:605–7.

7. Morgan AG, McAdam WAF, Pascoo C, Darnborough A. Comparison between cimetidine and Caved-S in the treatment of gastric ulceration, and subsequent maintenance therapy. *Gut* 1982;23:545–51.

8. Threlkeld DS, ed. Central Nervous System Drugs, Nonsteroidal Anti-Inflammatory Agents. In *Facts and Comparisons Drug Information*. St. Louis, MO: Facts and Comparisons, Feb 1992, 251i.

9. Threlkeld DS, ed. Central Nervous System Drugs, Nonsteroidal Anti-Inflammatory Agents. In *Facts and Comparisons Drug Information*. St. Louis, MO: Facts and Comparisons, Feb 1992, 251i.

Naproxen

Naproxen Sodium

1. Sorenson JRJ. Copper chelates as possible active forms of the antiarthritic agents. *J Medicinal Chem* 1976;19:135–48.

2. Bjarnason I, Macpherson AJ. Intestinal toxicity of non-steroidal anti-inflammatory drugs. *Pharmacol Ther* 1994;62:145–57.

3. Threlkeld DS, ed. Blood Modifiers, Iron-Containing Products. In *Facts and Comparisons Drug Information*. St. Louis, MO: Facts and Comparisons, Jun 1998, 62–69a.

4. Bailie GR. Acute renal failure. In *Applied Therapeutics: The Clinical Use of Drugs*, 6th ed. Vancouver, WA: Applied Therapeutics, 1995, 29–33.

5. Threlkeld DS, ed. Central Nervous System Drugs, Nonsteroidal Anti-Inflammatory Agents. In *Facts and Comparisons Drug Information*. St. Louis, MO: Facts and Comparisons, Mar 1993, 251n–251o.

6. Rees WDW, Rhodes J, Wright JE, et al. Effect of deglycyrrhizinated liquorice on gastric mucosal damage by aspirin. *Scand J Gastroenterol* 1979;14:605–7.

7. Morgan AG, McAdam WAF, Pascoo C, Darnborough A. Comparison between cimetidine and Caved-S in the treatment of gastric ulceration, and subsequent maintenance therapy. *Gut* 1982;23:545–51.

8. Threlkeld DS, ed. Central Nervous System Drugs, Nonsteroidal Anti-Inflammatory Agents. In *Facts and Comparisons Drug Information.* St. Louis, MO: Facts and Comparisons, Feb 1992, 251n–251o.

9. Threlkeld DS, ed. Central Nervous System Drugs, Nonsteroidal Anti-Inflammatory Agents. In *Facts and Comparisons Drug Information.* St. Louis, MO: Facts and Comparisons, Feb 1992, 251n–251o.

Nefazodone

1. Dockens RC, Greene DS, Barbhaiya RH. Assessment of pharmacokinetic and pharmacodynamic drug interactions between nefazodone and digoxin in healthy male volunteers. *J Clin Pharmacol* 1996;36:160–67.

2. Dockens RC, Greene DS, Barbhaiya RH. The lack effect of food on the bioavailability of nefazodone tablets. *Biopharm Drug Dispos* 1996;17:135–43.

3. Threlkeld DS, ed. Central Nervous System Drugs, Antidepressants, Trazodone. In *Facts and Comparisons Drug Information.* St. Louis, MO: Facts and Comparisons, Mar 1995, 263i–263k.

Neomycin

1. Roe DA. *Drug-Induced Nutritional Deficiencies,* 2d ed. Westport, CT: Avi Publishing, 1985, 157–58 [review].

2. Holt GA. *Food & Drug Interactions.* Chicago: Precept Press,1998, 183.

3. Holt GA. *Food & Drug Interactions.* Chicago, Precept Press, 1998, 183–84.

Nicotine

1. Threlkeld DS, ed. Miscellaneous Products, Smoking Deterrents, Lobeline. In *Facts and Comparisons Drug Information.* St. Louis, MO: Facts and Comparisons, Mar 1993, 736i.

2. Davison GC, Rosen RC. Lobeline and reduction of cigarette smoking. *Psychol Rep* 1972;31:443–56.

3. Threlkeld DS, ed. Miscellaneous Products, Smoking Deterrents, Nicotine. In *Facts and Comparisons Drug Information.* St. Louis, MO: Facts and Comparisons, Aug 1993, 736a–736h.

Nifedipine

1. Bailey DG, Arnold MO, Strong HA, Munoz C, Spence JD, et al. Effect of grapefruit juice and naringin on nisoldipine pharmacokinetics. *Clin Pharmacol Ther* 1993;54:589–94.

2. Reitberg DP, Love SJ, Quercia GT, Zinny MA. Effect of food on nifedipine pharmacokinetics. *Clin Pharmacol Ther* 1987;42:72–75.

3. Threlkeld DS, ed. Diuretics and Cardiovasculars, Calcium Channel Blocking Agents. In *Facts and Comparisons Drug Information*. St. Louis, MO: Facts and Comparisons, Mar 1996, 149m–149n.

4. Deanfield J, Wright C, Krikler S, et al. Cigarette smoking and the treatment of angina with propranolol, atenolol, and nifedipine. *N Engl J Med* 1984;310:951–54.

Nitrofurantoin

1. Naggar VF, Khalil SA. Effect of magnesium trisilicate on nitrofurantoin absorption. *Clin Pharmacol Ther* 1979;25:857–63.

2. Naggar VF, Khalil SA. Effect of magnesium trisilicate on nitrofurantoin absorption. *Clin Pharmacol Ther* 1979;25:857–63.

3. Soci MM, Parrott EL. Influence of viscosity on absorption from nitrofurantoin suspensions. *J Pharm Sci* 1980;69:403–6.

4. Rosenberg HA, Bates TR. The influence of food on nitrofurantoin bioavailability. *Clin Pharmacol Ther* 1976;20:227–32.

5. Threlkeld DS, ed. Systemic Anti-Infectives, Urinary Anti-Infectives, Nitrofurantoin. In *Facts and Comparisons Drug Information*. St. Louis, MO: Facts and Comparisons, Oct 1994, 431–433.

Nitroglycerin

1. Ghio S, de Servi S, Perotti R, et al. Different susceptibility to the development of nitroglycerin tolerance in the arterial and venous circulation in humans—Effects of *N*-acetylcysteine administration. *Circulation* 1992;86:798–802.

2. May DC, Popma JJ, Black WH, et al. In vivo induction and reversal of nitroglycerin tolerance in human coronary arteries. *N Engl J Med* 1987;317:805–9.

3. Iversen HK. N-acetylcysteine enhances nitroglycerin-induced headache and cranial artery response. *Clin Pharmacol Ther* 1992;52:125–33.

4. Ardissino D, Merlini PA, Savonitto S, et al. Effect of transdermal nitroglycerin or N-acetyl cysteine, or both, in the long-term treatment of unstable angina pectoris. *J Am Coll Cardiol* 1997;29:941–47.

5. Hogan JC, Lewis MJ, Henderson AH. N-acetylcysteine fails to attenuate haemodynamic tolerance to glycerol trinitrate in healthy volunteers. *Br J Clin Pharmacol* 1989;28:421–26.

6. Hogan JC, Lewis MJ, Henderson AH. Chronic administration of N-acetylcysteine fails to prevent nitrate tolerance in patients with stable angina pectoris. *Br J Clin Pharmacol* 1990;30:573–77.

7. Thelkeld DS, ed. Diuretics and Cardiovasculars, Antianginal Agents, Nitrates. In *Facts and Comparisons Drug Information*. St. Louis, MO: Facts and Comparisons, Apr 1992, 143f–144a.

Nitrous Oxide

1. Ermens AA, Refsum H, Rupreht J, et al. Monitoring cobalamin inactivation during nitrous oxide anesthesia by determination of

homocysteine and folate plasma and urine. *Clin Pharmacol Ther* 1991;49:385–93.

2. Flippo TS, Holder WD Jr. Neurologic degeneration associated with nitrous oxide anesthesia in patients with vitamin B12 deficiency. *Arch Surg* 1993;128:1391–95.

3. Nunn JF, Chanarin I, Tanner AG, Owen ER. Megaloblastic bone marrow changes after repeated nitrous oxide anesthesia. Reversal with folic acid. *Br J Anaesth* 1986;58:1469–70.

4. Amos RJ, Amess JA, Hinds CJ, Mollin DL. Investigations into the effect of nitrous oxide anesthesia on folate metabolism in patient receiving intensive care. *Chemioterapia* 1985;4:393–99.

5. Koblin DD, Tomerson BW, Waldman FM, et al. Effect of nitrous oxide on folate and vitamin B12 metabolism in patients. *Anesth Analg* 1990;71:610–17.

6. Amos RJ, Amess JAL, Hinds CJ, Mollin DL. Incidence and pathogenesis of acute megaloblastic bone-marrow change in patients receiving intensive care. *Lancet* 1982;ii:835–39.

Nizatidine

1. Aymard JP, Aymard B, Netter P, et al. Haematological adverse effects of histamine H2-receptor antagonists. *Med Toxicol Adverse Drug Exp* 1988;3:430–48.

2. Bachmann KA, Sullivan TJ, Jauregui L, et al. Drug interactions of H2-receptor antagonists. *Scand J Gastroenterol Suppl* 1994;206:14–19.

3. Aymard JP, Aymard B, Netter P, et al. Haematological adverse effects of histamine H2-receptor antagonists. *Med Toxicol Adverse Drug Exp* 1988;3:430–48.

4. Russell RM, Krasinski SD, Samloff IM. Correction of impaired folic acid (Pte Glu) absorption by orally administered HCl in subjects with gastric atrophy. *Am J Clin Nutr* 1984;39:656.

5. Tompsett SL. Factors influencing the aborption of iron and copper from the alimentary tract. *Biochem J* 1940;34:961–69.

6. Spiegel JE, Thoden WR, Pappas K, et al. A double-blind, placebo-controlled study of the effectiveness and safety of nizatidine in the prevention of postprandial heartburn. *Arch Intern Med* 1997;157:1594–99.

7. Duroux P, Emde C, Bauerfeind P, et al. Early evening nizatidine intake with a meal optimizes the antisecretory effect. *Aliment Pharmacol Ther* 1993;7:47–54.

8. Cerulli MA, Cloud ML, Offen WW, et al. Nizatidine as maintenance therapy of duodenal ulcer disease in remission. *Scand J Gastroenterol Suppl* 1987;136:79–83.

Ofloxacin

1. Lomaestro BM, Bailie GR. Quinolone-cation interactions: a review. *DICP* 1991;25:1249–58.

2. Threlkeld DS, ed. Systemic Anti-Infectives, Fluoroquinolones. In *Facts and Comparisons Drug Information.* St. Louis, MO: Facts and Comparisons, Feb 1994, 340q–340r.

3. Verho M, Malerczyk V, Rosenkranz B, Grotsch H. Absence of interaction between ofloxacin and phenprocoumon. *Curr Med Res Opin* 1987;10:474–79.

4. Dudley MN, Marchbanks CR, Flor SC, Beals B. The effect of food or milk on the absorption kinetics of ofloxacin. *Eur J Clin Pharmacol* 1991;41:569–71.

5. Neuvonen PJ, Kivisto KT. Milk and yoghurt do not impair the absorption of ofloxacin. *Br J Clin Pharmacol* 1992;33:346–48.

6. Dudley MN, Marchbanks CR, Flor SC, Beals B. The effect of food or milk on the absorption kinetics of ofloxacin. *Eur J Clin Pharmacol* 1991;41:569–71.

Omeprazole

1. Marcuard SP, Albernaz L, Khazanie PG. Omeprazole therapy causes malabsorption of cyanocobalamin (Vitamin B12). *Ann Intern Med* 1994;120:211–15.

2. Termanini B, Gibril F, Sutliff VE, et al. Effect of long-term gastric acid suppressive therapy on serum vitamin B12 levels in patients with Zollinger-Ellison syndrome. *Am J Med* 1998;104:422–30.

3. Koop H, Bachem MG. Serum iron, ferritin, and vitamin B12 during prolonged omeprazole therapy. *J Clin Gastroenterol* 1992;14:288–92.

4. Schenk BE, Festen HP, Kuipers EJ, et al. Effect of short-and long-term treatment with omeprazole on the absorption and serum levels of cobalamin. *Aliment Pharmacol Ther* 1996;10:541–45.

5. Saltzman JR, Kemp JA, Golner BB, et al. Effect of hypochlorhydria due to omeprazole treatment or atrophic gastritis on protein-bound vitamin B12 absorption. *J Am Coll Nutr* 1994;13:584–91.

6. Saltzman JR, Kemp JA, Golner BB, et al. Effect of hypochlorhydria due to omeprazole treatment or atrophic gastritis on protein-bound vitamin B12 absorption. *J Am Coll Nutr* 1994;13:584–91.

Oral Contraceptives

1. Lindenbaum J, Whitehead N, Reyner F. Oral contraceptive hormones, folate metabolism, and the cervical epithelium. *Am J Clin Nutr* 1975;28:346–53.

2. Frassinelli-Gunderson EP, Margen S, Brown JR. Iron stores in users of oral contraceptive agents. *Am J Clin Nutr* 1985;41(4):703.

3. Olatunbosum DA, Adeniyi FA, Adadevoh BK. Effect of oral contraceptives on serum magnesium levels. *Int J Fertil* 1974;19:224–26.

4. Blum M, Kitai E, Ariel Y, et al. Oral contraceptive lowers serum magnesium. *Harefuah* 1991;121:363–64.

5. Adams PW, Wynn V, Rose DP, et al. Effect of pyridoxine hydrochloride (vitamin B6) upon depression associated with oral contraception. *Lancet* 1973;I:897–904.

6. Werbach MR. *Foundations of Nutritional Medicine*. Tarzana, CA: Third Line Press, 1997, 210–11 [review].

7. Wynn V. Vitamins and oral contraceptive use. *Lancet* 1975;1:561–64.

8. Holt GA. *Food & Drug Interaction*. Chicago: Precept Press, 1998, 197–98.

9. Werbach MR. *Foundations of Nutritional Medicine*. Tarzana, CA: Third Line Press, 1997, 210–11 [review].

10. Wynn V. Vitamins and oral contraceptive use. *Lancet* 1975;1:561–64.

11. Holt GA. *Food & Drug Interaction*. Chicago: Precept Press, 1998, 197.

12. Threlkeld DS, ed. Hormones, Oral Contraceptives. In *Facts and Comparisons Drug Information*. St. Louis, MO: Facts and Comparisons, Jul 1994, 107b–108f.

13. Threlkeld DS, ed. Hormones, Oral Contraceptives. In *Facts and Comparisons Drug Information*. St. Louis, MO: Facts and Comparisons, Jul 1994, 107b–108f.

Oxaprozin

1. Sorenson JRJ. Copper chelates as possible active forms of the antiarthritic agents. *J Medicinal Chem* 1976;19:135–48.

2. Bjarnason I, Macpherson AJ. Intestinal toxicity of non-steroidal anti-inflammatory drugs. *Pharmacol Ther* 1994;62:145–57.

3. Threlkeld DS, ed. Blood Modifiers, Iron-Containing Products. In *Facts and Comparisons Drug Information*. St. Louis, MO: Facts and Comparisons, Jun 1998, 62–69a.

4. Bailie GR. Acute renal failure. In *Applied Therapeutics: The Clinical Use of Drugs*, 6th ed. Vancouver, WA: Applied Therapeutics, 1995, 29–33.

5. Threlkeld DS, ed. Central Nervous System Drugs, Nonsteroidal Anti-Inflammatory Agents. In *Facts and Comparisons Drug Information*. St. Louis, MO: Facts and Comparisons, Mar 1993, 252g.

6. Rees WDW, Rhodes J, Wright JE, et al. Effect of deglycyrrhizinated liquorice on gastric mucosal damage by aspirin. *Scand J Gastroenterol* 1979;14:605–7.

7. Morgan AG, McAdam WAF, Pascoo C, Darnborough A. Comparison between cimetidine and Caved-S in the treatment of gastric ulceration, and subsequent maintenance therapy. *Gut* 1982;23:545–51.

8. Threlkeld DS, ed. Central Nervous System Drugs, Nonsteroidal Anti-Inflammatory Agents. In *Facts and Comparisons Drug Information*. St. Louis, MO: Facts and Comparisons, Feb 1992, 252g.

9. Threlkeld DS, ed. Central Nervous System Drugs, Nonsteroidal Anti-Inflammatory Agents. In *Facts and Comparisons Drug Information*. St. Louis, MO: Facts and Comparisons, Feb 1992, 252g.

Oxycodone/Acetaminophen
Oxycodone/Aspirin

1. Threlkeld DS, ed. Central Nervous System Drugs, Narcotic Agonist Analgesics. In *Facts and Comparisons Drug Information*. St. Louis, MO: Facts and Comparisons, Feb 1990, 242–243v.

2. Threlkeld DS, ed. Central Nervous System Drugs, Narcotic Agonist Analgesics. In *Facts and Comparisons Drug Information*. St. Louis, MO: Facts and Comparisons, Feb 1990, 242–243v.

3. Threlkeld DS, ed. Central Nervous System Drugs, Narcotic Agonist Analgesics. In *Facts and Comparisons Drug Information*. St. Louis, MO: Facts and Comparisons, Feb 1990, 242–243v.

Paclitaxel

1. Savarese D, Boucher J, Corey B. Glutamine treatment of paclitaxel-induced myalgias and arthralgias. *J Clin Oncol* 1998;16:3918–19 [letter].

2. Boyle FM, Monk R, Davey R, et al. Prevention of experimental paclitaxel neuropathy with glutamate. *Proc AACR* 1996;37:290 [abstract].

Paroxetine

1. Threlkeld DS, ed. Central Nervous System Drugs, Antidepressants, Selective Serotonin Reuptake Inhibitors. In *Facts and Comparisons Drug Information*. St. Louis, MO: Facts and Comparisons, Apr 1997, 264q–264r.

2. Walinder J, Carlsson A, Persson R. 5-HT reuptake inhibitors plus tryptophan in endogenous depression. *Acta Psych Scand Suppl* 1981;290:179–90.

3. Spigset O, Hedenmalm K, Mortimer O. Hyponatremia as a side effect of serotonin uptake inhibitors. *Lakartidningen* 1998;95:3537–39 [Swedish].

4. Strachan J, Shepherd J. Hyponatraemia associated with the use of selective serotonin re-uptake inhibitors. *Aust N Z J Psychiatry* 1998;32:295–98.

5. Bouman WP, Pinner G, Johnson H. Incidence of selective serotonin reuptake inhibitor (SSRI) induced hyponatraemia due to the syndrome of antidiuretic hormone (SIADH) secretion in the elderly. *Int J Geriatr Psychiatry* 1998;13:12–15.

6. Cohen AJ. Long term safety and efficacy of *Ginkgo biloba* extract in the treatment of anti-depressant-induced sexual dysfunction. *Psychiatry On-Line* http://www.priory.com/ginkgo.html.

7. Sohn M, Sikora R. *Ginkgo biloba* extract in the therapy of erectile dysfunction. *J Sex Educ Ther* 1991;17:53–61.

8. Demott K. St. John's wort tied to serotonin syndrome. *Clinical Psychiatry News* 1998;26:28.

9. Gordon JB. SSRIs and St. John's Wort: possible toxicity? *Am Fam Physician* 1998;57:950.

10. Nemeroff CB. Paroxetine: an overview of the efficacy and safety of a new selective serotonin reuptake inhibitor in the treatment of depression. *J Clin Psychopharmacol* 1993;13(6 suppl 2):10S–17S [review].

11. Threlkeld DS, ed. Central Nervous System Drugs, Antidepressants, Selective Serotonin Reuptake Inhibitors. In *Facts and Comparisons Drug Information.* St. Louis, MO: Facts and Comparisons, Apr 1997, 264q–264r.

Penicillamine

1. Threlkeld DS, ed. Miscellaneous Products, Penicillamine. In *Facts and Comparisons Drug Information.* St. Louis, MO: Facts and Comparisons, Aug 1996, 714–716b.

2. Harkness JAL, Blake DR. Penicillamine nephropathy and iron. *Lancet* 1982;ii:1368–69.

3. Holt GA. *Food & Drug Interactions.* Chicago: Precept Press, 1998, 203.

4. Rothschild B. Pyridoxine deficiency. *Arch Intern Med* 1982;142:840.

5. Holt GA. *Food & Drug Interactions.* Chicago: Precept Press, 1998, 201.

6. Holt GA. *Food & Drug Interactions.* Chicago: Precept Press, 1998, 202

7. Threlkeld DS, ed. Miscellaneous Products, Penicillamine. In *Facts and Comparisons Drug Information.* St. Louis, MO: Facts and Comparisons, Aug 1996, 714–716b.

Penicillin V

1. Neubauer RA. A plant protease for potentiation of and possible replacement of antibiotics. *Exp Med Surg* 1961;19:143–60.

2. Huupponen R, Seppala P, Iisalo E. Effect of guar gum, a fibre preparation, on digoxin and penicillin absorption in man. *Eur J Clin Pharmacol* 1984;26:279–81.

3. Finkel Y, Bolme P, Eriksson M. The effect of food on the oral absorption of penicillin V preparations in children. *Acta Pharmacol Toxicol (Copenh)* 1981;49:301–4.

4. Guggenbichler JP, Kienel G. Bioavailability of orally administered antibiotics: influences of food on resorption. *Padiatr Padol* 1979;14:69–74 [German].

Pentoxifylline

1. Threlkeld DS, ed. Blood Modifiers, Hemorheologic Agent, Pentoxifylline. In *Facts and Comparisons Drug Information.* St. Louis, MO: Facts and Comparisons, Mar 1997, 89f–89g.

Phenelzine

1. Heller CA, Friedman PA. Pyridoxine deficiency and peripheral neuropathy associated with long-term phenelzine therapy. *Am J Med* 1983;75:887–88.

2. Threlkeld DS, ed. Central nervous system drugs, antidepressants, monoamine oxidase inhibitors. In *Facts and Comparisons Drug Information*. St. Louis, MO: Facts and Comparisons, Apr 1997, 264y.

3. Shader RI, Greenblatt DJ. Phenelzine and the dream machine-ramblings and reflections. *J Clin Psychopharmacol* 1985;5:65.

4. Jones BD, Runikis AM. Interaction of ginseng with phenelzine. *J Clin Psychopharmacol* 1987;7:201–2.

5. St. John's wort, *Hypericum perforatum*. In *American Herbal Pharmacopoeia and Therapeutic Compendium*, ed. R Upton. Santa Cruz, CA: AHP, 1997.

6. Brinker F. Interactions of pharmaceutical and botanical medicines. *J Naturopathic Med* 1997;7(2):14–20.

7. Threlkeld DS, ed. Central Nervous System Drugs, Antidepressants, Monoamine Oxidase Inhibitors. In *Facts and Comparisons Drug Information*. St. Louis, MO: Facts and Comparisons, Apr 1997, 264y.

8. Shader RI, Greenblatt DJ. Phenelzine and the dream machine-ramblings and reflections. *J Clin Psychopharmacol* 1985:5:65.

Phentermine

1. Threlkeld DS, ed. Central Nervous System Drugs, Anorexiants. In *Facts and Comparisons Drug Information*. St. Louis, MO: Facts and Comparisons, Mar 1989, 239.

2. Threlkeld DS, ed. Central Nervous System Drugs, Anorexiants. In *Facts and Comparisons Drug Information*. St. Louis, MO: Facts and Comparisons, Mar 1989, 239.

Phenylpropanolamine

1. Threlkeld DS, ed. Respiratory Drugs, Sympathomimetics. In *Facts and Comparisons Drug Information*. St. Louis, MO: Facts and Comparisons, May 1994, 173a–173h.

2. Hoffman BB, Lefkowitz RL. Catecholamines, sympathomimetic drugs, and adrenergic receptor antagonists. In *Goodman and Gilman's The Pharmcological Basis of Therapeutics*, 9th ed. New York: McGraw-Hill, 1996, 223.

3. Threlkeld DS, ed. Respiratory Drugs, Sympathomimetics. In *Facts and Comparisons Drug Information*. St. Louis, MO: Facts and Comparisons, Apr 1993, 173a–173h

4. Brown NJ, Ryder D, Branch RA. A pharmacodynamic interaction between caffeine and phenylpropanolamine. *Clin Pharmacol Ther* 1991;50:363–71.

5. Lake CR, Rosenberg DB, Gallant S, et al. Phenylpropanolamine increases plasma caffeine levels. *Clin Pharmacol Ther* 1990;47:675–85.

Potassium Chloride

1. Threlkeld DS, ed. Nutritional Products, Minerals and Electrolytes, Oral. Potassium Replacement Products. In *Facts and Compar-*

isons Drug Information. St. Louis, MO: Facts and Comparisons, Jul 1992, 15–16c.

2. Threlkeld DS, ed. Nutritional Products, Minerals and Electrolytes, Oral. Potassium Replacement Products. In *Facts and Comparisons Drug Information.* St. Louis, MO: Facts and Comparisons, Jul 1992, 15–16c.

3. Threlkeld DS, ed. Nutritional Products, Minerals and Electrolytes, Oral. Potassium Replacement Products. In *Facts and Comparisons Drug Information.* St. Louis, MO: Facts and Comparisons, Jul 1992, 15–16c.

4. Threlkeld DS, ed. Nutritional Products, Minerals and Electrolytes, Oral. Potassium Replacement Products. In *Facts and Comparisons Drug Information.* St. Louis, MO: Facts and Comparisons, Jul 1992, 15–16c.

5. Threlkeld DS, ed. Nutritional Products, Minerals and Electrolytes, Oral. Potassium Replacement Products. In *Facts and Comparisons Drug Information.* St. Louis, MO: Facts and Comparisons, Jul 1992, 15–16c.

Pravastatin

1. Mortensen SA, Leth A, Agner E, Rohde M. Dose-related decrease of serum coenzyme Q10 during treatment with HMG-CoA reductase inhibitors. *Mol Aspects Med* 1997;18(suppl):S137–44.

2. Bargossi AM, Grossi G, Fiorella PL, et al. Exogenous CoQ10 supplementation prevents plasma ubiquinone reduction induced by HMG-CoA reductase inhibitors. *Molec Aspects Med* 1994;15(suppl):s187–93.

3. Paloma'ki A, Malminiemi K, Solakivi T, Malminiemi O. Ubiquinone supplementation during lovastatin treatment: Effect of LDL oxidation ex vivo. *J Lipid Res* 1998;39:1430–7.

4. Gardner SF, Marx MA, White LM, et al. Combination of low-dose niacin and pravastatin improves the lipid profile in diabetic patients without compromising glycemic control. *Ann Pharmacother* 1997;31:677–82.

5. O'Keefe JH Jr, Harris WS, Nelson J, Windsor SL. Effects of pravastatin with niacin or magnesium on lipid levels and postprandial lipemia. *Am J Cardiol* 1995;76:480–84.

6. Garnett WR. Interactions with hydroxymethylglutaryl-coenzyme A reductase inhibitors. *Am J Health Syst Pharm* 1995;52:1639–45.

7. Heber D, Yip I, Ashley Jm, et al. Cholesterol-lowering effects of a proprietary Chinese red-yeast-rice dietary supplement. *Am J Clin Nutr* 1999;69:231–36.

8. Muggeo M, Zenti MG, Travia D, et al. Serum retinol levels throughout two years of cholesterol-lowering therapy. *Metabolism* 1995;44:398–403.

9. Threlkeld DS, ed. Diuretics and Cardiovasculars, Antihyperlipidemic Agents, HMG-CoA Reductase Inhibitors. In *Facts and Compar-*

isons Drug Information. St. Louis, MO: Facts and Comparisons, Sep 1998, 172.

10. Kantola T, Kivisto KT, Neuvonen PJ. Grapefruit juice greatly increases serum concentrations of lovastatin and lovastatin acid. *Clin Pharmacol Ther* 1998;63:397–402.

Prazosin

1. Jaillon P. Clinical pharmacokinetics of prazosin. *Clin Pharmacokinet* 1980;5:365–76 [review].

Promethazine

1. Blumenthal M, ed. *The Complete German Commission E Monographs.* Austin, TX: American Botanical Council, 1998, 146.

2. Threlkeld DS, ed. Respiratory Drugs, Antihistamines. In *Facts and Comparisons Drug Information.* St. Louis, MO: Facts and Comparisons, May 1998, 192b–192c.

3. Threlkeld DS, ed. Respiratory Drugs, Antihistamines. In *Facts and Comparisons Drug Information.* St. Louis, MO: Facts and Comparisons, May 1998, 192b–192c.

Propoxyphene

1. Threlkeld DS, ed. Central Nervous System Drugs, Narcotic Agonist Analgesics. In *Facts and Comparisons Drug Information.* St. Louis, MO: Facts and Comparisons, Feb 1990, 242–243v.

2. Threlkeld DS, ed. Central Nervous System Drugs, Narcotic Agonist Analgesics. In *Facts and Comparisons Drug Information.* St. Louis, MO: Facts and Comparisons, Feb 1990, 242–243v.

3. Threlkeld DS, ed. Central Nervous System Drugs, Narcotic Agonist Analgesics. In *Facts and Comparisons Drug Information.* St. Louis, MO: Facts and Comparisons, Feb 1990, 242–243v.

Propranolol

1. Hamada M, Kazatain Y, Ochi T, et al. Correlation between serum CoQ10 level and myocardial contractility in hypertensive patients. In *Biomedical and Clinical Aspects of Coenzyme Q,* vol 4, ed. K Folkers, Y Yamamura. Amsterdam: Elsevier, 1984, 263–70.

2. Bano G, Raina RK, Zutshi U, et al. Effect of piperine on bioavailability and pharmacokinetics of propranolol and theophylline in healthy volunteers. *Eur J Clin Pharmacol* 1991;41:615–17.

3. Threlkeld DS, ed. Diuretics and Cardiovasculars, Beta-Adrenergic Blocking Agents. In *Facts and Comparisons Drug Information.* St. Louis, MO: Facts and Comparisons, Feb 1993, 159a–159c.

4. Holt GA. *Food & Drug Interactions.* Chicago: Precept Press, 1998, 225.

5. Threlkeld DS, ed. Diuretics and Cardiovasculars, Beta-Adrenergic Blocking Agents. In *Facts and Comparisons Drug Information.* St. Louis, MO: Facts and Comparisons, Feb 1993, 159a–159c.

6. Deanfield J, Wright C, Krikler S, et al. Cigarette smoking and the treatment of angina with propranolol, atenolol, and nifedipine. *N Engl J Med* 1984;310:951–54.

Quinapril

1. Good CB, McDermott L, McCloskey B. Diet and serum potassium in patients on ACE inhibitors. *JAMA* 1995;274:538.

2. Golik A, Zaidenstein R, Dishi V, et al. Effects of captopril and enalapril on zinc metabolism in hypertensive patients. *J Am Coll Nutr* 1998;17:75–78.

3. Threlkeld DS, ed. Diuretics and Cardiovasculars, Antihypertensives, Angiotensin Converting Enzyme Inhibitors. In *Facts and Comparisons Drug Information.* St. Louis, MO: Facts and Comparisons, Apr 1998, 165q.

4. Ferry JJ, Horvath AM, Sedman AJ, et al.. Influence of food on the pharmacokinetics of quinapril and its active diacid metabolite, CI-928. *J Clin Pharmacol* 1987;27:397–99.

Ramipril

1. Good CB, McDermott L, McCloskey B. Diet and serum potassium in patients on ACE inhibitors. *JAMA* 1995;274:538.

2. Golik A, Zaidenstein R, Dishi V, et al. Effects of captopril and enalapril on zinc metabolism in hypertensive patients. *J Am Coll Nutr* 1998;17:75–78.

3. Threlkeld DS, ed. Diuretics and Cardiovasculars, Antihypertensives, Angiotensin Converting Enzyme Inhibitors. In *Facts and Comparisons Drug Information.* St. Louis, MO: Facts and Comparisons, Apr 1998, 165j.

Ranitidine

1. Aymard JP, Aymard B, Netter P, et al. Haematological adverse effects of histamine H2-receptor antagonists. *Med Toxicol Adverse Drug Exp* 1988;3:430–48.

2. Bachmann KA, Sullivan TJ, Jauregui L, et al. Drug interactions of H2-receptor antagonists. *Scand J Gastroenterol Suppl* 1994;206:14–19.

3. Aymard JP, Aymard B, Netter P, et al. Haematological adverse effects of histamine H2-receptor antagonists. *Med Toxicol Adverse Drug Exp* 1988;3:430–48.

4. Threlkeld DS, ed. Gastrointestinal Drugs, Histamine H2 Antagonists. In *Facts and Comparisons Drug Information.* St. Louis, MO: Facts and Comparisons, Sep 1995, 305d–305e.

5. Schurer-Maly CC, Varga L, Koelze HR, Halter F. Smoking and pH response to H2-receptor antagonists. *Scand J Gastroenterol* 1989;24:1172–78.

Risperidone

1. Threlkeld DS, ed. Central Nervous System Drugs, Antipsychotic Agents. In *Facts and Comparisons Drug Information*. St. Louis, MO: Facts and Comparisons, May 1998, 267f–268.

2. Threlkeld DS, ed. Central Nervous System Drugs, Antipsychotic Agents. In *Facts and Comparisons Drug Information*. St. Louis, MO: Facts and Comparisons, May 1998, 267f–268.

3. Threlkeld DS, ed. Central Nervous System Drugs, Antipsychotic Agents. In *Facts and Comparisons Drug Information*. St. Louis, MO: Facts and Comparisons, May 1998, 267f–268.

Senna

1. Threlkeld DS, ed. Gastrointestinal Drugs, Laxatives. In *Facts and Comparisons Drug Information*. St. Louis, MO: Facts and Comparisons, May 1991, 318a–319.

2. Threlkeld DS, ed. Gastrointestinal Drugs, Laxatives. In *Facts and Comparisons Drug Information*. St. Louis, MO: Facts and Comparisons, May 1991, 318a–319

3. Newall CA, Anderson LA, Phillipson JD. *Herbal Medicines: A Guide for Healthcare Professionals*. London: Pharmaceutical Press, 1996, 244.

Sertraline

1. Threlkeld DS, ed. Central Nervous System Drugs, Antidepressants, Selective Serotonin Reuptake Inhibitors. In *Facts and Comparisons Drug Information*. St. Louis, MO: Facts and Comparisons, Apr 1997, 264q.

2. Walinder J, Carlsson A, Persson R. 5-HT reuptake inhibitors plus tryptophan in endogenous depression. *Acta Psych Scand Suppl* 1981;290:179–90.

3. Spigset O, Hedenmalm K, Mortimer O. Hyponatremia as a side effect of serotonin uptake inhibitors. *Lakartidningen* 1998;95:3537–39 [Swedish].

4. Strachan J, Shepherd J. Hyponatraemia associated with the use of selective serotonin re-uptake inhibitors. *Aust N Z J Psychiatry* 1998;32:295–98.

5. Bouman WP, Pinner G, Johnson H. Incidence of selective serotonin reuptake inhibitor (SSRI) induced hyponatraemia due to the syndrome of antidiuretic hormone (SIADH) secretion in the elderly. *Int J Geriatr Psychiatry* 1998;13:12–15.

6. Cohen AJ. Long term safety and efficacy of *Ginkgo biloba* extract in the treatment of anti-depressant-induced sexual dysfunction. *Psychiatry On-Line* http://www.priory.com/ginkgo.html.

7. Sohn M, Sikora R. *Ginkgo biloba* extract in the therapy of erectile dysfunction. *J Sex Educ Ther* 1991;17:53–61.

8. Demott K. St. John's wort tied to serotonin syndrome. *Clinical Psychiatry News* 1998;26:28.

9. Gordon JB. SSRIs and St. John's wort: possible toxicity? *Am Fam Physician* 1998;57:950.

10. Ronfeld RA, Wilner KD, Baris BA. Sertraline. Chronopharma-cokinetics and the effect of coadministration with food. *Clin Pharmacokinet* 1997;32(suppl 1):50–55.

11. Threlkeld DS, ed. Central Nervous System Drugs, Antidepressants, Selective Serotonin Reuptake Inhibitors. In *Facts and Comparisons Drug Information*. St. Louis, MO: Facts and Comparisons, Apr 1997, 264q.

Simvastatin

1. Laaksonen R, Jokelainen K, Sahi T, et al. Decreases in serum ubiquinone concentrations do not result in reduced levels in muscle tissue during short-term simvastatin treatment in humans. *Clin Pharmacol Ther* 1995;57:62–66.

2. Laaksonen R, Ojala JP, Tikkanen MJ, et al. Serum ubiquinone concentrations after short- and long-term treatment with HMG-CoA reductase inhibitors. *Eur J Clin Pharmacol* 1994;46:313–17.

3. Bargossi AM, Grossi G, Fiorella PL, et al. Exogenous CoQ10 supplementation prevents plasma ubiquinone reduction induced by HMG-CoA reductase inhibitors. *Molec Aspects Med* 1994;15(suppl):s187–93.

4. Garnett WR. Interactions with hydroxymethylglutaryl-coenzyme A reductase inhibitors. *Am J Health Syst Pharm* 1995;52:1639–45.

5. Yee HS, Fong NT. Atorvastatin in the treatment of primary hypercholesterolemia and mixed dyslipidemias. *Ann Pharmacother* 1998;32:1030–43.

6. Jacobson TA, Amorosa LF. Combination therapy with fluvastatin and niacin in hypercholesterolemia: a preliminary report on safety. *Am J Cardiol* 1994;73:25D–29D.

7. Jokubaitis LA. Fluvastatin in combination with other lipid-lowering agents. *Br J Pract Suppl* 1996;77A:28–32.

8. Davignon J, Roederer G, Montigny M, et al. Comparative efficacy and safety of *pravastatin, nicotinic acid* and the two combined in patients with hypercholesterolemia. *Am J Cardiol* 1994;73:339–45.

9. Jacobson TA, Jokubaitis LA, Amorosa LF. Fluvistatin and niacin in hypercholesterolemia: a preliminary report on gender differences in efficacy. *Am J Med* 1994;96(suppl 6A):64S–68S.

10. Muggeo M, Zenti MG, Travia D, et al. Serum retinol levels throughout 2 years ofcholesterol-lowering therapy. *Metabolism* 1995;44:398–403.

11. Neunteufl T, Kostner K, Katzenschlager R, et al. Additional benefit of vitamin E supplementation to simvastatin therapy on vasoreactivity of the brachial artery of hypercholesterolemic men. *J Am Coll Cardiol* 1998;32:711–16.

12. Threlkeld DS, ed. Diuretics and Cardiovasculars, Antihyperlipidemic Agents, HMG-CoA Reductase Inhibitors. In *Facts and Comparisons Drug Information*. St. Louis, MO: Facts and Comparisons, Sep 1998, 172.

Sodium Bicarbonate

1. O'Neil-Cutting MA, Crosby WH. The effect of antacids on the absorption of simultaneously ingested iron. *JAMA* 1986;255:1468–70.

Spironolactone
Spironolactone/Hydrochlorothiazide

1. Devane J, Ryan MP. The effects of amiloride and triamterene on urinary magnesium excretion in conscious saline-loaded rats. *Br J Pharmacol* 1981;72:285–89.

2. Brinker F. *Herb Contraindications and Drug Interactions*. Sandy, OR: Eclectic Institute, 1997, 102–3.

3. Threlkeld DS, ed. Diuretics and Cardiovasculars, Potassium-Sparing Diuretics, Spironolactone. In *Facts and Comparisons Drug Information*. St. Louis, MO: Facts and Comparisons, Jul 1993, 138h–138j.

Stanozolol

1. Taberner DA. Iron deficiency and stanozolol therapy. *Lancet* 1983;I:648 [letter].

Sulfamethoxazole
Trimethoprim/Sulfamethoxazole

1. Holt GA. *Food & Drug Interactions*. Chicago: Precept Press, 1998, 248–49, 250–51.

2. Holt GA. *Food & Drug Interactions*. Chicago: Precept Press,1998, 248–49, 251–52.

3. Alappan R, Perazella MA, Buller GK. Hyperkalemia in hospitalized patients treated with trimethoprim-sulfamethoxazole. *Ann Intern Med* 1996;124:316–20.

4. Threlkeld DS, ed. Anti-Infectives, Sulfonamides. In *Facts and Comparisons Drug Information*. St. Louis, MO: Facts and Comparisons, Sep 1997, 364.

5. Holt GA. *Food & Drug Interactions*. Chicago: Precept Press, 1998, 249.

Sulfasalazine

1. Longstreth GF, Green R. Folate status in patients receiving maintenance doses of sulfasalazine. *Arch Intern Med* 1983;143:902–4.

2. Halsted CH, Gandhi G, Tamura T. Sulfasalazine inhibits the absorption of folates in ulcerative colitis. *N Engl J Med* 1981;305:1513–17.

3. Swinson CM, Perry J, Lumb M, Levi AJ. Role of sulphasalazine in the aetiology of folate deficiency in ulcerative colitis. *Gut* 1981;22:456–61.

4. Longstreth GF, Green R. Folate levels in inflammatory bowel disease. *N Engl J Med* 1982;306:1488 [letter].

5. Heimburger DC, Alexander B, Birch R, et al. Improvement in bronchial squamous metaplasia in smokers treated with folate and vitamin B12. *JAMA* 1988;259:1525–30.

6. Ma J, Stampfer MJ, Giovannucci E, et al. Methylenetetrahydrofolate reductase polymorphism, dietary interactions, and risk of colorectal cancer. *Cancer Res* 1997;57:1098–102.

7. Mason JB. Folate and colonic carcinogenesis: Searching for a mechanistic understanding. *J Nutr Biochem* 1994;5:170–75.

8. Lashner BA, Provencher KS, Seidner DL, et al. The effect of folic acid supplementation on the risk for cancer or dysplasia in ulcerative colitis. *Gastroenterol* 1997;112:29–32.

9. Lashner BA, Heidenreich PA, Su GL, et al. Effect of folate supplementation on the incidence of dysplasia and cancer in chronic ulcerative colitis. *Gastroenterol* 1989;97:255–59.

10. Dukes GE Jr, Duncan BS. Inflammatory bowel disease. In *Applied Therapeutics: The Clinical Use of Drugs*, 6th ed. Vancouver, WA: Applied Therapeutics, 1995, 24–27.

11. Threlkeld DS, ed. Gastrointestinal Drugs, Sulfasalazine. In *Facts and Comparisons Drug Information*. St. Louis, MO: Facts and Comparisons, Sep 1997, 326e–326h.

Sumatriptan

1. Threlkeld DS, ed. Central Nervous System Drugs, Agents for Migraine, Serotonin 5-HT$_1$ Receptor Agonists. In *Facts and Comparisons Drug Information*. St. Louis, MO: Facts and Comparisons, Jun 1996, 256a.

2. Holt GA. *Food & Drug Interactions*. Chicago: Precept Press, 1998, 253.

Tamoxifen

1. Lissoni P, Barni S, Meregalli S, et al. Modulation of cancer endocrine therapy by melatonin: A phase II study of tamoxifen plus melatonin in metastatic breast cancer patients progression under tamoxifen alone. *Br J Cancer* 1995;71:854–56.

Terbinafine

1. Nedelman J, Cramer JA, Robbins B, et al. The effect of food on the pharmacokinetics of multiple-dose terbinafine in young and elderly healthy subjects. *Biopharm Drug Dispos* 1997;18:127–38.

Tetracycline

1. Holt GA. *Food & Drug Interactions*. Chicago: Precept Press, 1998, 256–58.

2. Freinberg N, Lite T. Adjunctive ascorbic acid administration in antibiotic therapy. *J Dental Res* 1957;36:260–2.

3. Khin-Maung-U, Myo-Khin, Nyunt-Nyunt-Wai, et al. Clinical trial of berberine in acute watery diarrhoea. *Br Med J* 1985;291:1601–05.

4. Rabbani GH, Butler T, Knight J, et al. Randomized controlled trial of berberine sulfate therapy for diarrhea due to enterotoxigenic *Escherichia coli* and *Vibrio cholerae*. *J Infect Dis* 1987;155:979–84.

5. Threlkeld DS, ed. Anti-Infectives, Tetracyclines. In *Facts and Comparisons Drug Information*. St. Louis, MO: Facts and Comparisons, Dec 1989, 341–342f.

Theophylline
Aminophylline

1. Rayssiguier Y. Hypomagnesemia resulting from adrenaline infusion in ewes: Its relation to lipolysis. *Horm Metab Res* 1977;9:309–14.

2. Smith SR, Gove I, Kendall MJ. Beta agonists and potassium. *Lancet* 1985;1:1394.

3. Shimizu T, Maeda S, Arakawa H, et al. Relation between theophylline and circulating vitamin levels in children with asthma. *Pharmacology* 1996;53:384–89.

4. Martinez de Haas MG, Poels PJ, de Weert CJ, et al. Subnormal vitamin B6 levels in theophylline users. *Ned Tijdschr Geneeskd* 1997;141:2176–79 [in Dutch].

5. Ubbink JB, Delport R, Becker PJ, Bissbort S. Evidence of a theophylline-induced vitamin B6 deficiency caused by noncompetitive inhibition of pyridoxal kinase. *J Lab Clin Med* 1989;113:15–22.

6. Bano G, Raina RK, Zutshi U, et al. Effect of piperine on bioavailability and pharmocokinetics of propranolol and theophylline in healthy volunteers. *Eur J Clin Pharmacol* 1991;41:615–17.

7. Brinker F. Interactions of pharmaceutical and botanical medicines. *J Naturopathic Med* 1997;7(2):14–20.

8. Threlkeld DS, ed. Respiratory Drugs, Bronchodilators, Xanthine Derivatives. In *Facts and Comparisons Drug Information*. St. Louis, MO: Facts and Comparisons, Feb 1991, 178–179a.

9. Holt GA. *Food & Drug Interactions*. Chicago: Precept Press, 1998, 260.

10. Threlkeld DS, ed. Respiratory Drugs, Bronchodilators, Xanthine Derivatives. In *Facts and Comparisons Drug Information*. St. Louis, MO: Facts and Comparisons, Feb 1991, 178–179a.

11. Threlkeld DS, ed. Respiratory Drugs, Bronchodilators, Xanthine Derivatives. In *Facts and Comparisons Drug Information*. St. Louis, MO: Facts and Comparisons, Feb 1991, 178–179a.

12. Threlkeld DS, ed. Respiratory Drugs, Bronchodilators, Xanthine Derivatives. In *Facts and Comparisons Drug Information*. St. Louis, MO: Facts and Comparisons, Feb 1991, 178–179a.

13. Threlkeld DS, ed. Respiratory Drugs, Bronchodilators, Xanthine Derivatives. In *Facts and Comparisons Drug Information*. St. Louis, MO: Facts and Comparisons, Feb 1991, 178–179a.

Thiazide Diuretics

1. Threlkeld DS, ed. Diuretics and Cardiovasculars, Thiazides and Related Diuretics. In *Facts and Comparisons Drug Information*. St. Louis, MO: Facts and Comparisons, Jul 1993, 135a–137c.

2. Martin B, Milligan K. Diuretic-associated hypomagnesiumia in the elderly. *Arch Intern Med* 1987;147:1768–71.

3. Kroenke K, Wood DR, Hanley JF. The value of serum magnesium determination in hypertensive patients receiving diuretics. *Arch Intern Med* 1987;147:1553–56.

4. Whang R, Whang DD, Ryan MP. Refractory potassium repletion—a consequence of magnesium deficiency. *Arch Intern Med* 1992;152:40–45.

5. Riis B, Christiansen C. Actions of thiazide on vitamin D metabolism: A controlled therapeutic trial in normal women early in the postmenopause. *Metabolism* 1985;34:421–24.

6. Reyes AJ, Leary WP, Lockett CJ, et al. Diuretics and zinc. *S Afr Med J* 1982;62:373–75.

7. Brinker F. *Herb Contraindications and Drug Interactions*. Sandy, OR: Eclectic Institute, 1997, 102–3.

8. Threlkeld DS, ed. Diuretics and Cardiovasculars, Thiazides and Related Diuretics. In *Facts and Comparisons Drug Information*. St. Louis, MO: Facts and Comparisons, Apr 1993, 135a–137c.

9. Shaw D et al. Traditional remedies and food supplements: a 5-year toxicological study (1991–1995). *Drug Safety* 1997;17:342–56.

10. Shintani S, Murase H, Tsukagoshi H, Shiigai T. Glycyrrhizin (licorice)-induced hypokalemic myopathy. Report of two cases and review of the literature. *Eur Neurol* 1992;32:44–51.

11. Threlkeld DS, ed. Diuretics and Cardiovasculars, Thiazides and Related Diuretics. In *Facts and Comparisons Drug Information*. St. Louis, MO: Facts and Comparisons, Jul 1993, 135a–137c.

Thyroid Hormones

1. Kung AWC, Pun KK. Bone mineral density in premenopausal women receiving long-term physiological doses of levothyroxine. *JAMA* 1991;265:2688–91.

2. Schneider DL, Barrett-Connor EL, Morton DJ. Thyroid hormone use and bone mineral density in elderly men. *Arch Intern Med* 1995;155:2005–7.

3. Franklyn JA, Betteridge J, Daykin J, et al. Long-term thyroxine treatment and bone mineral density. *Lancet* 1992;340:9–13.

4. Beard J, Borel M, Peterson FJ. Changes in iron status during weight loss with very-low-energy diets. *Am J Clin Nutr* 1997;66:104–10.

5. Beard JL, Borel MJ, Derr J. Impaired thermoregulation and thyroid function in iron deficiency anemia. *Am J Clin Nutr* 1990;52:813–19.

6. Beard JL, Borel MJ, Derr J. Impaired thermoregulation and thyroid function in iron-deficiency anemia. *Am J Clin Nutr* 1990;52:813–19.

7. Campbell NR, Hasinoff BB. Iron supplements: A common cause of drug interactions. *Brit J Clin Pharmacol* 1991;31:251–55.

8. Jabbar MA, Larrea J, Shaw RA. Abnormal thyroid function tests in infants with congenital hypothyroidism: The influence of soy-based formulas. *J Am Coll Nutr* 1997;16:280–82.

9. Brinker F. *Herb Contraindications and Drug Interactions.* Sandy, OR: Eclectic Institute, 1997, 21, 29–30.

10. Threlkeld DS, ed. Hormones, Thyroid Hormones. In *Facts and Comparisons Drug Information.* St. Louis, MO: Facts and Comparisons, Jun 1991, 132–133c.

11. Threlkeld DS, ed. Hormones, Thyroid Hormones. In *Facts and Comparisons Drug Information.* St. Louis, MO: Facts and Comparisons, Jun 1991, 132–133c.

Ticlopidine

1. Hopkins MP, Androff L, Benninghoff AS. Ginseng face cream and unexplained vaginal bleeding. *Am J Obstet Gynecol* 1988;159(5):1121–22.

2. Greenspan EM. Ginseng and vaginal bleeding. *JAMA* 1983;249(15):2018.

3. Janetzky K, Morreale AP. Probable interaction between warfarin and ginseng. *Am J Health-Syst Pharm* 1997;54:692–93.

4. Yu CM, Chan JCN, Sanderson JE. Chinese herbs and warfarin potentiation by "danshen." *J Intern Med* 1997;241:337–39.

5. Tam LS, Chan TYK, Leung WK, Critchley JAJH. Warfarin interactions with Chinese traditional medicines: Danshen and methyl salicylate medicated oil. *Aust NZ J Med* 1995;25:258.

6. Shaw D, Leon C, Kolev S, Murray V. Traditional remedies and food supplements: a 5-year toxicological study (1991–1995). *Drug Safety* 1997;17(5):342–56.

7. Rose KD, Croissant PD, Parliment CF, Levin MB. Spontaneous spinal epidural hematoma with associated platelet dysfunction from excessive garlic ingestion: A case report. *Neurosurg* 1990;26:880–82.

8. Gadkari JV, Joshi VD. Effect of ingestion of raw garlic on serum cholesterol level, clotting time and fibrinolytic activity in normal subjects. *J Postgrad Med* 1991;37:128–31.

9. Burnham BE. Garlic as a possible risk for postoperative bleeding. *Plast-Reconst-Surg* 1995;95:213.

10. Newall CA, Anderson LA, Phillipson JD. *Herbal Medicines: A Guide for Health-Care Professionals.* London: The Pharmaceutical Press, 1996, 135–37.

11. Kleijnen J, Knipschild P. *Ginkgo biloba. Lancet* 1992;340:1136–39.

12. Kim YS, Pyo MK, Park KM. Antiplatelet and antithrombotic effects of a combination of ticlopidine and *Ginkgo biloba* ext (EGb 761). *Thrombosis Res* 1998;91:33–38.

13. Rosenblatt M, Mindel J. Spontaneous hyphema associated with ingestion of *Ginkgo biloba* extract. *New Engl J Med* 1997;336:1108.

14. Rowin J, Lewis SL. Spontaneous bilateral subdural hematoma with chronic *Gingko biloba* ingestion. *Neurology* 1996;46:1775–76.

15. Tatro D, ed. Anticoagulants-quinine derivatives. In *Drug Interaction Facts*. St. Louis, MO: Facts and Comparisons, Jul 1993.

16. Wichtl M, Bisset NG, eds. *Herbal Drugs and Phytopharmaceuticals* Stuttgart: Medpharm GmBH Scientific Publishers. 1994.

17. Janssen PL, Katan MB, van Staveren WA, et al. Acetylsalicylate and salicylates in foods. *Cancer Lett* 1997:114(1–2):163–64.

18. McGuffin M, Hobbs C, Upton R, Goldberg A, eds. *American Herbal Product Association's Botanical Safety Handbook*. Boca Raton, FL: CRC Press, 1997, 154–55.

19. Threlkeld DS, ed. Blood Modifiers, Antiplatelet Agents, Ticlopidine HCl. In *Facts and Comparisons Drug Information*. St. Louis, MO: Facts and Comparisons, Jan 1992, 85c–85g.

Timolol
Timolol/Hydrochlorothiazide

1. Takahashi N, Iwasaka T, Sugiura T, et al. Effect of coenzyme Q10 on hemodynamic response to ocular timolol. *J Cardiovasc Pharmacol* 1989;14:462–68.

2. Mantyla R, Mannisto P, Nykanen S, et al. Pharmacokinetic interactions of timolol with vasodilating drugs, food and phenobarbitone in healthy human volunteers. *Eur J Clin Pharmacol* 1983;24:227–30.

3. Threlkeld DS, ed. Diuretics and Cardiovasculars, Beta-Adrenergic Blocking Agents. In *Facts and Comparisons Drug Information*. St. Louis, MO: Facts and Comparisons, Feb 1993, 158q.

Tobramycin
Tobramycin/Dexamethasone

1. Slayton W, Anstine D, Lakhdir F, et al. Tetany in a child with AIDS receiving intravenous tobramycin. *South Med J* 1996;89:1108–10.

2. Keating MJ, Sethi MR, Bodey GP, Samaan NA. Hypocalcemia with hypoparathyroidism and renal tubular dysfunction associated with aminoglycoside therapy. *Cancer* 1977;39:1410–14.

3. Rhodes EG, Harris RI, Welch RS, et al. Empirical treatment of febrile, neutropenic patients with tobramycin and latamoxef. *J Hosp Infect* 1987;9:278–84.

4. Baxter JG, Marble DA, Whitfield LR, et al. Clinical risk factors for prolonged PT/PTT in abdominal sepsis patients treated with moxalactam or tobramycin plus clindamycin. *Ann Surg* 1985;201:96–102.

Tramadol

1. Mason BJ, Blackburn KH. Possible serotonin syndrome associated with tramadol and sertraline coadministration. *Ann Pharmacother* 1997;31:175–77.

2. Hernandez AF, Montero MN, Pla A, Villanueva E. Fatal moclobemide overdose or death caused by serotonin syndrome? *J Forensic Sci* 1995;40:128–30.

3. Threlkeld DS, ed. Central Nervous System Drugs, Central Analgesics, Tramadol HCl. In *Facts and Comparisons Drug Information*. St. Louis, MO: Facts and Comparisons, May 1995, 246b–246f.

4. Threlkeld DS, ed. Central Nervous System Drugs, Central Analgesics, Tramadol HCl. In *Facts and Comparisons Drug Information*. St. Louis, MO: Facts and Comparisons, May 1995, 246b–246f.

Trazodone

1. Rauch PK, Jenike MA. Digoxin toxicity possibly precipitated by trazodone. *Psychosomatics* 1984;25:334–35.

2. Threlkeld DS, ed. Central Nervous System Drugs, Antidepressants, Trazodone. In *Facts and Comparisons Drug Information*. St. Louis, MO: Facts and Comparisons, Apr 1990, 263i–263k.

3. Threlkeld DS, ed. Central Nervous System Drugs, Antidepressants, Trazodone. In *Facts and Comparisons Drug Information*. St. Louis, MO: Facts and Comparisons, Apr 1990, 263i–263k.

Tretinoin

1. Threlkeld DS, ed. Antineoplastics, Miscellaneous Antineoplastics, Tretinoin. In *Facts and Comparisons Drug Information*. St. Louis, MO: Facts and Comparisons, Jul 1996, 685w–685z.

Triamterene
Triamterene/Hydrochlorothiazide

1. Werbach WR. *Foundations of Nutritional Medicine*. Tarzana, CA: Third Line Press, 1997, 246 [review].

2. Jackson EK. Diuretics. In *Goodman & Gilman's The Pharmacological Basis of Therapeutics*, 9th ed. New York: McGraw Hill, 1996, 706.

3. Mason JB, Zimmerman J, Otradovec CL, et al. Chronic diuretic therapy with moderate doses of triamterene is not associated with folate deficiency. *J Lab Clin Med* 1991;117:365–69.

4. Brinker F. *Herb Contraindications and Drug Interactions*. Sandy, OR: Eclectic Institute, 1997, 102–3.

5. Threlkeld DS, ed. Diuretics and Cardiovasculars, Potassium-Sparing Diuretics, Triamterene. In *Facts and Comparisons Drug Information*. St. Louis, MO: Facts and Comparisons, Jul 1993, 138k–139.

Tricyclic Antidepressants

1. Bell IR, Edman JS, Morrow FD, et al. Brief communication: Vitamin B1, B2, and B6 augmentation of tricyclic antidepressant treatment in geriatric depression with cognitive dysfunction. *J Am Coll Nutr* 1992;11:159–63.

2. Chouinard G, Young SN, Annable L, Sourkes TL. Tryptophan-nicotinamide, imipramine and their combination in depression. *Acta Psychiatr Scand* 1979;59:395–414.

3. Walinder J, Skott A, Carlsson A, et al. Potentiation of the anti-depressant action of clomipramine by tryptophan. *Arch Gen Psychiatry* 1976;33:1384–89.

4. Shaw DM, MacSweeney DA, Hewland R, Johnson AL. Tricyclic antidepressants and tryptophan in unipolar depression. *Psychol Med* 1975;5:276–78.

5. Kishi T, Makino K, Okamoto T, Kishi H, Folkers K. Inhibition of myocardial respiration by psychotherapeutic drugs and prevention by coenzymeQ. In Y Yamamura, K Folkers, Y Ito, eds. *Biomedical and Clinical Aspects of Coenzyme Q,* Vol. 2. Amsterdam: Elsevier/North-Holland Biomedical Press,1980:139–54.

6. Lasswell WL Jr, Weber SS, Wilkins JM. In vitro interaction of neuroleptics and tricyclic antidepressants with coffee, tea, and gallotannic acid. *J Pharm Sci* 1984;73:1056–58.

7. Threlkeld DS, ed. Central Nervous System Drugs, Antidepressants, Tricyclic Compounds. In *Facts and Comparisons Drug Information.* St. Louis, MO: Facts and Comparisons, Apr 1990, 2621–263.

Trimethoprim

Trimethoprim/Sulfamethoxazole

1. Holt GA. *Food & Drug Interactions.* Chicago: Precept Press, 1998, 248–49, 250–51.

2. Holt GA. *Food & Drug Interactions.* Chicago: Precept Press, 1998, 248–49, 251–52.

3. Sahai J. Urinary tract infections. In *Applied Therapeutics: The Clinical Use of Drugs,* 6th ed. Vancouver, WA: Applied Therapeutics, 1995, 63–66.

4. Kahn SB, Fein SA, Brodsky I. Effects of trimethoprim on folate metabolism in man. *Clin Pharmacol Ther* 1968;9:550–60.

5. Threlkeld DS, ed. Systemic Anti-Infectives, Miscellaneous Anti-Infectives, Trimethoprim. In *Facts and Comparisons Drug Information.* St. Louis, MO: Facts and Comparisons, Aug 1992, 408–408a.

6. Sahai J. Urinary tract infections. In *Applied Therapeutics: The Clinical Use of Drugs,* 6th ed. Vancouver, WA: Applied Therapeutics, 1995, 63–66.

7. Alappan R, Perazella MA, Buller GK. Hyperkalemia in hospitalized patients treated with trimethoprim-sulfamethoxazole. *Ann Intern Med* 1996;124:316–20.

Trimethoprim/Sulfamethoxazole, TMP/SMX

1. Young LY, Koda-Kimble MA, eds. *Applied Therapeutics: The Clinical Use of Drugs.* Vancouver, WA: Applied Therapeutics, 1988, 911.

2. Kahn SB, Fein SA, Brodsky I. Effects of trimethoprim on folate metabolism in man. *Clin Pharmacol Ther* 1968;9:550–60.

3. Young LY, Koda-Kimble MA, eds. *Applied Therapeutics: The Clinical Use of Drugs.* Vancouver, WA: Applied Therapeutics, 1988, 911.

4. Safrin S, Lee BL, Sande MA. Adjunctive folinic acid with trimethoprim-sulfamethoxazole for pneumocystis carinii pneumonia in AIDS patients is associated with an increased risk of therapeutic failure and death. *J Infect Dis* 1994;170:912–17.

5. Alappan R, Perazella MA, Buller GK. Hyperkalemia in hospitalized patients treated with trimethoprim-sulfamethoxazole. *Ann Intern Med* 1996;124:316–20.

Valproic Acid
Divalproex Sodium
Sodium Valproate

1. Nurge ME, Anderson CR, Bates E. Metabolic and nutritional implications of valproic acid. *Nutr Res* 1991;11:949–60.

2. Van Wouwe JP. Carnitine deficiency during valproic acid treatment. *Internat J Vit Nutr Res* 1995;65:211–14.

3. Castro-Gago M, Camina F, Rodriguez-Segade S. Carnitine deficiency caused by valproic acid. *J Pediatr* 1992;120:496 [letter].

4. Gidal BE, Inglese CM, Meyer JF, et al. Diet-and valproate-induced transient hyperammonemia: Effect of L-carnitine. *Pediatr Neurol* 1997;16:301–5.

5. Freeman JM, Vining EPG, Cost S, Singhi P. Does carnitine administration improve the symptoms attributed to anticonvulsant medications? A double-blinded, crossover study. *Pediatr* 1994;93:893–95.

6. Kelley RI. The role of carnitine supplementation in valproic acid therapy. *Pediatr* 1994;93:891–92 [editorial].

7. Kaji M, Ito M, Okuno T, et al. Serum copper and zinc levels in epileptic children with valproate treatment. *Epilepsia* 1992;33:555–57.

8. Lerman-Sagie T, Statter M, Szabo G, Lerman P. Effect of valproic acid therapy on zinc metabolism in children with primary epilepsy. *Clin Neuropharmacol* 1987;10:80–86.

9. Sozuer DT, Barutcu UB, Karakoc Y, et al. The effects of antiepileptic drugs on serum zinc and copper levels in children. *J Basic Clin Physiol Pharmacol* 1995;6:265–69.

10. Sozuer DT, Barutcu UB, Karakoc Y, et al. The effects of antiepileptic drugs on serum zinc and copper levels in children. *J Basic Clin Physiol Pharmacol* 1995;6:265–69.

11. Lerman-Sagie T, Statter M, Szabo G, Lerman P. Effect of valproic acid therapy on zinc metabolism in children with primary epilepsy. *Clin Neuropharmacol* 1987;10:80–86.

12. Kaji M, Ito M, Okuno T, et al. Serum copper and zinc levels in epileptic children with valproate treatment. *Epilepsia* 1992;33:555–57.

13. Lerman-Sagie T, Statter M, Szabo G, Lerman P. Effect of valproic acid therapy on zinc metabolism in children with primary epilepsy. *Clin Neuropharmacol* 1987;10:80–86.

14. Threlkeld DS, ed. Central Nervous System Drugs, Anticonvulsants, Valproic Acid and Derivatives. In *Facts and Comparisons Drug Information*. St. Louis, MO: Facts and Comparisons, May 1997, 284b–284g.

15. Threlkeld DS, ed. Central Nervous System Drugs, Anticonvulsants, Valproic Acid and Derivatives. In *Facts and Comparisons Drug Information*. St. Louis, MO: Facts and Comparisons, May 1997, 284b–284g.

16. Threlkeld DS, ed. Central Nervous System Drugs, Anticonvulsants, Valproic Acid and Derivatives. In *Facts and Comparisons Drug Information*. St. Louis, MO: Facts and Comparisons, May 1997, 284b–284g.

Venlafaxine

1. Brubacher JR, Hoffman RS, Lurin MJ. Serotonin syndrome from venlafaxine-tranylcypromine interaction. *Vet Hum Toxicol* 1996;38:358–61.

2. Weiner LA, Smythe M, Cisek J. Serotonin syndrome secondary to phenelzine-venlafaxine interaction. *Pharmacotherapy* 1998;18:399–403.

3. Bhatara VS, Magnus RD, Paul KL, Preskorn SH. Serotonin syndrome induced by venlafaxine and fluoxetine: a case study in polypharmacy and potential pharmacodynamic and pharmacokinetic mechanisms. *Ann Pharmacother* 1998;32:432–36.

4. Diamond S, Pepper BJ, Diamond ML, et al. Serotonin syndrome induced by transitioning from phenelzine to venlafaxine: four patient reports. *Neurology* 1998;51:274–76.

5. Ranieri P, Franzoni S, Rozzini R, Trabucchi M. Venlafaxine-induced reset osmostat syndrome: case of a 79-year-old depressed woman. *J Geriatr Psychiatry Neurol* 1997;10:75–78.

6. Threlkeld DS, ed. Central Nervous System Drugs, Antidepressants, Venlafaxine. In *Facts and Comparisons Drug Information*. St. Louis, MO: Facts and Comparisons, Mar 1995, 263r–263x.

7. Threlkeld DS, ed. Central Nervous System Drugs, Antidepressants, Venlafaxine. In *Facts and Comparisons Drug Information*. St. Louis, MO: Facts and Comparisons, Mar 1995, 263r–263x.

8. Threlkeld DS, ed. Central Nervous System Drugs, Antidepressants, Venlafaxine. In *Facts and Comparisons Drug Information*. St. Louis, MO: Facts and Comparisons, Mar 1995, 263r–263x.

Verapamil

1. Haft JI, Habbab MA. Treatment of atrial arrhythmias. Effectiveness of verapamil when preceded by calcium infusion. *Arch Intern Med* 1986;146:1085–89.

2. Weiss AT, Lewis BS, Halon DA, et al. The use of calcium with verapamil in the management of supraventricular tachyarrhythmias. *Int J Cardiol* 1983;4:275–80.

3. Kuhn M, Schriger DL. Low-dose calcium pretreatment to prevent verapamil-induced hypotension. *Am Heart J* 1992;124:231–32.

4. Threlkeld DS, ed. Diuretics and Cardiovasculars, Calcium Channel Blocking Agents. In *Facts and Comparisons Drug Information.* St. Louis, MO: Facts and Comparisons, Nov 1992, 150–150b.

5. Threlkeld DS, ed. Diuretics and Cardiovasculars, Calcium Channel Blocking Agents. In *Facts and Comparisons Drug Information.* St. Louis, MO: Facts and Comparisons, Nov 1992, 150–150b.

6. Holt GA. *Food & Drug Interactions.* Chicago: Precept Press, 1998, 274–75.

Warfarin

1. Harris JE. Interaction of dietary factors with oral anticoagulants: Review and applications. *J Am Dietet Assoc* 1995;95:580–84 [review].

2. Spigset O. Reduced effect of warfarin caused by ubidecarenone. *Lancet* 1994;344:1372–73 [letter].

3. Holt GA. *Food & Drug Interactions.* Chicago: Precept Press, 1998, 284.

4. Harris JE. Interaction of dietary factors with oral anticoagulants: Review and applications. *J Am Dietet Assoc* 1995;95:580–84 [review].

5. Schrogie JJ. Coagulopathy and fat soluble drugs. *JAMA* 1975;232:19 [letter].

6. Corrigan J, Marcus FI. Coagulopathy associated with vitamin E ingestion. *JAMA* 1974;230:1300–01.

7. Kim JM, White RH. Effect of vitamin E on the anticoagulant response to warfarin. *Am J Cardiol* 1996;77:545–46.

8. Harris JE. Interaction of dietary factors with oral anticoagulants: Review and applications. *J Am Dietet Assoc* 1995;95:580–84 [review].

9. Weibert RT, Le DT, Kayser SR, et al. Correction of excessive anticoagulation with low-dose oral vitamin K1. *Ann Intern Med* 1997;125:959–62.

10. Hopkins MP, Androff L, Benninghoff AS. Ginseng face cream and unexplained vaginal bleeding. *Am J Obstet Gynecol* 1988;159(5):1121–22.

11. Greenspan EM. Ginseng and vaginal bleeding. *JAMA* 1983;249(15):2018.

12. Janetzky K, Morreale AP. Probable interaction between warfarin and ginseng. *Am J Health-Syst Pharm* 1997;54:692–93.

13. Yu CM, Chan JCN, Sanderson JE. Chinese herbs and warfarin potentiation by "danshen." *J Intern Med* 1997;241:337–39.

14. Tam LS, Chan TYK, Leung WK, Critchley JAJH. Warfarin interactions with Chinese traditional medicines: Danshen and methyl salicylate medicated oil. *Aust NZ J Med* 1995;25:258.

15. Shaw D, Leon C, Kolev S, Murray V. Traditional remedies and food supplements: a 5-year toxicological study (1991–1995). *Drug Safety* 1997;17(5):342–56.

16. Rose KD, Croissant PD, Parliment CF, Levin MB. Spontaneous spinal epidural hematoma with associated platelet dysfunction from excessive garlic ingestion: A case report. *Neurosurg* 1990;26:880–82.

17. Gadkari JV, Joshi VD. Effect of ingestion of raw garlic on serum cholesterol level, clotting time and fibrinolytic activity in normal subjects. *J Postgrad Med* 1991;37:128–31.

18. Burnham BE. Garlic as a possible risk for postoperative bleeding. *Plast-Reconst-Surg* 1995;95:213.

19. Sunter WH. Warfarin and garlic. *Pharm J* 1991;246:722 [letter].

20. Newall CA, Anderson LA, Phillipson JD. *Herbal Medicines: A Guide for Health-Care Professionals.* London: The Pharmaceutical Press, 1996, 135–37.

21. Kleijnen J, Knipschild P. *Ginkgo biloba. Lancet* 1992;340:1136–39.

22. Rosenblatt M, Mindel J. Spontaneous hyphema associated with ingestion of *Ginkgo biloba* extract. *New Engl J Med* 1997;336:1108.

23. Rowin J, Lewis SL. Spontaneous bilateral subdural hematoma with chronic *Gingko biloba* ingestion. *Neurology* 1996;46:1775–76.

24. Mathews MK. Association of *Ginkgo biloba* with intracerebral hemorrhage. *Neurology* 1998;50:1934.

25. Miller LG, Murray WJ, eds. *Herbal Medicinals: A Clinician's Guide.* New York: Pharmaceutical Products Press, 1999, 313–15.

26. Tatro D, ed. Anticoagulants-quinine derivatives. In *Drug Interaction Facts.* St. Louis, MO: Facts and Comparisons, Jul 1993.

27. Harris JE. Interaction of dietary factors with oral anticoagulants: Review and application. *J Am Diet Assoc* 1995;95:580–84 [review].

28. Holt GA. *Food & Drug Interactions.* Chicago: Precept Press, 1998, 293.

29. Holt GA. *Food & Drug Interactions.* Chicago, Precept Press, 1998, 284–85.

30. Shaw D, Leon C, Kolev S, Murray V. Traditional remedies and food supplements: a 5-year toxicological study (1991–1995). *Drug Safety* 1997;17(5):342–56.

31. Holt GA. *Food & Drug Interactions.* Chicago: Precept Press, 1998, 282.

Zolpidem

1. Elko CJ, Burgess JL, Robertson WO. Zolpidem-associated hallucinations and serotonin reuptake inhibition: a possible interaction. *J Toxicol Clin Toxicol* 1998;36:195–203.

2. Threlkeld DS, ed. Central Nervous System Drugs, Sedatives and Hypnotics, Nonbarbiturate, Imidazopyridines. In *Facts and Comparisons Drug Information.* St. Louis, MO: Facts and Comparisons, Feb 1993, 269h–269m.

3. Threlkeld DS, ed. Central Nervous System Drugs, Sedatives And Hypnotics, Nonbarbiturate, Imidazopyridines. In *Facts and Comparisons Drug Information.* St. Louis, MO: Facts and Comparisons, Feb 1993, 269h–269m.

Index

About the Authors

SCHUYLER W. "SKYE" LININGER, JR., D.C., CONTRIBUTOR AND EDITOR-IN-CHIEF

Dr. Skye Lininger is an acknowledged expert and popular speaker on nutritional therapeutics, computer technology, and the Internet. He has authored or coauthored a dozen computer books, and written numerous technology-related and health-related articles. Healthnotes, Inc., which he founded in 1986, is the publisher of *Healthnotes Newsletter, Healthnotes Review of Complementary and Integrative Medicine*, and Healthnotes Online, and is the leading provider of high-quality, scientifically based information on natural medicine. A former instructor in nutrition, he gives regular seminars in both the United States and England and serves on the boards of several natural medicine colleges. He is also the editor-in-chief of *The Natural Pharmacy, 2nd Edition* (Prima Health and Healthnotes, Inc., 1999).

ALAN R. GABY, M.D., CONTRIBUTOR

Dr. Alan Gaby, an expert in nutritional therapies, is the Contributing Medical Editor of the *Townsend Letter for Doctors*. He served as a member of the Ad-Hoc Advisory Panel of the National Institutes of Health Office of Alternative Medicine. He is the author of *B6: The Natural Healer* (Keats, 1987), *Preventing and Reversing Osteoporosis* (Prima, 1994), and *The Patient's Book of Natural Healing* (Prima, 1999). He is also coauthor of *The Natural Pharmacy, 2nd Edition* (Prima Health and Healthnotes, Inc., 1999). He is past-president of the American Holistic Medical Association. He has, along with Dr. Jonathan Wright, conducted nutritional seminars for physicians and has collected over 30,000 scientific papers related to the field of nutritional and natural medicine. He is currently the Endowed Professor of Nutrition at

Bastyr University, Bothell, Washington, and is a frequent contributor to Healthnotes.

STEVE AUSTIN, N.D., CONTRIBUTOR

Dr. Steve Austin is a licensed naturopathic physician in Portland, Oregon. He is former Professor of Nutrition at the National College of Naturopathic Medicine. Dr. Austin has also headed the nutrition departments at Bastyr University and Western States Chiropractic College. He is the coauthor of *Breast Cancer: What You Should Know (But May Not Be Told) About Prevention, Diagnosis, and Treatment* (Prima, 1994) and *The Natural Pharmacy, 2nd Edition* (Prima Health and Healthnotes, Inc., 1999), a contributor to the *Textbook of Natural Medicine,* and nutrition editor for the *Healthnotes Review of Complementary and Integrative Medicine.*

FORREST BATZ, PHARM.D., CONTRIBUTOR

Dr. Forrest Batz received a doctor of pharmacy degree from the University of California, San Francisco, and completed a Clinical Pharmacy Residency at the Tucson VA Medical Center. As a drug information pharmacist he noted the difficulties involved for non-herbally trained healthcare professionals in easily locating accurate herbal information. With this in mind he developed materials and presentations to assist healthcare professionals integrate herbal information into their practices. He is the author of articles for consumers and healthcare professionals, continuing education materials, and is co-editor of the *Pharmacist's Letter* and Prescriber's Letter Natural Medicines Comprehensive Database. Dr. Batz is an Assistant Clinical Professor in the School of Pharmacy, University of California, San Francisco.

ERIC YARNELL, N.D., CONTRIBUTOR

Dr. Eric Yarnell works as a naturopathic physician and is chair of the department of botanical medicine at the Southwest College of Naturopathic Medicine. He is treasurer of the board of the Botanical Medicine Academy and research editor for the *Journal of Naturopathic Medicine.* He is a contributor to the *Healthnotes Review of Complementary and Integrative Medicine* and coauthor of *The Natural Pharmacy, 2nd Edition* (Prima Health and Healthnotes, Inc., 1999).

DONALD J. BROWN, N.D., CONTRIBUTOR

Dr. Donald Brown is a naturopathic physician and one of the leading authorities in the United States on evidence-based herbal medicine. A graduate and former associate professor of the Bastyr University of

Natural Health Sciences in Seattle, he is the founder and director of Natural Product Research Consultants, Inc., and serves on the Advisory Board of the American Botanical Council and the President's Advisory Board of Bastyr University. Dr. Brown has served as an adviser to the Office of Dietary Supplements at the National Institutes of Health. He is the editor-in-chief of the *Healthnotes Review of Complementary and Integrative Medicine* (formerly the *Quarterly Review of Natural Medicine*), author of *Herbal Prescriptions for Better Health* (Prima, 1996), and coauthor of *The Natural Pharmacy, 2nd Edition* (Prima Health and Healthnotes, Inc., 1999).

GEORGE CONSTANTINE, R.PH., PH.D., CONTRIBUTOR

Dr. George Constantine, a faculty member at the College of Pharmacy, Oregon State University, has extensive knowledge of natural products and herbal medicine. Licensed in California and Oregon, his primary teaching responsibilities include drug information services, natural products chemistry, gerontology, pharmacy history, and medical ethics. Dr. Constantine also teaches Continuing Education programs to pharmacists throughout the United States and lectures regularly at the National College of Naturopathic Medicine and Western States Chiropractic College. A past president of the American Society of Pharmacognosy, he has authored 38 professional and scientific articles and currently is a reviewer for the American Herbal Pharmacopoeia. Dr. Constantine is cofounder of the Benton Hospice in Corvallis, Oregon, which has helped over 8,000 patients and their families.

EDITORIAL STAFF

Victoria Dolby Toews, M.P.H., Managing Editor

Mrs. Victoria Dolby Toews writes about health issues, with a special focus on nutritional supplements. Her articles appear regularly in several magazines. She is the coauthor of *The Common Cold Cure* (Avery, 1999) and *The Green Tea Book* (Avery, 1998). She is the managing editor for Healthnotes Online and *The Natural Pharmacy, 2nd Edition* (Prima Health and Healthnotes, Inc., 1999) and the editor-in-chief of the *Healthnotes Newsletter*.

Rick Wilkes, Chief Technology Officer

Mr. Rick Wilkes is an Internet and electronic publishing specialist from Deep Creek Lake, Maryland. For over 20 years he has focused on building supportive, interactive online communities; and publishing enabling software and newsletters to help clients apply complex computer technology more effectively. He graduated from Johns Hopkins University, Baltimore, Maryland, where he now serves on the Computer Science Advisory Board.

HEALTHNOTES, INC. TEAM

Skye Lininger (President/CEO), Tim O'Connor (General Manager), Cheryl Bottger (Director of Marketing and Product Development), Mike Shriner (Director of Business Development), Rick Wilkes (Chief Technology Officer), Rachel Gaffney (Accounting Manager), Geoff Lay (Internet Product Manager), Tara Schweig (National Retail Sales Manager), Cindy Hambly (National Accounts Manager), Brent Blomgren (National Accounts Manager), Karen Considine (Inside Sales Representative), Caroline Petrich (Marketing Manager), Janet Jaffee (Marketing Assistant), Autumn Moore (Customer Care Manager), Jim Garner (Customer Care Specialist), Dan Widger (Technical Support Specialist), JoAnn DeVischer (Office Manager), Debbie Cheney (Fulfillment Specialist), Annette LaBarge (Accounts Receivable Specialist), Sally S. K. Lee (Bookkeeper) Judy Robinson (Executive Assistant), Marcia Barrentine (Creative Services Manager), Nichole Klaes (Graphic Designer); Loren Jenkins (Programmer), Marianne Bhonslay (Editorial Manager), Victoria Dolby Toews, M.P.H. (Managing Editor), Jenny Morrison and Richard Walsh (Copy Editors); Legal and Accounting: Curt Gleaves and Jim Baker; U.K. Team: Michael Peet, Taylor, Gareth Zeal, and Nigel Perkins.

Also Available from Healthnotes

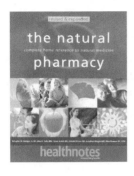

The Natural Pharmacy, *2nd Edition* (Prima Health and Healthnotes, Inc., 1999), by Schuyler W. Lininger, Jr, D.C., (editor-in-chief), Alan R. Gaby, M.D., Steve Austin, N.D., Donald J. Brown, N.D., Jonathan V. Wright, M.D., and Alice Duncan, D.C., CCH.

Imagine being able to have the world's most respected natural health experts talk to you about your health concerns. Now, with *The Natural Pharmacy, 2nd Edition* you can! In this one volume, some of the world's most highly regarded clinical practitioners in the field have teamed together to offer timely, practical, and fully integrated advice on treating troublesome conditions the natural way.

Inside, you will find complete coverage of the most common conditions, together with useful guidance on how to treat them. In addition, this essential guide gives you up-to-date, fully referenced, reliable information on a world of supplements that can improve your health. Clearly, *The Natural Pharmacy, 2nd Edition* is your most trusted guide to conditions, supplements, herbs, and homeopathic remedies. (*$24.95*)

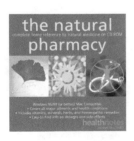

The Natural Pharmacy: Complete Home Reference to Natural Medicine CD-ROM (Healthnotes, Inc., 1999). With this companion to *The Natural Pharmacy,* you'll have a wealth of information literally at your fingertips. This Macintosh or Windows compatible CD-ROM has fully referenced information on Health Concerns, Nutritional Supplements, Herbal Remedies, Homeopathic Remedies, and Diets and Therapies.

Take home—for personal or family use—this fascinating and comprehensive database, and increase your understanding of herbs and vitamin supplements. Requires an Internet browser (such as Microsoft Internet Explorer version 3.x or later, or Netscape 3.x or later) and a CD-ROM drive. Does not require Internet access. (*$24.95*.)

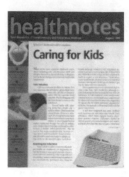

Healthnotes Newsletter (Healthnotes, Inc. 1999) This four-page, monthly newsletter focuses on specific health concerns and related natural remedies. Fully referenced articles are easy to understand and informative. Topics for 2000 include: Managing Medications for Seniors; Sports Nutrition; Women and Hormones (PMS and Menopause); Digestive Health; Antibiotic Overuse; Cold and Flu Prevention; and Thyroid Health. To register online to receive the newsletter via e-mail every month go to http://www.healthnotes.com, and click on "*Healthnotes Newsletter.*"